THE SELLING OF DSM
The Rhetoric of Science in Psychiatry

D0209831

SOCIAL PROBLEMS AND SOCIAL ISSUES
An Aldine de Gruyter Series of Texts and Monographs

SERIES EDITOR

Joel Best, *University of Southern Illinois, Carbondale*

Images of Issues:
Typifying Contemporary Social Problems
Joel Best (Editor)

Intimate Enemies:
Moral Panics in Contemporary Great Britain
Philip Jenkins

The Selling of *DSM*:
The Rhetoric of Science in Psychiatry
Stuart A. Kirk and Herb Kutchins

Mirrors of Madness:
Patrolling the Psychic Border
Bruce Luske

The New Pediatrics:
A Profession in Transition
Dorothy Pawluch

Juvenile Gang Violence and Grounded Culture
William B. Sanders

The Politics of Readjustment:
Vietnam Veterans Since the War
Wilbur J. Scott

Constructing Social Problems
Malcolm Spector and John I. Kitsuse

THE SELLING OF DSM

The Rhetoric of Science in Psychiatry

Stuart A. Kirk
Herb Kutchins

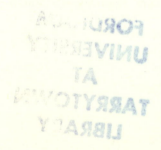

ALDINE DE GRUYTER
New York

ABOUT THE AUTHORS

Stuart A. Kirk is Professor of Social Work at Columbia University. He earned his doctorate from the University of California at Berkeley. Dr. Kirk was Dean of the School of Social Welfare at the State University of New York at Albany from 1980–1987. He is the author of many publications on deinstitutionalization and chronic mental illness, research utilization, service delivery and on labeling in mental health. With Herb Kutchins, he has coauthored many articles about psychiatric diagnosis.

Herb Kutchins is Professor of Social Work at California State University, Sacramento. He earned his doctorate from the University of California at Berkeley. In addition to his articles about psychiatric diagnosis, he has written about the fiduciary relationship, advocacy, and other issues involving law and social reform. He is currently doing research on prescription of psychotropic medication by nonphysicians.

ALDINE DE GRUYTER
A division of Walter de Gruyter, Inc.
200 Saw Mill River Road
Hawthorne, New York 10532

The paper used in this publication meets the minimum requirements of American National Standard for Information Sciences—Permanence of Paper for Printed Library Materials, ANSI Z39.48-1984. ⊗

Library of Congress Cataloging-in-Publication Data
Kirk, Stuart A., 1945–
    The selling of DSM : the rhetoric of science in psychiatry / Stuart A. Kirk and Herb Kutchins.
        p.   cm. — (Social problems and social issues)
    Includes bibliographical references and index.
    ISBN 0-202-30431-0 (cloth : alk. paper). — ISBN 0-202-30432-9 (paper)
    1. Diagnostic and statistical manual of mental disorders.
2. Mental illness—Classification—Political aspects.   3. Mental illness—Classification—Social aspects.   4. Mental illness—Diagnosis—Political aspects.   5. Mental illness—Diagnosis—Social aspects.   I. Kutchins, Herb.   II. Title.   III. Series.
RC455.2.C4K57   1922
616.89'0012—dc20   92-16376
                                                      CIP

Manufactured in the United States of America

10   9   8   7   6   5   4   3   2   1

To
Victor and Irene Kirk
Regina Siciliano-Kutchins
Po Kutchins

"What's the use of their having names," the Gnat said, "if they won't answer to them?" "No use to *them*," said Alice, "but it's useful to the people that name them, I suppose."

—Lewis Carroll
Through the Looking Glass

CONTENTS

ACKNOWLEDGMENTS

In the early 1980s we began to notice that an unusually large number of our graduate social work students every semester were lugging around copies of a huge green book. We were unaccustomed to seeing such dedication to scholarship. We also increasingly spotted the green book on the desks or bookshelves of many of our colleagues at the university and in human service agencies. The book's omnipresence piqued our interest. Although the color changed to blue in 1987 at the time of a revision, it continues to be ubiquitous. In fact, it is now without doubt the most frequently used book among all mental health profesionals.

That book, the *Diagnostic and Statistical Manual of Mental Disorders, Third Edition* (DSM-III), became an object of our interest as soon as we began to read it. What struck us were the claims about DSM-III's development, content, and scientific basis. Given the popularity of the book, the claims deserved careful scrutiny. Our examination of some of those claims has taken us much longer than we ever expected, has pushed us in directions we did not anticipate and has resulted in a book that we had never planned to write.

Along the way, we incurred many debts to colleagues, family, and friends. We have imposed on various people whose judgment we respected by asking them to read at least some parts of this manuscript or to aid us in some other way. They include Rita Black, Ron Boltz, Mary Burger, Susan Einbinder, Donald Gerth, Ronald Feldman, Linda Freeman, Walter Hudson, Nancy Kirk, Brenda McGowan, Carol Meyer, Ed Mullen, Barbara Simon, Wesley Sokolosky, Victor Van Beuren and Jerry Wakefield. They have given us aid and comfort when we were discouraged, advice when we needed it, and criticism where it was deserved. Mark Mattaini served as our ever-helpful bilingual translator, allowing us to collaborate long distance on two different computer systems. Partial support for some of our research was provided by the Faculty Professional Development Program at California State University, Sacramento, and by the Columbia University School of Social Work. We have also had the benefit of comments received when we have presented aspects of our work at Case Western Reserve University, the

Rutgers-Princeton Program in Mental Health Research, the Psychiatric Epidemiological Training Program at the School of Public Health of Columbia University and at numerous professional conferences. There are also several individuals whose thoughtful critiques of the entire manuscript were very helpful, but whose identities were protected through the normal peer review system. We have tried to heed their advice, sometimes more successfully than at others.

Portions of Chapter 6 have been adapted from "The reliability of DSM-III: A critical review," *Social Work Research & Abstracts*, 22(4), 3–12, copyright © 1986, National Association of Social Workers, Inc. Portions of Chapter 9 have similarly been adapted from a published article, "Deliberate misdiagnosis in mental health practice," *Social Service Review*, 62, 225–237, copyright © 1988, University of Chicago Press; and from a chapter of an edited volume published this same year: "Diagnosis and Uncertainty in Mental Health Organizations," in Yeheskel Hasenfeld, *Human Services as Complex Organizations*, copyright © 1992, Sage Publications, Inc. We gratefully acknowledge the permission granted by these publishers to make use of our materials in this book.

Unlike our professional colleagues who are partially obliged to assist when asked, our intimate associates have been dragged unwillingly into DSM land. They deserve credit for hanging in there with us throughout this process. Carol Ann Koz and Gina Siciliano-Kutchins have been unfailingly tolerant in listening to endless DSM-speak and lovingly supportive for so many years in so many ways. They also happen to be fearless critics of our prose. Our children, Brandon, Allison, and Po, have endured our efforts with amused good humor, similar to their response to our parenting. Mike Fitzgibbons has administered two-wheel therapy when needed and when weather permitted. Finally, without the unrequested help of Lily—a feline with an Oppositional Defiant Disorder—who insisted on participating on the word processor, the book would have been finished much sooner.

To write about DSM, two old friends had to learn to become coauthors as well. Many friendships are never tested so severely. Fortunately, with friendship intact, we have overcome differences in work style, perspective, habits of mind, writing style, computer programs, and time zones to complete this task. We both deserve credit. We disagree on who deserves the most.

Stuart A. Kirk
Herb Kutchins

PSYCHIATRIC DIAGNOSIS
AND THE NEW BIBLE

A photograph in *The New York Times* on Monday, January 29, 1990, showed an attractive, groomed, well-dressed young couple sitting at a kitchen table graced by flowers and candles, dining on *gnocchi alla Gorgonzola* that the 33-year-old husband had just prepared. Both he and his 25-year-old wife had serious and determined expressions that matched their attire. Dining without his suit coat, he sported a fashionable striped shirt with tie and suspenders. He and his wife looked like any upper-middle-class young couple on their way up in the corporate and social world.

In fact, the husband had grown up surrounded by wealth and privilege as an heir to the duPont family. Both he and his wife have been active in political affairs; he had contributed handsomely to political causes. He himself had run for a New Hampshire seat in the United States House of Representatives in 1988, but had been defeated in the primary.

This news story did not appear in the home or food or society section of the *Times*; it appeared in the national news section because the couple was not headed to a charity event, but was returning to court to ask a judge to reverse a 1986 court decision that the husband was mentally ill and legally incompetent. That early decision, the couple explained to the news reporter (Hinds, 1990), has meant that the husband is not allowed to manage his own money, was unable to vote when he lived in Virginia, needed the court to validate his marriage three years before and has affected their plans to have children. The wife explained that the court action, prompted by her husband's parents, was a stigma on their marriage and terribly humiliating. They were afraid to have children for fear that his family would try to take them away. It was reported that the parents had already sought to have a guardian appointed for their unborn children.

The precipitating events in this family struggle are the son's political activities and financial contributions to the conservative political organizations of Lyndon H. LaRouche. The parents apparently feared that their son would give away his family inheritance to a disfavored organization.

From the news account, the critical issue for the court in the case is the husband's legal competence as evaluated by psychiatric experts. Although legal competence is not determined solely by psychiatric diagnosis, psychiatric experts usually build their testimony around their diagnostic conclusions. In this case, as often happens, both sides in the dispute hired psychiatrists to give testimony. As often happens, the psychiatrists disagreed. Manhattan psychiatrist Dr. David A. Halperin, hired by the parents in 1985, testified that the son was mentally ill and suffered from a "schizoaffective disorder." Further, the doctor claimed, the son had joined the LaRouche organization "as an expression of his mental illness." A psychiatrist hired by the son testified that the son was mentally competent, but did have a "mixed personality disorder." Both psychiatrists drew their diagnoses from the American Psychiatric Association's (APA) *Diagnostic and Statistical Manual of Mental Disorders, Third Edition* (1980)—DSM-III—the official "bible" for categorizing mental disorders.

Anyone who cared to go beyond the *Times* account by looking up the description of these diagnoses of mental disorders in DSM-III would discover a novel world of categories and criteria. Schizoaffective Disorder is found in a residual section titled "Psychotic Disorders Not Elsewhere Classified." The opening sentence about Schizoaffective Disorder is candidly enlightening:

> The term Schizoaffective Disorder has been used in many different ways since it was first introduced, and at the present time there is no consensus on how this category should be defined. (p. 202)

The few sentences that follow this opening more than confirm the general confusion.

What does DSM-III reveal about the diagnostic judgment of the defense psychiatrist? The description of that diagnosis in its entirety is:

> *Mixed Personality Disorder* should be used when the individual has a Personality Disorder that involves features from several of the specific Personality Disorders, but does not meet the criteria for any one Personality Disorder. (p. 330, emphasis in original)

The diagnostician is confronted with the perplexing task of first determining that the individual has a personality disorder even though the individual does not meet the criteria for any of the defined personality disorders. The clinician may pick and choose features for a tailor-made "mixed personality disorder.'

This family struggle is newsworthy in part because it pits some cherished American values against each other: political freedom versus state intervention; personal liberty versus protection from self-inflicted harm; parental responsibility versus filial independence. These conflicts find their way into the judicial system from many sources and directions. In the duPont case, however, the outcome appears to rest on the accuracy of a psychiatric diagnosis and what that diagnosis implies about an individual's capacities to manage his life. The diagnosis in this case is clearly consequential—it affects the personal and civil liberties of an individual. But just as clearly, the accurate diagnosis is in dispute among reputable psychiatrists.

This is not a rare occurrence. A few months later, *The New York Times* reported (Shulruff, 1990) that a Wisconsin man was facing charges of sexually assaulting an acquaintance who had been diagnosed as having a "multiple personality disorder." The prosecutor suggested that the woman had 21 personalities, not all of which consented to sexual relations. Lawyers and psychiatrists debated whether different personalities would be sworn to testify, whether each had different sexual histories and whether the diagnosis was valid. A National Public Radio report on November 9, 1990, indicated that the man had been convicted and that three of the victim's personalities had testified against him. By December, a circuit court judge had ordered a new trial because of several irregularities (*New York Times*, 1990), including the fact that the defense attorney had not been allowed to conduct a psychiatric examination of the victim before the trial. Some medical experts by then had claimed that the victim had 46 personalities. Will newly identified personalities testify at the second trial?

Since diagnosis guides decisions about treatment, diagnostic confusion can have profound consequences for both patient and practitioner. A decade ago, diagnostic and treatment controversies concerning Raphael J. Osheroff's psychiatric condition led to a famous malpractice suit against Chestnut Lodge, a well-respected private psychiatric hospital near Washington, D.C. Although the case was eventually settled out of court, the issues it raised struck close to the heart of the status of psychiatry as a scientifically grounded profession, as it highlighted the ideological divisions between psychoanalytic and psychopharmacological psychiatrists (Shuchman & Wilkes, 1990; Klerman, 1990; Stone, 1990). Debate about what constituted the appropriate treatment hinged on what constituted the appropriate diagnosis. Over the course of his treatment, Osheroff was diagnosed at various times and by various psychiatrists as having a psychotic depressive reaction; manic-depressive illness, depressed type; major depressive episode with psychotic features; and narcissistic personality disorder. Part of the diagnostic dispute was ideological, reflecting very different theoretical views held among psychiatrists who treated Osheroff. Part of the confusion was over determining which official diagnostic manual was being used. During the course of the patient's treatment, the APA adopted a new diagnostic manual and some of the shifting diagnoses depended on which manual was being used. Narcissistic Personality Disorder, for example, one of the controversial diagnoses in this famous case, appears in the manual used until 1968, but is missing from the manual used from 1968 until 1980 (during which period the diagnosis was used by Chestnut Lodge), and reappears again in the manual used since 1980. Is a diagnosis of Narcissistic Personality Disorder an invalid one in 1979, but valid a few months later? The Osheroff case raised questions about the validity of diagnoses in the face of shifting diagnostic systems and ideological conflicts about the proper methods of understanding and treating clinical conditions.

To some observers, these recent cases suggest that psychiatrists are merely hired guns, paid to say whatever will help their clients. In this view, psychiatrists' testimony is predictably divergent; their professional status as experts serves merely to cloak their paid performances in respectability. Any detailed analysis of the scientific basis for their testimony would be irrelevant. To others, psychiatrists are objective, scientific practitioners trying to bring their best professional judgment as competent mental health experts to bear on difficult cases. Their sharply divergent opinions, therefore, must be due to the uncertain state of psychiatric knowledge or the uncertain art of psychiatric diagnosis (Faust & Ziskin, 1988). Neither of these explanations would please the APA, which has invested the better part of two decades trying to remedy such diagnostic problems, or at least trying to keep them from full public view. The major vehicle in this campaign to rebuild public respect for psychiatric diagnosis and practice was a revolutionary revision of the diagnostic manual—DSM-III.

A New Diagnostic Manual

The year 1856 was a momentous one for modern psychiatry; it marked the births of the leaders of two modern traditions in psychiatry, Sigmund Freud and Emil Kraepelin. Freud, the father of psychoanalysis, has influenced not only psychiatry, but the course of modern thought about human psychology and the role of child development. His theories about mental disorders are psychodynamic and developmental. Childhood experiences in the family, including sexual attractions during the earliest years of life, profoundly influence psychological and emotional development. Childhood experiences, recorded in something that Freud called the unconscious, shape the way we think, feel, and act throughout the rest of our lives. Although Freud was initially an outsider and rejected by the medical establishment of Vienna (he was trained as a neurologist, not a psychiatrist), his dramatic, highly literate writing and his fascinating descriptions of cures captured the public imagination. Eventually his theories came to dominate psychological treatment in many countries. Nowhere was his influence greater than in the United States, a country he detested and refused to visit after his initial sojourn in 1911 to give the famous Clark lectures.

Freud's dynamic theories of the substructures of mental disorders have been contrasted with Kraepelin's approach, which is primarily descriptive. Kraepelin is virtually unknown, even to most mental health professionals. He was a respected professor and a tireless researcher in Germany. He established one of the first psychiatric laboratories and was the author of several important texts. Both his books, *Psychiatry* and an *Introduction to Clinical Psychiatry*, went through many editions during his lifetime. Whereas Freud was primarily concerned with the etiological dynamics of mental disorders, Kraepelin throughout his career attempted to classify, categorize, and describe psychiatric disorders as discrete entities. Kraepelin's descriptive efforts are the basis for the current approach to the identification of mental disorders. Although his books are now outdated, and seldom read even by his adherents, it is his approach that has come to dominate modern psychiatry and to eclipse Freud's work, if not his fame. The growing Kraepelian shadow is currently cast by the *Diagnostic and Statistical Manual of Mental Disorders, Third Edition*, DSM-III.

In 1980, the APA officially adopted a new classification system of mental disorders. The previous classification system, familiar as an old shoe to most clinicians, was of little practical consequence to most mental health professionals and, under most circumstances, was of no more concern to the public than any other technical manual used by professionals. A revised diagnostic system in and of itself would virtually never be a candidate for the sustained attention of anyone other than classification specialists with a special fondness for categorizing behavioral deviance. The development of a new psychiatric taxonomy is rarely momentous. And yet, the system adopted in 1980 received unprecedented attention and is widely believed to have marked a significant milestone in American psychiatry. In influence alone, it may be one of the most significant events in psychiatry in the last half of the 20th century.

Certainly the manual's principal architect does not underestimate its impact. In an article about the development of the DSM-III, its principal author and an associate (Bayer & Spitzer, 1985) characterized it in the following manner:

> The adoption of DSM-III by the American Psychiatric Association (APA) has been viewed as marking a signal achievement for psychiatry. Not only did the new diagnostic manual represent an advance toward the fulfillment of the scientific aspirations of the profession, but it indicated an emergent professional consensus over procedures that would eliminate the disarray that has characterized psychiatric diagnosis. (p. 187)

Gerald Klerman, who was the highest ranking psychiatrist in the federal government at the time that DSM-III was developed and published, was even more forceful. In a debate sponsored by the APA at its 1982 national convention between proponents and critics of DSM-III, Klerman asserted:

> In my opinion, the development of DSM-III represents a fateful point in the history of the American psychiatric profession. . . . The decision of the APA first to develop DSM-III and then to promulgate its use represents a significant reaffirmation on the part of American psychiatry to its medical identity and its commitment to scientific medicine. (Klerman, 1984, p. 539)

He went on to say:

> The theme of this meeting is "science in the service of healing." In my opinion, DSM-III embodies this theme to a greater extent than any other achievement in American psychiatry since the advent of the new drugs. (p. 541)

And he concluded:

> the judgment is in; DSM-III has already been declared a victory. There is not a textbook of psychology or psychiatry that does not use DSM-III as the organizing principle for its table of contents and for classification of psychopathology.
>
> This debate is already an anachronism. The victory of DSM-III has been acknowledged by our colleagues and adversaries in psychology, in the other mental health professions and in other countries. (p. 542)

An even less restrained description of the achievements of DSM-III was written for the general public in a popular softcover, *The New Psychiatrists*, by Gerald Maxmen, who proclaimed in oracular fashion:

> On July 1, 1980, the ascendance of scientific psychiatry became official. For on this day, the APA (APA) published a radically different system for psychiatric diagnosis called . . . DSM-III. By adopting the scientifically based DSM-III as its official system for diagnosis, American psychiatrists broke with a fifty year tradition of using psychoanalytically based diagnoses. Perhaps more than any other single event, the publication of DSM-III demonstrated that American Psychiatry had indeed undergone a revolution. (1985, p. 35)

This revolution in psychiatry was not a popular uprising. It was not spurred on by widespread public interest in the new developments, as had happened when Freudian psychoanalysis came to dominate psychiatry 50 years earlier. Nor were mental health clinicians themselves clamoring loudly for radical changes in diagnoses. Those who created DSM-III did not call on the rich heritage of Greek legends and other literature that Freud used to invent what he referred to as his mythology. The creators of this revolution were far less colorful officials in government agencies, professional associations, and university research centers whose motives were as much bureaucratic and political as scientific. And what is most remarkable about their revolution is that they did not discover a single new disorder, they proposed no new treatments, and they provided no new explanation for mental illness. In fact, one of the things that they prided themselves on was that they carefully avoided any etiological explanations for mental disorders that did not already have widely recognized, well-established organic causes.

What was the nature of the revolution signaled by the appearance of DSM-III? Maxmen claims scientific psychiatry replaced psychoanalytic psychiatry and that the contrasts between the two are profound: "Psychoanalytic psychiatry bases truth on authority; something is true because Freud said so. Scientific psychiatry bases truth on scientific experimentation. . . . The old psychiatry derives from theory, the new psychiatry from fact" (p. 31).

It is often a debater's trick to claim that one's position is accurate because it is factual, in contrast to that of one's opponent, who has invented justifications for his or her position. The strategy may be obvious, but the stakes were much greater than are usually the case in academic disputes. What was at stake was the fate of the psychiatric profession and the enormous, multibillion dollar mental health industry. DSM-III and "the new psychiatry" that it reflected were important features in the effort made by a new generation of psychiatrists to gain control over the infrastructure of the psychiatric profession and to reverse the diffusion of power to other professions in the mental health enterprise.

The Mental Health Enterprise

The new diagnostic manual provides the official justification for psychiatry's expanding control over what some have labeled the "medicalization of deviance" (Conrad & Schneider, 1980). The influence of the manual radiates out beyond the state asylum or the private physician's office, affecting many sectors of American life in subtle and at times controversial ways. The diagnostic manual is used in the judicial system when questions are raised about a defendant's mental capacities, intentional states, or cognitive abilities. Legal problems involving guardianship, criminal liability, fitness to stand trial, and the extent to which defendants have the capacity to appreciate the consequences of their acts are common circumstances in which testimony about diagnostic categories is invited. Psychiatrists and other mental health professionals frequently are asked to make judgments on the health status of various private behaviors such as homosexuality or substance use. Psychiatrists even claim that tobacco use falls within their purview. Furthermore, psychiatric classification affects how society allocates millions of dollars of health funds. Psychiatric diagnoses directly affect which human problems will be covered by public funds and private insurance. Inevitably, psychiatric concepts seep deeply into our art, fiction, theater, movies, language, humor, and our views of ourselves and our neighbors.

Numbers tell part of the story of how rapidly the mental health enterprise has grown. Mental health treatment in the United States has become a major industry both in terms of the expansion in the number of professionals employed and in the growth of government and private insurance expenditures for problems of mental disorder. From 1975 to 1990, the number of psychiatrists increased from 26 to 36 thousand, clinical psychologists from 15 to 42 thousand, clinical social workers from 25 to 80 thousand, and marriage and family counselors from 6 to 40 thousand. In aggregate, the increase in 15 years has been from 72 to 198 thousand professionals in just those four professions (Goleman, 1990). Similarly, in NIMH-surveyed psychiatric facilities, the number of personnel increased from 375 thousand in 1976 to 441 thousand by 1984 (Schulberg & Manderscheid, 1989:16).

There are no reliable figures on the total cost of mental health care. In 1981, inpatient treatment for mental disorders was estimated to be almost $12 billion (Kiesler & Sibulkin, 1987) and the costs for all forms of treatment were estimated a decade ago to consume one tenth of all health care expenditures or over $20 billion (Mechanic, 1980). A more recent government estimate is that the direct economic costs of mental health care is close to $55 billion per year (NIMH, 1991:29). Estimates of the number of people suffering from mental disorders vary directly with the broadness of the definition, but range from a few percent to one third of the population (Cleary, 1989; Robins & Regier, 1991).

People receiving help from mental health organizations have contact with a variety of agencies. After a decade of shift from inpatient to outpatient settings, by 1975 approximately 70% of all psychiatric episodes (initial contacts) involved ambulatory care, 27% occurred in inpatient facilities, and 3% in partial care settings (Schulberg & Manderscheid, 1989:15–16). But the total number of caregiving episodes of all types mushroomed by almost 300% during the two previous decades (Schulberg & Manderscheid, 1989:16).

There has been a parallel explosion in the number of mental health organizations. From 1970 to 1984 the increase was almost 50%. The number of private psychiatric hospitals grew by 47%; the number of general hospitals operating separate psychiatric services by 59%; equally significant growth occurred among community mental health centers. By contrast, the number of state and county hospitals declined by 10% (Schulberg & Manderscheid, 1989). But not all psychiatric services are provided in these organizational settings. By 1980, by one estimate, 75% of outpatients were seen in the private offices of psychiatrists, psychologists, social workers or primary care physicians (Schulberg & Manderscheid, 1989).

The mental health enterprise has been transformed in three decades from a system of large public mental hospitals where most psychiatric services took place—supplemented by a few outpatient clinics and private psychiatrists—to an array of public, not-for-profit, and for-profit inpatient facilities and an explosion of clinics and private psychotherapists from many disciplines. From a system in which the majority of treatment facilities were public institutions of last resort for the impoverished, elderly, and mentally disabled, where admission was by involuntary civil commitment and resulted in lengthy stays at public expense, we now have a fragmented, multitiered, diversely sponsored and financed array of services for less impaired clients who voluntarily seek help from those who dispense what has been dubbed the "popular psychotherapies" (Specht, 1990).

American psychiatrists sit precariously on top of this expanding business in the profession that provides the intellectual and programmatic leadership to the field. Their position is precarious for at least two reasons. First, having won cultural jurisdiction over personal problems from the clergy and from neurologists by the middle of this century, psychiatrists so successfully promoted outpatient psychotherapy that when widespread third-party funding for such services became available so did widespread competition from psychologists, social workers, nurses, and marriage and family counselors (Abbott, 1988). Today, psychiatrists constitute less than 20% of all mental health professionals. As mental health practice became multiprofessional and located in community mental health centers rather than in the state hospitals, it became less "medical" in orientation. Thus, by the late 1960s, outpatient psychotherapists from various professions started to look indistinguishable and community psychiatrists looked like social workers or community psychologists. Psychiatrists, by partially abandoning their claim to special expertise rooted in medicine, were able to promote psychotherapy as a cultural institution, but they also spawned their own professional competition.

The second reason for psychiatry's precariousness is its marginal status within the medical profession. Although trained as physicians, psychiatrists sit at the bottom of the totem pole of medical specialties. Providing services that were similar to those offered by nonmedical professions, especially when the scientific basis for many psychotherapeutic theories and techniques was uncertain, did not help their image with their medical brethren over the last several decades.

What would help with both the nonmedical competition and with colleagues in medicine was the development of biopsychiatry, an ambitious attempt by psychiatry to reposition itself professionally. The biopsychiatry project involves the search for physiological, genetic, and chemical bases for mental disorders and the development and use of psychopharmacological agents for treatment. Both elements emphasize the medical aspects of psychiatric knowledge and distinguish psychiatrists' professional contributions from those of their psychotherapeutic competitors. Biopsychiatry is an attempt to secure a more powerful base for psychiatry within the jurisdiction of both medicine and mental health.

This context provides a backdrop for the attempts of psychiatrists to assert leadership in developing an official language about mental disorders. Psychiatric diagnosis provides the fundamental rubric for discourse about mental illness. The publication of DSM-III in 1980 marked a major turning point for American psychiatry (Sabshin, 1990). It abruptly shifted emphasis from the etiological psychodynamic perspective that had dominated psychiatry since World War II, it introduced an official definition of mental disorder, it brought a philosophy of empiricism to the nosology that had heretofore been absent, it proposed that mental disorders be considered along multiple axes, it attempted to describe in behavioral terms the criteria that must be present for the use of each diagnostic category, and it self-consciously asserted that the new classification manual represented the best that psychiatric research had to offer. By intent and careful plan, the developers of DSM-III sought to bring about a revolution in how mental health professionals thought about and practiced psychiatric diagnosis.

On many levels, the revolution succeeded remarkably well. The new manual was strikingly different than its predecessor (DSM-II; APA, 1968) and its popularity as measured by sales was unprecedented. It immediately shaped almost all discussion of diagnosis not only in the United States, but throughout the world. References to it are ubiquitous in the mental health journals, where by 1990 over 2,300 scientific articles explicitly referred to it in the title or abstract. Most clinical discourse and psychiatric research are conducted within its confines. Many psychiatrists welcomed the new approach as redefining psychiatry in ways that were more compatible with the emerging biological models of mental disorder and thereby moving psychiatry closer to mainstream medicine, from which it had wandered during the decades of the sixties and seventies.

Any revolution, however, has its skeptics and naysayers. DSM-III has had its share. There are many views of what the development of DSM-III meant to the mental health enterprise in America, in addition to the pronouncements of its developers that it was a triumph of science over clinical ideology. Not surprisingly, psychologists have been among the most vociferous critics. They worried that DSM-III was an attempt by psychiatrists to medicalize more human problems, laying claim to professional territory that was being hotly contested by them and others (Goleman, 1990; Salzinger, 1986). A few viewed the new manual as the misguided triumph of empirical research and logical positivism in psychiatry (Faust & Miner, 1986). Other critics labeled DSM-III as "scientifically disastrous," the outcome of efforts "to reconcile different power groups" through large-scale committee work (Eysenck, 1986). And from the political left came a stinging critique that the manual was "basically a political and social device for protecting the status quo, for maintaining a social order that supports exploitation and injustice" (Rothblum, Solomon, & Albee, 1986).

Whatever the true significance of DSM-III and regardless of which of its characteristics embodied that essence, no one claims that the appearance of DSM-III was a trivial event. To the contrary, its publication is often described as a landmark, revolutionary, a tour de force and a major achievement. Perhaps no way of gauging DSM-III's impact is more revealing than the fact that the APA's diagnostic manual itself became an object of intense discussion in a way that no previous manual had. An abundance of journal articles were written about it, symposia were held, debates were arranged, training materials were disseminated, DSM-III workshops proliferated, and conference sessions were scheduled to discuss it or its revision. The APA's diagnostic manual was transformed from an obscure desk reference—a peripheral clinical tool—into an omnipresent, huge compendium that became the center of attention in American psychiatry for a decade. Most strikingly, despite being controversial, the approach it introduced has survived two major revisions of the manual.

The sustained attention was justified. An official classification system of mental disorders embodies fundamental aspects of how psychiatry views the nature of its enterprise. To classify is to arrange and group some phenomena according to some system or principle. DSM-III contains the official classification system of psychiatric disorders and as such sets the boundaries of the domain in which psychiatry claims expertise and exclusive authority. The manual specifies the kind of behaviors and problems for which the profession's counsel should be sought and its voice heard. DSM-III is making a claim regarding psychiatry's authority within the broader community.

Equally important, DSM-III, as a classification system, asserts how knowledge about mental disorders should be organized. Here the claim is not on the external community about authority, but on the internal community of scholars about how best to advance knowledge. This latter claim asserts how behaviors should be grouped and interpreted. It implicitly suggests how knowledge should be organized and how it should be accumulated. Thus, a classification system of disorders inevitably structures the research and knowledge development activities of a profession, including the evolution of the theoretical understanding that will emerge from them. DSM-III, then, by providing a revised structure for the conceptual development of psychiatry, offered more than a series of revised labels for diseases; it asserted a new paradigm for the advancement of psychiatry.

Overview

Surprisingly, among the vast literature about DSM-III, virtually nothing has been written about how this revolution occurred. In fact, most commentary on DSM-III treats its development as somehow inevitable, an overdue breakthrough for scientific psychiatry. The achievement, whether applauded or occasionally decried, is frequently described but rarely critically analyzed. DSMs proponents are frequently heard describing its major achievements, its unique features, and its developmental stages, and offering examples of its impact on mental health research and practice. But nowhere can one find a serious examination of how the making and selling of DSM came about. Although there are many scientific and political threads to the full story, *The Selling of DSM* concentrates on the most salient scientific problem—diagnostic reliability—and traces how the developers of DSM-III created, managed, and used this problem to reform the official diagnostic manual.

Our approach to this story grows out of a sociological tradition that views social problems and social issues as phenomena that are created through collective definition rather than as conditions that objectively exist to be studied and remedied (Spector & Kitsuse, 1987). This approach emphasizes the study of claim-making activities in which individuals or groups make assertions and complaints about something that they consider harmful and try to mobilize other people or institutions to do something about them (Best, 1989). Thus, the focus is on claim-makers and their activities, how the problematic conditions get defined, how approaches to ameliorating the problem are promoted, and how various contingencies shape the success of the claim-makers' efforts.

The "problem" of diagnostic reliability that will occupy much of our attention became a problem because influential researchers were able to use a historical moment to claim effectively that diagnostic inconsistency was a serious matter that should be attended to. Our analysis makes no concerted attempt to determine whether diagnostic reliability really was or is a problem, how serious it was or is, or how it should be remedied. Rather, we focus primarily on how claims were made about reliability, what those claims implied, how those claims were used, and what consequences those claims had. In the process of examining these phenomena, we are forced to attend to the language and methods of science as well as to the political processes that surrounded the creation of DSM-III (Gusfield, 1981). Thus, our analytical focus is on the creation and management of a scientific problem that played an important role in the development of a revolutionary, new diagnostic manual.

In Chapters 2 and 3 we describe the scientific and political context from which DSM-III developed. We emphasize the variety of problems that confronted American psychiatry in the 1950s and 1960s. We explore how the unreliability of psychiatric diagnoses became symbolic of the profession's self-doubts and of its vulnerability to public and scientific criticism. This conundrum partially explains why diagnostic reliability became the focus for sustained scientific attention. We argue that through the creation and use of a new statistic, the kappa statistic, the problem of reliability was transformed from a seriously threatening conceptual and practical problem into a technical problem, best left to experts who promised technical solutions. Redefined as a technical problem, diagnostic reliability lost its simple, intuitive meaning to practitioners and became, in the hands of a few teams of research psychiatrists, complex and mystified. This particular rendering of the problem allowed these teams of investigators to assume virtual control over both the problem and the terms of its solution. More importantly, their work on the reliability problem provided them with critical leverage to position themselves to initiate a broader paradigmatic shift in American psychiatry.

The way that these psychiatric researchers achieved such remarkable influence is explained in Chapter 4, where we describe their role in the development of DSM-III. The problem of reliability, as well as the simultaneous controversy over the psychiatric status of homosexuality as a diagnosis, were used as entry points by some of these investigators to reshape the psychiatric nomenclature. Just before the revision of the manual started, dissatisfaction over psychiatric diagnosis came to a climax in a highly publicized and acrimonious debate over the legitimacy of homosexuality as a psychiatric diagnosis. This controversy was resolved by an embarrassing plebiscite of the APA membership.

In order to avoid a repetition of this type of political decision-making about diagnosis, research psychiatrists tried to create a manual that was based on scientific principles and data. This transformation was spearheaded by the DSM-III Task Force, appointed by the APA and composed primarily of a few select members from small research teams. The members, particularly the Task Force's chair, used the problem of reliability to achieve a powerful position in American psychiatry. By developing a massive superstructure consisting of dozens of committees, and involving hundreds of participants, the Task Force created the illusion that the development of the manual was the result of a enormous research effort. Despite the widespread participation of psychiatrists and other mental health professionals, actual decisions were made by a small group of participants in the Task Force. Research, including the data generated from a large federally supported study, was used selectively to support the goals of the Task Force and to undermine the objections of their opponents, particularly psychotherapists with a Freudian orientation, who constituted the majority of the APA. The eventual coup, led by psychiatric researchers, successfully used the language, paradigms, and technology of research to gain influence over clinical language and practice. Thus, DSM-III was presented not only as a solution to the problem of psychiatric reliability, but as the embodiment of a new science of psychiatry.

In Chapters 5 and 6, we critically examine the frequently made claim that DSM-III greatly resolved the reliability problem. In particular, we review whether the data gathered in the original DSM-III field trials actually support the claims of the developers. These studies have often been the object of adoration, but infrequently the subject of careful scrutiny. These chapters offer a thorough reanalysis of the methodology and data. Even using the modest standards suggested by the developers, we find that the studies so frequently cited to claim success in resolving the reliability problem were flawed, incompletely reported, and inconsistent. The interpretation of the data was often partially misleading. Data from other reliability studies that appeared at the time also raise serious questions about the reliability of the new manual. Because the interpretation of diagnostic reliability had become mystified, would-be critics found themselves persuaded by the sanguine interpretations offered by the developers of DSM-III. Despite the apparent weaknesses of the scientific evidence supporting the bold claims of its developers, DSM-III capped a successful revolution in psychiatry.

In Chapter 7, we explore the paradox of how a successful revolution occurred when its success had been tied so closely to its ability to solve the reliability problem, even though the problem was not, in fact, greatly ameliorated. We examine how the rhetorical language of scientific psychiatry in important journal articles made bold claims about equivocal data. Moreover, we reveal how the standards for interpreting reliability data were dramatically shifted over 15 years in a direction that made it easy for sophisticated and respected investigators to control the strategic use of these data. To appreciate the uncommon success of DSM-III fully, we argue that one must understand the politics and management of science that are important ingredients of the DSM-III story.

Once the manual had been published and accepted, the revolution that it represented had to be protected. In Chapter 8, we place the development of DSM-III in historical perspective by reviewing the patterns through which the manual has been revised during the last 40 years. We look carefully at how the developers of DSM-III strategically managed the processes of revising the manual in ways to protect its future. In part, the strategy of the developers depends, paradoxically, on continuing revisions that leave critics off balance when they attempt to criticize a constantly moving target. It also depends on a strategy in which the developers of each revision publicly claim that only minor changes will be made, while privately developing major ones. We document these maneuvers in the most recent revisions of the manual. Such tactics have institutionalized the DSM-III revolution in nosology and largely protected it through the next two revisions of the manual.

In the final chapter, we place the reliability problem in a broader sociological context and suggest that the meaning of diagnostic reliability as defined and approached by the developers of DSM-III is inadequate for an understanding of diagnosis and diagnostic errors as they occur in clinical practice. While reliability had been a salient problem for investigators, clinicians and the organizations in which they work approach diagnosis with different concerns. The needs and routines of psychiatric researchers for "technical rationality" are remarkably different than those of clinical practitioners who must cope with the uncertainties of patients, third-party reimbursement, and their own mental health organizations. On the surface, DSM-III was successful in appearing to impose a rigorous research solution on clinicians. Clinicians, however, appear to use the new diagnostic system in a variety of ways, some of which are neither scientific nor anticipated.

Our analysis of the development and selling of DSM-III offers an unconventional interpretation of the circumstances, activities, and research that produced a revolutionary change in the way psychiatrists and other mental health professionals approach mental illness. We challenge the generally accepted understanding about the research data and the process that led to DSM-III. Some major institutions and professional associations have a stake in the conventional view, but many mental health professionals and others may be interested in how that conventional view was created and maintained. This book examines that process.

2

THE TRANSFORMATION
OF PSYCHIATRIC TROUBLES

The real revolution in medicine . . . did not begin with the introduction of science into medicine. That came years later. Like a good many revolutions, this one began with the destruction of dogma. It was discovered, sometime in the 1830s, that the greater part of medicine was nonsense.

Lewis Thomas, *The Medusa and the Snail*

Certainly the failure of both psychiatrists and psychologists to develop a satisfactory classification of their subject matter . . . is a most serious barrier to fruitful research into the aetiology of mental illness and even into the efficacy of therapeutic regimes. It is more exciting to develop explanatory theories, or to claim impressive results for this or that treatment, than it is to define the critical characteristics of the patients on whom one's research was based. It is probably more exciting to an architect to design parabolic canopies or baroque facades than it is to calculate the size and shape of the concrete slab on which his building will rest. But theories and therapeutic claims have no more chance of surviving than buildings if they are not built on secure foundations. Developing reliable diagnostic criteria and a valid classification may be as tedious as filling muddy holes with concrete but both provide the foundation on which all else depends.

R.E. Kendell, *The Role of Diagnosis in Psychiatry*

Perhaps there has been no period in American psychiatry when the profession was not confronted by serious problems. For psychiatry, or for that matter for any profession, there is always room, and often a public demand, for improvement. Inhuman conditions in state asylums periodically aroused the public's concern and their medical superintendents were expected to take corrective action. New knowledge opens doors to what appears momentarily to be a path to more effective treatment. Shifting social values or new social problems, such as homelessness, family violence, or sexual abuse, emerge and the profession is asked to address conditions that it is ill prepared to handle. Moreover, social critics from the political right suspect that psychiatry is peddling a liberal social ideology, while those on the political left sense that mental health is a modern method for the state to suppress dissent and maintain order. Other critics simply lie in wait for the profession to overstep its bounds or inflate its abilities. From its earliest days, American psychiatry has been sensitive to these shifting currents of American social thought (Rothman, 1971).

Some of psychiatry's special sensitivity to public opinion stems from the fact that it lies on the outskirts of American life. Insanity describes those furthest from acceptable and expectable behavior. Those who minister to the insane or dispossessed tend to become marginal as well, subject to the fluctuating standards of public life and decorum. When society shifts its philosophy, values or direction, those on the periphery are the first to feel the effects. Trouble is no stranger to psychiatry.

Normal Troubles

By the early 1950s, American psychiatry as a profession was confronted with an array of serious problems. Both psychiatric institutions and psychiatric technologies were under fire. The predominant mental health treatment facilities—state asylums—originally constructed as retreats for those adversely affected by the stresses of industrial society (Rothman, 1971), were the target of exposés alleging inhuman conditions, brutal treatment, and overcrowding. Furthermore, the fact that most "patients" were confined involuntarily conveyed asylums' similarity to prisons rather than to medical hospitals. The steadily increasing operating costs of these facilities were causing enormous concern among state officials, particularly the projections of the need for new hospitals to be built in the near future, which were expected to consume enormous state fiscal resources.

Psychiatry's primary therapeutic orientation, based on psychodynamic theory, while enormously influential in intellectual and cultural circles for nearly a half-century, was hopelessly impotent in confronting what were being recognized as the public mental health needs of the nation. However effective individual, long-term, outpatient psychotherapy was with people with neuroses, psychiatry was ill equipped to handle the problems of those crowded into state facilities.

Psychiatric medications, first widely used in the mid-1950s to control the florid symptoms of psychosis, offered a ray of hope that a new treatment technology would alleviate the problem of custodialism in state hospitals and would equip psychiatrists with indisputably effective treatments. It was a scientific breakthrough that created a more positive public image for the profession. Psychiatry's public image was very poor and there was an acknowledged difficulty in attracting well-trained professionals into its ranks (Joint Commission, 1961). Psychiatry, like its clientele, had been stigmatized and socially neglected (Joint Commission, 1961; Star, 1955). Ironically, the advent of psychiatric medications, which provided one justification for discharging masses of patients from state hospitals, exposed psychiatry, two decades later, to renewed public criticism as former hospital patients wandered around city streets, unkept, ill housed, and untreated. Deinstitutionalization was a shortsighted and costly success (Johnson, 1990). By the 1980s, the public did not have to depend on newspaper exposés to learn about the shameful neglect of the seriously mentally ill, they could witness it themselves on the streets of every major city.

By midcentury, problems for psychiatry were not only coming from the press, public, and policymakers, but also from social and behavioral scientists, who were raising new and equally ominous concerns about psychiatry's effectiveness as a helping profession. The troubling suggestion heard more frequently was that psychiatric treatment itself, particularly as it existed in state hospitals, violated the Hippocratic admonition to do no harm. The cloak of rehabilitation that had covered the essentially custodial functions of state asylums was removed, exposing the stark reality of the iatrogenic effects of institutionalization. Goffman's brilliant and widely read essays epitomized this critique (Goffman, 1961). These criticisms, in combination with other concerns, played a powerful role in reshaping mental health care in the decades that followed.

Institutional care was not the only aspect of psychiatric treatment to be criticized. Outpatient treatment, which grew in importance and prominence as institutional care diminished, came under critical scrutiny. For example, evidence accumulated that the preferred treatment of choice— psychoanalytic psychotherapy—was ineffective (Eysenck, 1952) or, at best, no more effective than other forms of therapy. Equally damaging in the socially conscious 1960s when poverty and disenfranchised minorities were reluctantly recognized, it appeared that psychotherapists preferred clients who were young, attractive, verbal, intelligent, and successful—what came to be labeled the YAVIS syndrome. Psychotherapy was described as the purchase of friendship (Schofield, 1964). Psychotherapists were accused of creating demands for services from those who were not really ill, but were merely discontent—the worried well—and neglecting the more needy.

While these criticisms threatened psychiatry, they pointed to problems that could be managed. New psychiatric treatment facilities could be built and staffed with better trained professionals. New community-based mental health clinics could be developed to provide services in the community. Social insurance could be extended to assist those who were unable to afford private psychiatrists. Social and legal policies could be altered to safeguard the mentally ill from unwarranted involuntary hospitalization. More research could be undertaken to uncover the etiology of mental illness and the differential effectiveness of alternative treatments.

For the most part, the various criticisms of psychiatry could be managed through enlightened and progressive reforms. As badly bruised as psychiatry may have appeared from this pummeling, the attacks could be used to stimulate needed correctives to professional practice. At the core, the attacks were not on the fundamental assumptions of the profession, but rather on the failure of psychiatric practice to live up to its ideals. All professions, of course, are subject to these accusations. But psychiatry's troubles became far more serious.

Fundamental Problems

More fundamental and troublesome attacks on psychiatry emerged. Some of them came from within the profession itself. By far, the most serious assaults came from those who questioned the concept of mental illness or the aims of psychiatry. There were many different directions from which such attacks came in the 1950s and 1960s.

Thomas Szasz (1960, 1961) was one of the most prolific, controversial, and persistent critics of psychiatric theory and practice. A psychiatrist and psychoanalyst by training, Szasz argued that what were called mental illnesses were not illnesses, but merely socially devalued behaviors. Real mental illnesses, he argued, are those abnormalities of behavior and thought that are clearly linked to an underlying physiological dysfunction. With many of those behaviors diagnosed as mental illnesses, however, such physical bases do not exist or at least have not been established. In fact, he argued, the criteria for determining what constitute mental illnesses are social and ethical, not medical. They are similar to illnesses only by metaphor, not by fact. Mental illnesses are myths, concepts derived from an inappropriate metaphor. These myths function "to disguise and thus render more palatable the bitter pill of moral conflicts in human relations" (p. 118). Mental illness, he claimed, was a fancy name for problems in living.

The attack by Szasz reverberated throughout the mental health field. Its power to disturb the profession of psychiatry came not only from Szasz's persistence and prodigious writings, but from the fact that he attacked psychiatry's ties to medicine, ties that were historically weak and vulnerable. Psychiatry's claim to preeminence in the mental health industry was already under siege from clinical psychology, psychiatric social work, psychiatric nursing, and other emerging professions like marriage and family counseling, and from the proliferation of new non-medical therapies that emerged from the counterculture of the sixties (Castel, Castel, & Lovell, 1982). Equally important, Szasz's attack suggested that in identifying and treating the mentally ill, psychiatrists had more in common with ministers and police than with physicians. In making these accusations, he threatened the intellectual and political foundations of psychiatry as a profession.

Sociologists, who adopted the spirit of the times, developed a particularly unsettling view of mental illness and psychiatric practice, at least as far as the psychiatric establishment perceived it. Emerging from a theoretical perspective known as symbolic interactionism, sociologists viewed *mental illness* as they would any other label for deviant behavior (Spitzer & Denzin, 1968). Mental illness, they suggested, told us not so much about internal, individual pathology, as about the social processes through which certain behaviors became defined by people in authority as instances of insanity. Mental illness was viewed as an arbitrary social label, conveying more about the structure of authority in a particular social situation than about pathology. This view spawned an active sociological literature on the conditions and processes by which some people were labeled as mentally ill and the consequences of such labeling for self-attitudes and the reactions of others. To many sociologists, mental illness was merely another instance of how society labels and controls those who behave badly.

One widely read sociologist (Scheff, 1966) went several steps further in debunking psychiatry by arguing that behaviors that are labeled mental illness are simply behaviors for which other explanations were unconvincing. Mental illness is merely a residual category of behavior, an explanation of last resort. From this perspective, mental disorder is viewed as a label behind which psychiatrists and the public hide their ignorance. Furthermore, Scheff argued that the act of labeling "residual deviants" played an important part in encouraging the individual to meet the role expectations of someone who is "insane." Other authors also raised similar concerns about the iatrogenic effects of diagnostic labels themselves (Stuart, 1970). Ironically, intervention in the form of diagnosis was viewed as a self-fulfilling prophecy.

Lawyers, like those involved in the duPont case described in the introduction, routinely pitted psychiatrists against each other in widely publicized criminal trials where their contradictory testimony did little to convince the public that the profession of psychiatry knew what it was talking about. As recently as 1988, extensive reviews of the empirical evidence raised serious questions about whether psychiatrists and psychologists meet legal standards for expertise in courtroom testimony (Faust & Ziskin, 1988). On much more general grounds, other legal scholars have criticized the trend toward the medicalization of a variety of forms of deviant behavior (Kittrie, 1972).

Broader historical and cultural critiques of psychiatry appeared. Some argued that psychiatric labels served functional purposes for society by demarcating the boundaries between sanity and madness (e.g., Foucault, 1965). Others (e.g., Ivan Illich, 1975) criticized medicine and the professions for usurping authority under the guise of knowledge and technology, and inappropriately extending their influence throughout modern life. R. D. Laing's (1967) critique turned mental illness on its head by suggesting the schizophrenia was an adaptive response to a chaotic and disordered society. And even as psychiatrists left the much criticized confines of the state asylum to practice in the community, they were accused of being skilled specialists supervising a world where they would manipulate people to accept the constraints of society (Castel et al., 1982:320), a radical critique that continues today (Cohen, 1990). These criticisms found receptive audiences in the 1960s and 1970s when so many American institutions, values, and practices were subjected to critical scrutiny and reassessment.

These pointed attacks constituted a much more fundamental challenge to psychiatry than criticisms of its clinical effectiveness or its hospitals. Services can always be improved, access to them for the poor arranged, and patients' rights protected. On the other hand, if mental illness does not exist, if psychiatric symptoms have little to do with medical science, if the entire mental health enterprise is a carefully structured fiction about life's normal troubles, and if psychiatrists are policemen in white coats, then psychiatry confronts a much more serious challenge. That is why these latter criticisms so threatened psychiatry as a profession; they questioned the *conceptual* integrity of the entire enterprise. Did mental illness exist? What was its conceptual definition? On what basis could diagnostic judgments be made? Could psychiatrists recognize mental illness when it exists? It was increasingly apparent that the system for determining and classifying psychiatric disorders was in serious trouble. So vulnerable was the classification system that, even from respectable quarters within psychiatry, calls were made to abandon diagnoses altogether (for a review, see Zigler & Phillips, 1961, and Kendell, 1975). By the early 1970s, some psychiatrists argued that psychiatry and the medical model were dying and deserved a good Irish wake (Torrey, 1974).

Although invitations to the wake were premature, psychiatry was viewed by many to be in critical condition. Nothing is more basic to a profession or a science than the validity of its core concepts. Concepts are the building blocks for organizing and advancing knowledge. The problems that psychiatry addresses must be named, defined, and distinguished from each other. Scientific respectability requires this ability from a profession. And in medicine, clinical knowledge and effective intervention are supposed to flow from such differentiation. As criticisms mounted, the definition and classification of mental disorders emerged as an enormously important problem for psychiatry.

Transformation of the Problem

Psychiatry and the other mental health professions aspire to be professions using science to help people. As a science-based profession, psychiatry is expected to have a scheme for organizing knowledge of mental illness and developing methods of intervening effectively. Making a diagnosis is a pivotal clinical decision that summarizes the practitioner's understanding of the disorder and guides the clinician to select a disorder-specific treatment. Psychiatric diagnosis and treatment, and the vast sums of money that support them, are presented by the profession as firmly grounded in natural and behavioral science.

Every profession's wish for scientific respectability is understandable. All the mental health professions aspire to it. Psychiatrists, clinical psychologists, social workers, nurses, and others are expected to apply the knowledge and skills of their respective professions in assisting clients. Among the hallmarks of many professions is the claim that their practitioners will consciously and carefully apply specialized scientific knowledge to specific cases and circumstances with the objective of solving particular problems. Professional knowledge is specialized, firmly bounded by purpose, rooted in science, and standardized in application. Professional practice is service through the application of science. Schon (1983) refers to this process of instrumental problem solving made rigorous by the application of scientific theory and technique as *technical rationality*. Mental health professionals and the organizations in which they work explain many of their decisions and behaviors as the expression of technical rationality. The process of diagnosing mental disorder provides a powerful framework for mental health professionals to demonstrate the connection between science and practice.

Although the value of diagnosis is rarely questioned in most branches of medicine, it has been disputed in psychiatry for decades, because the therapeutic and prognostic implications were viewed as weak and the diagnoses themselves as unreliable (Kendell, 1975). Many psychiatrists, however, took little interest in this problem, feeling that it was merely an academic matter without any practical importance. A few psychiatrists, on the other hand, continued to argue that the nature of mental illness and diagnosis were of fundamental importance and could not be ignored or dismissed. Despite the wavering and flawed definitions of disease, the uncertain knowledge of etiology, the diverse bases for classification, and the fact that all concepts have a tendency to become reified as if they refer to real entities, there was no reasonable alternative to developing a diagnostic classification system (Kendell, 1975).

Classification

A profession whose sole mission is understanding and treating a particular form of illness must show convincingly that it can describe and recognize the illness when it occurs. Further, if there are different varieties of the illness, the profession needs to identify what those subtypes are and how they are distinguished. If one were to claim to be an expert healer of "skyitus," a rare disease presumably associated with the consumption of airplane food, one would be required to define skyitus, document its occurrence, and distinguish it from other illnesses, such as "fast-fooditus." Moreover, to acquire status and influence, one would need to show that the disease has serious consequences and that one's profession could effectively prevent or treat it. One would have to begin, however, with a convincing definition of the disease, a system for identifying its characteristics, and a procedure for locating it in some classification scheme that differentiates it from other similar phenomena.

Description and classification are basic to all science. That is precisely why attacks on the concept of mental disorder raised such serious questions for psychiatry. When critics suggested that psychiatric classification was invalid, the allegation could not go uncontested. Classification is essential to all science, and while there are inevitably losses of information as phenomena are grouped into categories, these processes are not in and of themselves problematic. The defenders of psychiatry used this line of argument to justify having and using classification systems and to rebut those who suggested abandoning psychiatric diagnoses altogether (Zigler & Phillips, 1961; Kendell, 1975).

Defending the legitimacy of the *need* for a classification system was not, however, the same as defending the *existing* classification system. While some jumped to the defense of the necessity for psychiatric diagnosis, by the early 1970s few jumped to defend the scientific merit of the then current system of diagnoses.

History of Classification Systems

Although descriptions of madness and its subtypes have been around since the ancient Greeks (Zilboorg, 1941; Alexander & Selesnick, 1966), until the last half of the 20th century a handful of unofficial, broad categories appeared to be sufficient for the task. By the 1990s, however, the count had grown to about three hundred and appears to be rising rapidly. Moreover, categories of disorders are all now carefully encrusted in a nationally approved classification system. How, in brief, did this evolve?

The context of this evolution is the linguistic legacy of 19th-century epidemiology, which pursued the causes of infectious diseases by plotting morbidity and death among various populations (Mirowsky & Ross, 1989a, 1989b). As epidemiology developed, it spawned a variety of methods of counting and sorting people who were at risk of having some disease. These methods presupposed that people could be sorted into two groups: those with the disease and those without it. Psychiatry, mimicking the approach of medicine, adopted this basic concept of "caseness" and pursued systems of classification into which cases of psychiatric disorders could be placed.

But psychiatry was slow to become enamored with diagnostic classifications, in part because psychiatrists recognized that any nosology, i.e., a classification of diseases, based on symptomatology rather than etiology presented formidable problems. Furthermore, while there were vigorous discussions about etiology in the 1800s, there was little consensus that enough was known about the causes of insanity to produce a nosology (Grob, 1991). Nevertheless, at the end of the 19th century, Emil Kraepelin, working with patients at his clinic in Heidelberg, developed a system of identifying diseases by focusing on certain groups of signs and tracking their eventual outcomes as a method of determining disease entities.

The development of psychiatric nosology in the United States has been shaped primarily by external demands and broad social forces, rather than by the desires or felt needs of practicing clinicians. The earliest classification systems of mental disorders in the United States were developed by the federal government for the U.S. census, which played a predominant role in psychiatric nosology for almost a century (Grob, 1991). In the 1840 census there was only one category: idiocy, which included insanity. By 1880, there were seven categories: mania, melancholia, monomania, paresis, dementia, dipsomania, and epilepsy. In 1904 and 1910, two special surveys were conducted enumerating the institutionalized insane. Neither census paid much attention to psychiatric nosology. The one in 1904 was particularly concerned with race and ethnicity, and the growing fear of the large-scale immigration of presumably inferior groups. The 1904 census was an attempt somehow to document that putative inferiority by statistical studies of patients in asylums (Grob, 1991).

In subsequent years census officials became more interested in the need for a standard nosology and asked the American Medico-Psychological Association, the forerunner to the APA, to appoint a committee on nomenclature to facilitate the collection of data. Psychiatrists, who were beginning to involve themselves in a broader array of community problems and adopting a broader vision of their social mission, began to see how better social statistics might be used to guide mental health planning. In 1913, the Association created a Committee on Statistics (Grob, 1991). By 1918, it produced, with the cooperation of the National Committee for Mental Hygiene, the first standardized psychiatric nosology, the *Statistical Manual for the Use of Institutions for the Insane*. The manual offered 22 principal categories that had a decidedly somatic or biological orientation. This perspective was congruent with the fact that most psychiatrists practiced in mental hospitals and many patients, perhaps a majority, had severe physical as well as mental problems. The somatic nosology reflected the nature of psychiatric care (Grob, 1991). Developed in 1918, the manual was adopted by the census and was used to survey mental institutions annually, a tradition that was continued by the National Institute of Mental Health after World War II.

The major opponent of the new nosology was Adolf Meyer, a prominent figure in American psychiatry, who said that "statistics will be most valuable if they do not attempt to solve all the problems of administration and psychiatry and sociology under one confused effort of a one-word diagnosis marking the individual. . . . The statistics published annually as they are now are a dead loss to the States that pay for them, and an annual ceremony misdirecting the interests of the staff" (as quoted in Grob, 1991, p. 426).

Despite such criticism, the new manual went through ten editions between 1918 and 1942, retaining its somatic orientation. In 1935, it was incorporated in the first publication of the American Medical Association's *Standard Classified Nomenclature of Disease* (Spitzer & Williams, 1983).

These advances in nosology, however, were of only marginal significance to psychiatrists or their patients. The categories were broad, and psychiatric treatment at the time was nonspecific. The struggles to develop a systematic nomenclature, from the earliest decades of the 19th century, were motivated by administrative and governmental needs, not by demands from practitioners (Grob, 1991). This is a pattern that has persisted.

World War II produced the next nosology. The experience of psychiatrists during the war was responsible for the first major change in psychiatric nosology. It was embodied in the *Diagnostic and Statistical Manual: Mental Diseases*, now commonly referred to as DSM-I. Published in 1952, it was the first edition of the *Diagnostic and Statistical Manual* published by the American Psychiatric Association. DSM-I reflected major political and theoretical shifts that had occurred in American psychiatry. The somatic tradition gave way to psychodynamic and psychoanalytic perspectives, which had achieved ascendancy in the profession by the middle of the 20th century. These new viewpoints (more so than the somatic theories) emphasized the role of environment and the variety of less severe forms of disturbance that could benefit from the attention of the psychiatric profession. Military and Veterans Administration psychiatrists, many of them physicians assigned to psychiatry during the war, had difficulty using the old nomenclature to describe the psychiatric casualties of battlefield stress because many of the casualties appeared to be helped by brief treatment in noninstitutional settings. Finally, following the war, there was a dramatic increase in the number of psychiatrists and a radical shift in the settings where psychiatry was practiced, away from mental hospitals to community clinics and private practice (Grob, 1991). Clinicians increasingly worked with noninstitutionalized populations and those suffering from less severe disorders, such as neuroses and personality disorders, rather than psychosis. These constituted some of the developments that resulted in the more "modern" nosology represented by DSM-I. This new manual was produced in one year by an appointed working group and published in 1952. DSM-I reflected this transformation of psychiatry and the ascendancy of new leadership in the profession.

DSM-II, published by the APA 16 years later in 1968, expanded the number of disease categories and continued the psychodynamic traditions of DSM-I. DSM-II, however, differed from its predecessor in several notable ways. It encouraged rather than discouraged the use of multiple diagnoses for a single patient and the DSM-I term *reaction*, as in *schizophrenic reaction*, a legacy of the influential psychiatrist Adolf Meyer, was largely dropped. The APA committee that was assigned the task of preparing the second edition took three years to complete its work. Robert Spitzer, who was to become a major spokesperson for psychiatric nosology for two decades, served as a consultant to the Committee on

Nomenclature and Statistics that developed DSM-II and he emerged after its publication as a major defender of it (Spitzer & Wilson, 1968, 1969). Again, as with earlier nosologies, DSM-II was intended primarily to reflect, not to change, the current practice of psychiatry.

Psychiatric classification has continued to change and at an accelerated rate since DSM-II. Many chapters in this book will examine the change to DSM-III in 1980 and some attention will be devoted to its revision (DSM-III-R) in 1987 and to DSM-IV, currently being developed. Several generalizations about these processes of revision will be made on the basis of the analysis to follow. First, none of the revisions are stimulated by clinical practitioners demanding a new classification system. Second, the writing of each revision has become more time consuming, elaborate, and politically complex. Third, the numerous changes made with each revision are justified explicitly or implicitly as improving the scientific credibility of the classification system, although the scientific basis for them is often questionable. Finally, the process of revision inevitably begins by attacking the current system, even when it has only recently been adopted and ends by claiming the superiority of the new one. Before examining in detail the transition to DSM-III, however, we need to review how the troubles confronting psychiatry were transformed.

The Validity Problem

The attacks on the conceptual foundations of psychiatry, much more than the attacks on its methods of delivering services or its treatment effectiveness, were assaults on the validity of its classification system as represented by DSM-I and DSM-II. Nosology, which had never assumed a prominent role in psychiatric research or practice, started to become the object of considerable professional concern. Could the profession withstand sharp criticisms from social and behavioral scientists if it continued to neglect the problem of the credibility of its nosology? DSM-I and DSM-II evolved largely in response to external administrative interests and through professional consensus. They stressed comprehensive coverage and clinical acceptance or compliance, much more than scientific validity or clinical usefulness (Barrett, 1987). Understandably, the end product did not fare well in a modern environment in which scientific standards of inquiry and evidence increasingly provided the structure for discourse. Psychiatry, by the last quarter of the 20th century, was not a strong contender in the scientific arena. It had drifted both from medicine and from the rapidly developing behavioral sciences. And nowhere was the profession as vulnerable as on issues of diagnostic validity.

The notion of validity is an important one in the social and behavioral sciences, particularly among psychologists concerned with measurement (Nunnally, 1978; Kerlinger, 1986) and diagnosis (Kendell, 1975; Barlow, 1991). Classification is, in the crudest way, a form of measurement, a method of determining whether phenomena have the particular characteristics for membership in a class. Questions about the meaningfulness of the concept of mental illness, just like questions about the substantive meaning of many relatively abstract concepts such as intelligence or anxiety, involve issues about the validity of scientific constructs. Construct validity is distinguished from other types of validity (such as content validity and predictive validity) in that it concerns basic questions about the nature of reality. Having an operational procedure for determining whether a phenomenon belongs in a class does not fully address the question of what that construct or class is. For example, intelligence tests have been used for generations, even though there is wide disagreement about the nature of the construct intelligence. The frequent response that intelligence is what is measured by the IQ test is an awkward way of avoiding the very difficult construct validity problem. It is a way of using a technical measure to solve, or rather to avoid essentially, a thorny conceptual problem.

Critics of psychiatry were asking about the construct validity of "mental illness." Can it be defined in a conceptually coherent and logical way to distinguish it clearly from "normality"? Are there subtypes of mental illness that can be defined and distinguished in meaningful ways? These are enormously difficult questions that continue to intrigue diagnostic theoreticians (for a review, see Wakefield, 1992a, 1992b).

Psychiatric nosology, as expressed by DSM-II, did not attempt to provide a conceptual definition of mental disorder. Instead, it offered general, vague descriptions of specific disorders that had evolved over the years through professional consensus. For example, one disorder, "inadequate personality," was defined as "ineffectual responses to emotional, social, intellectual and physical demands . . . inadaptability, ineptness, poor judgment, social instability, and lack of physical and emotional stamina" (APA, 1968:44). Even though such a description survived the scrutiny of those involved in developing DSM-II, it hardly silenced those who raised questions about construct validity. This description of inadequate personality had, at best, a form of validity that is called *face validity*. Robert Spitzer, who was a key consultant on DSM-II and who was the senior architect of DSM-III, quipped that face validity was "directly proportional to the number of approving faces and the wisdom of the people behind those faces" (Spitzer & Williams, 1983:593). To a great extent psychiatric nosology has been a product of committee meetings and smiling faces.

Nowhere was the issue of validity so poignantly raised as in the heated debates in the early 1970s about the psychiatric status of homosexuality, listed in DSM-II as a mental disorder (Bayer, 1981). The APA was unable to determine whether being gay was grounds for establishing a diagnosis of mental disorder. This controversy, which we discuss in greater detail in the next chapter, highlighted the existing confusion among psychiatrists about what constituted a mental disorder. Furthermore, the continuing public embarrassment for the APA as it tried to decide what was a mental disorder—amidst the political clamoring of various factions—gave the appearance that scientific psychiatry was an oxymoron. Even after the matter was temporarily resolved through negotiations, there were few smiling faces within the APA.

The debates about homosexuality could have been about most other diagnoses, had there been strong differences of opinions and hungry media. The debates had nothing to do with the ability of psychiatrists to identify homosexuals, but everything to do with a conceptual and theoretical problem, namely, whether homosexuality constituted a disorder. In order to address that question, psychiatrists would have to define disorder convincingly. On that question, no consensus existed. To make matters more complicated, there was also no consensus on the etiology of homosexuality or of many other putative mental disorders, leaving spokespersons for psychiatry to face a bewildering array of embarrassing questions. Hence, without a workable definition of mental disorder and without an established theory of pathology, psychiatry appeared to be confronting insurmountable conceptual problems that appeared to center on the system of classification. This is not to say that the evidence for the validity of specific diagnoses was nonexistent, but taken as a whole, according to a widely respected researcher, the evidence for the validity of diagnostic categories was "meagre" (Kendell, 1975).

The nosology itself appeared to limit the advance of empirical research that could clarify questions of construct validity. In order to make progress on this front, researchers and clinicians had to be able to determine consistently what disorders individual patients really had. Questions about validity were hampered by the inability of psychiatrists to agree on who was mentally ill and what type of illness they had. When psychiatrists regularly disagreed about the diagnosis of specific clients, it was very difficult to rebut outside critics or persuade them that the basic psychiatric concepts were valid or meaningful. Thus, as psychiatrists struggled with problems of validity, they also had to confront a more visible problem: reliability. Unlike problems of validity, however, reliability could be more readily transformed into a manageable problem that was less threatening to the profession. Unlike problems of validity, solutions to reliability problems appeared to be closer at hand and required no firm knowledge about etiology, treatment, or prognosis.

The Reliability Problem

The reliability of a psychiatric classification system refers to "the extent to which users can agree on diagnoses applied to a series of cases" (Spitzer & Williams, 1983:596). Can clinicians assessing a group of people sort them into the official diagnostic categories and agree with each other about who goes where? The intuitive meaning of reliability is quite simple: Can two clinicians independently identify the person with schizophrenia and distinguish that person from the one with, say, a personality disorder? This simple meaning of reliability can be understood quite easily by clinicians who often differ with colleagues about the proper diagnosis for particular clients. Even the lay public, which has little clinical or technical knowledge, can recognize the practical problems of clinicians disagreeing about diagnoses. The popularity of getting "second opinions" from medical experts attests to this recognition.

To researchers, however, unreliability poses a particularly difficult impediment to advancing knowledge. If diagnoses cannot be reliably made, it is nearly impossible to conduct research or make progress on etiology and treatment effectiveness or to engage in research across geographically different settings. Unreliability constrains the ability of scholars to enhance diagnostic validity; it sets a cap on the level of possible validity that can be achieved.

The commonsense simplicity of the concept of reliability made it particularly easy for critics to highlight this important weakness in psychiatric classification and practice. If the diagnostic system was unreliable, it was probably invalid as well. Since the official classification system in American psychiatry after World War II was deeply rooted in psychoanalytic concepts, the problem of reliability challenged the validity of the dominant theoretical perspective in the profession. No theory, just as no profession, can claim preeminence for long if it cannot firmly establish that its adherents agree on the use of its basic organizing concepts.

There is, however, one ironic advantage of problems of reliability: they make it possible to forget about the messy problems of validity. Preoccupation with the consistency of clinicians' judgments about the presence of mental illness or about the types of mental illness in a particular group of patients has the attraction of avoiding the issue of the general conceptual definition and meaning of disorder. Reliability problems can be reduced to questions about techniques of decision-making, in contrast to validity problems, which must answer complex philosophical and theoretical questions.

To illustrate how different reliability and validity problems are, consider what would have happened if psychiatrists had been accused in the early 1970s simply of not making the diagnosis of homosexuality reliably, i.e., not consistently determining who was homosexual. The APA could have appointed a small committee to establish and refine the observable criteria that had to be present to make the diagnosis of homosexuality, test the criteria to be sure that trained clinicians could apply them consistently, tinker some more with the criteria, and walk away from the matter with the problem more or less solved. It would have been comparatively easy to focus on the inconsistencies in diagnosis rather than to delve into the highly charged political and conceptual dilemmas about the validity of homosexuality as a mental disorder.

Not only do reliability problems appear much less threatening and much more resolvable than validity problems, they tend to attract attention away from serious dilemmas, while appearing to resolve them. Although the APA's drama over homosexuality forced attention on issues of validity, these issues are no less complex for less controversial categories of mental disorders, e.g., schizophrenia or personality disorders. But most categories of disorder do not have active constituencies of labelees raising tricky questions of meaning and social values. Most disorders can be sustained in the psychiatric nosology by mere incumbency.

The advantages of focusing on reliability were only relative to addressing the conundrum of validity. Reliability problems themselves presented potentially grave consequences for psychiatry. Reliability problems came to be viewed as so severe that they themselves also struck at the heart of the legitimacy of psychiatry as a scientific enterprise. Many authors have stressed the point that a classification system that is unreliable surely cannot be valid (Spitzer & Fleiss, 1974:341). However, the unintended false implication was that a reliable system would be valid. To the contrary, a perfectly reliable system can be completely invalid, as many authors have shown (for a cross-cultural example, see Kleinman, 1988). Although as a practical matter, diagnostic reliability was of much more concern to research psychiatrists and to the critics of psychiatry than to clinicians, weaknesses of reliability, once brought into the open, could not be ignored or left unresolved. Diagnostic reliability was the easily recognized glass jaw of psychiatry, and critics from many quarters came to take a swing at it.

Early Studies and the Beginning of Mystification

The authors of many of the early studies of diagnostic reliability—those conducted prior to 1970—were not as pessimistic about their findings or as quick to conclude that reliability was low as more recent reviewers have been. Reliability studies by teams of investigators in England (Kreitman, Sainsbury, Morrissey, Towers, & Scrivener, 1961) and in Philadelphia (Beck, Ward, Mendelson, Mock, & Erbaugh, 1962) presented rather upbeat interpretations of their findings. Both teams attempted to overcome some of the methodological problems of prior studies and both proudly reported what they clearly thought of as encouraging, but not perfect outcomes. Kreitman et al. report specific diagnostic agreement of 65% for 90 consecutive patients. Beck et al., using DSM-I, were pleased with diagnostic agreement of 54% among experienced psychiatrists assessing 153 outpatients, pointing out that the finding was statistically significant ($p<.001$) and "was higher than that obtained in other comparable studies" (p. 356). Other researchers (Sandifer et al., 1964) who found a 57% agreement rate judged it as "not generally satisfactory for scientific purposes" (p. 355), although their interpretation revealed more puzzlement than condemnation for this state of affairs.

Early reviews of multiple studies of diagnostic agreement reached no simple conclusions, certainly not that diagnostic reliability was disastrously low nor that the profession was in jeopardy. Kendell (1975) suggested that the pessimism that did arise was not completely justified. In 1961, Kreitman, writing in the forerunner of the *British Journal of Psychiatry*, found ample ambiguity in the existing reliability studies. He emphasized the difficulty of comparing reliability studies because of the variety of uncontrolled factors that could affect the results of each study, such as the experience and orientation of the psychiatrist, the purpose and setting of the diagnostic examination, the nomenclature used, the characteristics of the patients and way in which agreement was calculated. He concluded, "with so many variables haphazardly controlled, it is not surprising that there is little unanimity of results in the literature" (Kreitman, 1961:880). He summarized five studies that appeared between 1949 and 1959 and concluded, "Even though there is scant evidence that the present state of diagnosis is as uniformly bad as it is often reported to be, there is clearly room for improvement" (p. 884). While acknowledging the importance of improved reliability, he stressed that the problem of diagnosis is ultimately one of validity and that seeking high reliability did not ensure high validity. He warned, "It is enough to point out that blind adherence to reliability alone can be misleading whether applied to diagnosis or any other clinical assessment" (p. 884).

Later commentators came to view these early studies unambiguously as representing a very serious problem. For example, Matarazzo (1983), past president of the American Psychological Association, who has written about the reliability of psychiatric diagnoses for 25 years, made these summary comments on the early reliability studies that were conducted between 1930 and 1965: "In fact, until 1967, the number of research workers who found diagnostic judgments based on psychiatric interviews unreliable outnumbered those who reported studies showing that they were reliable" (p. 105). Since at the time of these early studies there were no standards by which to judge whether a study documented reliable or unreliable diagnoses, such judgments depended on the viewpoint of the reviewer. Matarazzo cited one of the important early studies conducted by Ash in 1949:

> In his study, 52 white males were evaluated in a government-related clinic in a joint interview by two or three psychiatrists who worked full time in this clinic. Typically, one of the psychiatrists conducted a physical examination of each man and then called his colleague(s) in for the psychiatric interview. The psychiatric interview was jointly conducted, each psychiatrist asking whatever questions he wished. However, each psychiatrist recorded his diagnosis independently. . . . An earlier, pre-1952 version of the official nomenclature of the American Psychiatric Association . . . was used for their diagnostic judgments. This involved five *major categories* (mental deficiency, psychosis, psychopathic personality, neurosis, and "normal range but with predominant personality characteristics") and some sixty *specific* diagnostic subcategories. Agreement levels among the three psychiatrists in the 35 cases (examined by all *three* in simultaneous conference) for the *major* category diagnosis was 45.7%; for *specific subcategory* diagnosis it was only 20%. (1983:106, emphasis in original)

This was clearly a disappointing finding. Even among psychiatrists who worked closely together and conducted joint interviews there was diagnostic disagreement just about as often as agreement. Agreement on specific diagnoses occurred only one out of five times. Such unreliability was embarrassing to the psychiatric community, which knew that the findings would be viewed as curious by the public on whose faith they depended. Although the findings could not have bolstered the confidence of psychiatrists in their craft, at the time there was clearly no agreed-upon standard to measure what degree of consistency *should* be expected. The ambiguity about what should be expected provided a fertile context for the later resolution of reliability problems.

More recent observers, like Matarazzo, who systematically reviewed reliability studies appearing before 1965, generally conveyed similar disappointment. Grove, in a 1987 review of some early studies in which he recomputed agreement rates, made no direct interpretation of their results, but the thrust of his overall review was to interpret more recent studies as indicating much better reliability than the pre-1965 studies, which, in his opinion, were "low." But here, as well, Grove neglected the issue of how to *interpret* the results of reliability studies, although it is at the core of the problem and, as we shall argue later, the core of the solution.

Concern about diagnostic reliability was also prompted by cross-national studies. Some research psychiatrists found that diagnostic practices varied across countries. In one early study, Sandifer, Hordern, Timbury, & Green (1968) discovered that psychiatrists in North Carolina, London, and Glasgow reached different diagnostic conclusions while viewing the same filmed patient interview. They raised concerns about improving comparative studies, but they expressed no disappointment about the within-group levels of diagnostic agreement, which ranged from 58 to 73%. Other studies found that some American psychiatrists used a broader definition of schizophrenia than some of their European counterparts, which made epidemiological studies across nations difficult. Cross-national research, such as the International Pilot Study of Schizophrenia (Wing, Cooper, & Sartorius, 1974; Wing & Nixon, 1975) and the United States–United Kingdom study (Kendell et al., 1971) led to the development of narrower definitions of schizophrenia in the United States and to the development of methods of standardizing approaches to diagnosis (Andreasen, 1989). Despite these efforts, cross-national differences in the definition of mental disorders, frequently one of the rationalizations for changing the official nosology, continue to this day.

No sooner had serious questions emerged about diagnostic reliability than both defenders of psychiatry and its critics agreed that the problem was much more complex than it had appeared at first. Through critiques of the methodologies used in the early studies, reinterpretations of their data, development of more complex measures of agreement, and identification of the various sources of error that could account for unreliability, the problem of reliability was further removed from the conceptual and political problem of defining mental illness. As research psychiatrists approached the problem of diagnostic reliability, they transformed it into a technical difficulty requiring technical solutions. Questions of validity were not solved, they were simply set aside.

As a technical problem, reliability had two major advantages: The first was that it appeared to be more solvable than problems of validity, at least in controlled research settings. The second advantage, an unintended by-product of many scientific advances, was that the technical solutions proposed and the gauge developed to measure their success were beyond the easy comprehension of clinicians and the public alike. To understand the implications of these dual advantages and how they transformed some of the problems confronting psychiatry, one has to follow how the seemingly simple matter of agreement between clinicians about a diagnosis became much more complex and difficult.

To begin, let us review one initial step in this transformation. In an early, rudimentary critique of reliability studies, Beck (1962) analyzed nine studies. He ignored data based on organic diagnoses because they generally had much higher rates of agreement and therefore masked the relatively low rates of other categories. He then concluded that methodological problems made "it difficult to draw *any* definite conclusions about the reliability of the present nomenclature" (pp. 212–213, emphasis added). The methodological problems he identified may have either inflated or reduced the levels of diagnostic agreement in any single study. They included:

- greatly varying degrees of training and experience among clinicians
- poorly defined, overlapping categories
- administrative or other extraneous considerations used in classifying patients
- different amounts and quality of information available on which to make diagnoses
- long time intervals between diagnostic appraisals in some cases, which raised the possibility that the patient's condition had actually changed
- awareness of the earlier diagnosis in some cases
- and too few or restricted ranges of clinical conditions in some studies.

To Beck, these obvious problems made "any comparison of the results . . . difficult to interpret" (p. 213). Nevertheless, when excluding the "organic" cases, he found diagnostic agreement ranging from 32 to 42%. He raised a simple, but crucial question: Is that acceptable? He continued:

> It is evident that any appraisal of the value of the system of diagnosis needs to take into account the specific purposes for which the system is to be used.
> It would seem that for research purposes a system of classification using the refined categories, which had an inter-judge agreement rate of no better than 42%, would be considered inadequate. On the other hand, if one is interested only in the broader categories (such as neurosis and psychosis), where the degree of agreement is substantially higher, then the present system is more acceptable. (p. 213)

He then pinpointed a significant issue that was generally ignored in the ensuing decades. He suggested that reliability was not that important to clinicians anyway. Although common sense suggested that clinicians were handicapped by unreliable diagnoses, in reality,

> the extent of this handicap is related to the degree to which the psychiatrist depends on the diagnostic label in actual clinical decision-making. It could be argued, for instance, that the psychiatrist is seldom bound exclusively by the actual diagnosis, (p. 213)

but bases his treatment recommendations on other factors. The distinction between diagnosis for research or clinical purposes is an important one, and it hovers over the reliability problem, but is never fully or squarely recognized in the subsequent reliability literature, where its implications are subtle and largely neglected. We will address some of these in the final chapter.

As a remedy for the methodological shortcomings of the early studies, Beck recommended that future studies use: (1) the most recent standard nomenclature; (2) psychiatrists with sufficient and comparable experience to make the diagnoses; (3) uniform conditions, e.g., setting, time allotted, and amount of information, to make the diagnoses; (4) studies to determine how much contamination occurs between psychiatrists in joint interviews and how much effect the passage of time has between interviews; (5) diagnoses made independently of the routine clinical decision-making of the institution. These were all reasonable and modest suggestions that psychiatric researchers provide better designed studies of reliability.

Beck's cautious critique contained the kernels of what later grew into a major research enterprise. While he was reluctant to conclude that reliability of psychiatric diagnoses was poor (a reluctance not shared by others a decade later), he sensed the ways that better research could be designed. His suggestions were simply attempts to bring studies of reliability up to accepted standards for psychological research. His primary message was that the whole reliability matter was much more complex and difficult to understand than many thought.

The Kappa Contortion

The transformation of psychiatry's classification problem into a technical problem is nowhere as well illustrated as by the emergence of a new statistic. This new statistic, called kappa (κ), rapidly became the coin of the reliability realm. Originally developed for other academic fields (Cohen, 1960) as a general measure of agreement for nominal (or categorical) scales, it found a welcoming economy within psychiatry. Like other coinage, it was pursued relentlessly, was used to assert authority, and was instrumental in transforming the language of diagnostic commerce.

By the 1960s, researchers recognized that interpreting the results of the early reliability studies was handicapped by the use of different statistical methods. For example, some studies would report the overall rate (percentage) of perfect agreement, others would report an overall measure of association (e.g., contingency coefficient), and still others would report the probability that given that one clinician had made a particular diagnosis, a second clinician would make the same diagnosis (Spitzer, Cohen, Heiss, & Endicott, 1967). Although each of these methods conveyed some information about reliability, because they presented different aspects of it they were not fully comparable. Consequently, while each approach was relatively simple and could be understood by a nontechnical professional reader, they impeded the ability of researchers to compare findings across studies or to assess whether progress was made in achieving greater diagnostic consistency.

There were other serious problems with some of these simple methods of calculating diagnostic agreement. The first was the serious problem of agreement that occurred by chance. Whenever two independent judges make a diagnosis of a patient, there is always the possibility that they might make the same diagnosis, even if neither had any actual knowledge of the patient. That is, they might *by chance alone* make the same guess. In actual studies, of course, diagnosticians all have some of the same information about a patient on which to base their independent judgments, but embedded in the likelihood of their agreement is some unspecified element of chance. This possibility of agreement by chance alone needed to be recognized in measures of reliability.

Here is the way in which the issue of chance agreement clouded the interpretation of reliability studies: Suppose we learned from two different studies of reliability, each involving 100 patients and 2 clinicians, that in one study the level of agreement between diagnosticians (i.e., interrater agreement) was 50% and in the second it was 68%. Is this "higher" rate of agreement in the second study a "better" rate of reliability?

In the simple situation of two clinicians independently diagnosing a series of persons as either having or not having a psychiatric disorder, a certain level of agreement could be expected by chance alone. In fact, it would be very difficult for two clinicians *not* to agree in any cases, especially if they were making dichotomous decisions. Let us see how this happens. In the hypothetical study above, where the two psychiatrists achieved 50% agreement, they could have reached that level of agreement in very different ways. For now, let us assume that the two psychiatrists knew absolutely nothing about each patient and that they each simply independently flipped a coin to decide if the patient had a mental disorder or not. This procedure would result in each clinician diagnosing about half the persons as having a mental disorder, half as

Table 2.1.   Diagnostic Agreement Between Two
           Clinicians for 100 Patients by Flipping a Coin

Judgments of Clinician B	Judgements of Clinician A	Yes	No	Total
Yes		25	25	50
No		25	25	50
Total		50	50	100

Note: Yes, presence of disorder; no, absence of disorder.

not. The clinicians would not have identified all the same persons as having a mental disorder. By chance alone, however, some of their random "guesses" would have coincided. In fact, the laws of probability allow us to estimate the extent of their overall diagnostic agreement in this situation (see Table 2.1). In this circumstance, we would expect that they would agree on specific individuals about 50% of the time by chance alone (25 of those judged jointly with a disorder and 25 of those judged without a disorder ($25 + 25 = 50/100 = 0.50$). We would interpret this 50% agreement as not better than chance or, more bluntly, as not exhibiting any meaningful agreement.

In the second study, where the two clinicians agreed 68% of the time about 100 patients, let us assume that these two clinicians were prone to see evidence of psychopathology in many people. In fact, let us assume that with any group of people they assessed, they both would find signs of psychiatric disorder in about 80% of the cases evaluated (see Table 2.2). In their independent assessments of the 100 test clients, they both found mental disorder in 80 of the 100 people. In this situation, by chance alone, we would expect them to agree diagnostically 68% of the time ($64 + 4 = 68/100 = 0.68$). Thus, the findings from the second study, although reporting a higher level of agreement, did not report a better

Table 2.2.   Diagnostic Agreement Between Two
           Clinicians for 100 Patients Where Both Clinicians
           Found Mental Disorder in 8 Out of 10 Cases

Judgments of Clinician B	Judgments of Clinician A	Yes	No	Total
Yes		64	16	80
No		16	4	20
Total		80	20	100

Note: Yes, presence of disorder; no, absence of disorder.

level of agreement. In both studies, the level of agreement could be explained by chance alone, rather than by professional skill.

Notice how intriguing and slippery the level-of-agreement problem becomes and how, while pondering it, the validity problem can easily escape notice. Agreement between clinicians is not necessarily grounded in any objective reality about the actual condition of the people being assessed. For example, the 50% agreement in Table 2.1 or the 68% agreement in Table 2.2 could be achieved even if all or none of the 100 people had a mental disorder. In fact, 100% agreement can be achieved as long as two clinicians both find mental disorders in everyone they see or never find disorder in anyone, independent of the actual or "real" condition of the cases. In other words, high agreement can be achieved even if diagnostic validity is completely absent.

The second serious problem with reports of reliability was with what are called *base rates*. A base rate is the proportion of a population that has a disease or disorder. The base rate problem involves the statistical problem of chance agreement played out in situations where there is great variation in the proportion of the study population who may have particular psychiatric disorders. It is particularly problematic when there are diseases with low prevalence, i.e., low base rates.

This problem was illustrated in a recent article (Shrout, Spitzer, & Fleiss, 1987). Suppose 100 people in a community are carefully assessed by two skilled clinicians, each of whom makes a diagnosis when he or she finds evidence of mental disorder. Let us assume that each clinician diagnoses a disorder in only 6% of the cases; the vast majority of people are viewed by both clinicians as not having a mental disorder. In this situation (see Table 2.3), in 94 (91 + 3 = 94) of the 100 cases the clinicians agreed. Given this 6% base rate, is 94% agreement better than chance? By chance alone (even if the clinicians never interviewed the people, but simply guessed that 94% would be without disorder and randomly chose which 6 people should be given a diagnosis), the clinicians would have guessed correctly on 88.4% of the noncases ($0.94 \times 0.94 = 0.8836$) and on 0.4% of the cases ($0.6 \times 0.6 = 0.36$), achieving an overall agree-

Table 2.3. Hypothetical Results from a Reliability Study

Clinician B \ Clinician A	Diagnosis Positive	Diagnosis Negative	Total No. of Cases
Diagnosis Positive	3	3	6
Diagnosis Negative	3	91	94
Total No. of Cases	6	94	100

Note: Adapted from Shrout et al. (1987).

ment rate of about 88.8% (88.4% + 0.4%). In the example, the clinicians agreed in 94% of the cases, which is a very high rate of agreement, but is at the same time only slightly better than chance. Thus, low base rates alone can make the percentage level of chance agreement very high.

These problems involving the possibility of chance agreement and base rates led to the introduction of a new method of quantifying agreement that attempted to solve these problems. In a very influential paper (Spitzer et al., 1967) titled "Quantification of Agreement in Psychiatric Diagnosis," the kappa statistic and its computation were introduced to the psychiatric audience. The formula for computing kappa is: $\kappa = (p_o - p_c)/(1 - p_c)$, where p_o is the observed proportion of agreement and p_c is the proportion of agreement expected by chance. For example, in Table 2.3, the clinicians actually do better than what would be expected by chance. The difference $94 - 88.8\% = 5.2\%$ represents their improvement over chance. The best improvement possible in this case is 11.2% $(100 - 88.8\% = 11.2\%)$. The kappa statistic is defined as the proportion of improvement actually obtained by the clinicians over and above chance; in this case, $\kappa = 5.2/11.2 = .46$. Thus, chance corrected agreement in Table 2.3 is almost half of what is theoretically possible (11.2%). In this particular case, a small 5.2 percentage point improvement over chance results in a kappa of .46. With other base rates, very different percentage point improvements—some lower, some much higher—might be needed to achieve a kappa of .46. Thus, kappa, by correcting for chance agreement, moved the focus away from simple agreement measured by percentages to a second-order statistic that had no immediate observable relationship to clinical activity.

The introduction of kappa into the reliability literature was not presented in a way that made the statistic immediately comprehensible to anyone other than researchers or statisticians. Part of this problem is inherent in the nature of statistical concepts and computations and part is in the inability of researchers to make their technical papers comprehensible to a general readership. Most researchers are clumsy science writers.

When kappa was introduced (Spitzer, Cohen, & Fleiss, 1967), it was embedded in an article that was marred by two interesting, but unnecessary complications. The first was the attempt to calculate degrees of agreement on the assumption that some psychiatric disagreements were better than others. There were shades of disagreement, it was argued, and some inconsistencies among diagnosticians were more profound than others. The promoters of kappa gave prominence in the article to a "weighted kappa" that distinguishes among degrees of disagreement. Weighted kappa provides for partial credit when there are levels of disagreement that can be predetermined. For example, if a classification of mental disorders allowed for three categories (No Disorder, Anxiety Disorder, Schizophrenic Disorder), a weighted kappa could be used to give partial credit if one clinician diagnosed anxiety disorder and a second one diagnosed schizophrenic disorder, instead of judging their conclusions as disagreement. The assumption would be that both clinicians found a "disorder," even if they disagreed about the type, and therefore their judgments should receive some reliability credit.

In introducing the weighted kappa in this important article, however, the authors offered no guidelines for how or when these weights should be assigned. Instead, considerable space was given to the more complex statistical formula that should be used in calculating a weighted kappa and to discussing an example of its use. The authors also did not propose any guidelines for properly interpreting it. Weighted kappa was simply presented as a complicated tool that was now available for use, although how exactly to use it was ambiguous. Ten years later, Helzer et al. (1977a:132) argued that using a weighted kappa would introduce confusion into interpretations of kappa since, clearly, weighted kappas would almost always be higher than unweighted ones using the same data. This would, of course, defeat the primary objective of using kappa to standardize levels of diagnostic agreement and, ironically, would lead to exactly the same interpretive confusion in the literature that kappa was introduced to remedy.

Despite the considerable emphasis in this article that was placed on weighted kappa, in subsequent decades weighted kappa has hardly made any appearance in the psychiatric reliability literature. In several instances, including the very important DSM-III field trial data that we will scrutinize later, there is some ambiguity about whether "partial" credit was given for near misses. However, the introduction and prominence of weighted kappa in this seminal paper added unnecessary complexity to the meaning and calculation of diagnostic reliability. It was an unintended warning to readers that reliability studies could be heady affairs, suitable only for the statistically sophisticated.

The second unnecessary complication introduced in the 1967 article was the introduction and description of a computerized program called KAPPA. Written in Fortran IV for an IBM 7094, this program, developed by the authors, was designed to compute weighted and unweighted kappas. Data from an unpublished study were presented to illustrate the results of this computerized analysis. Like the introduction of the weighted kappa, the use of the Fortran computer program hardly ever appeared subsequently in the psychiatric literature dealing with diagnostic reliability.

The article appeared to make a useful tool available to others and perhaps implied that they did not have to be statisticians to use kappa;

the computer would do the work. Although today the mention of a specialized, single-function software program would be considered mundane, the era when this article first appeared was very different. Not only were few psychiatrists interested in the finer points of nosology or reliability computation to begin with, but even fewer were familiar with the emerging capacities of computers. Personal computers did not exist, user-friendly software was not available, and statistical analysis was handled by huge mainframe computers in university computer centers or was done by hand. Thus, at the time, reference to the use of a computer in this article was not only an advertisement for a new reliability product, but also alerted clinicians that reliability problems henceforth were likely to be the province of a few research and statistical specialists who had the capability and resources to study these matters.

The full complexity of understanding and comparing reliability studies is still unfolding. Ten years after the introduction of kappa, Carey and Gottesman (1978) pointed out in the same journal that in some circumstances the pursuit of diagnostic reliability can result in *decreases* in validity. For example, in order to ensure that only those who have schizophrenia are diagnosed accurately, an attempt to reduce what is referred to as *false positives* (those who are diagnosed with schizophrenia but do not have it), the criteria for schizophrenia can be defined very specifically and narrowly. This may reduce the false positive errors and it may increase diagnostic reliability. But it would also simultaneously increase the number of false negatives, those with schizophrenia who failed to meet all the stringent criteria, and undermine the validity of the narrow definition of schizophrenia. In this example and other circumstances, higher reliability may not necessarily indicate high validity. Carey and Gottesman suggest that the term *reliability* often is misinterpreted as having some intrinsic merit all its own, rather than being subordinate to issues of validity. They conclude that pride in reliability, however well intentioned, may "give a false impression of advances in solving problems of nomenclature and taxonomy" (p. 1459).

Twenty years after its introduction, kappa is generating controversy about it uses and value. But significantly, clinicians are not involved at all in these discussions. The debates transpire among a small cluster of statisticians and research psychiatrists arguing over the validity of kappa and other statistics when dealing with low base rates (see Spitznagel & Helzer, 1985, 1987; Kraemer, 1987; Uebersax, 1987; Shrout et al., 1987). And when questions were raised in practitioner-oriented periodicals about kappa (Kutchins & Kirk, 1988b), the response was that the matter is "too complicated" to discuss (Williams & Spitzer, 1988). What began as a simple metric to deal with a common clinical problem became part of a highly specialized technique for research applications.

The introduction of kappa into the diagnostic literature had other subtle effects. By introducing statistical formulas, displaying computer prowess, and linking these capacities directly to the use of kappa, the authors (Spitzer, Cohen, & Fleiss, 1967), may have produced two other noteworthy effects. First, they moved the intuitive understanding of diagnostic agreement one step further from the ability of clinicians and the public to participate meaningfully in the interpretation of reliability studies. However potentially misleading the simple use of percentage agreement is, it was easily comprehended by others, even if their understanding was faulty. By introducing a modestly complex formula for kappa, by providing an additional statistical overlay for a weighted kappa, and by tying both to a relatively inaccessible computer technology, the reliability problem was removed from public prominence and ensconced in the private laboratories of research psychiatrists.

Second, these developments transformed the problem of reliability, which had become an additional threat to the conceptual foundations of psychiatry, into a technical problem to be solved by research specialists. The problem was embedded in a closely knit research community, which accepted responsibility for solving the problem, on its own terms and in its own territory.

This transformation had another characteristic that would become much more important later. The introduction of kappa offered no standard for its interpretation. Instead, it opened the door for a variety of interpretations, each at least one step removed from an intuitive sense of whether interrater agreement was good, better, or acceptable. The 1967 article that introduced kappa did not promulgate any guidelines for interpretation. In the transformation of reliability into a technical problem, no standards were explicitly established for what would constitute a technical solution. The lack of specificity about what standard of interpretation to use allowed psychiatric researchers to use fluctuating standards to criticize old paradigms and promote new ones. We will discuss this problem at greater length in later chapters. Since the nature of the problem had been defined as highly technical, even skeptics of the new nosologies found themselves dependent on the interpretations of researchers in matters of diagnostic reliability. This dependence proved helpful to those who championed DSM-III.

The introduction of kappa by psychiatric researchers appeared to provide a unifying method of comparing reliability studies, while eliminating the statistical problem of chance agreement. This was viewed as a major methodological advance. By itself, this advance, however, did nothing to solve the serious problem of clinicians arriving at different diagnoses for the same patient. However elegantly diagnostic decisions could be quantified by research psychiatrists, if clinicians continued to disagree, the reliability problem would not be solved. For example, if a physician wanted to help a patient lose weight, it would not matter how accurate, sophisticated, or technically advanced a new scale might be. If the patient lost no weight, the scale would only document the failure. The scale could not do anything about the excess pounds it recorded. Even if kappa could measure more accurately the degree of failure or success in achieving agreements about psychiatric diagnoses, it alone had no capacity to produce it.

Nevertheless, the mystification introduced through kappa provided an idiom for interpreting data about diagnostic reliability. The kappa coefficient reported diagnostic agreement in a new metric that was not readily translatable into anything familiar to the general reader. This unfamiliarity permitted certain liberties in interpretation. Kappa became a flexible device into which an eventual solution to the reliability problem could be fitted.

3

THE SOCIAL CONTROL
OF ERROR

The problem of diagnostic reliability lay with clinical practitioners who disagreed with one another about the nature of clients' problems. Fancy statistics could not easily mask clinical disagreements; that was the heart of the matter. To the researchers who began to study this issue, unreliability was the product, not of any one deficit, but of a confluence of errors made by clinicians. The typical clinical setting in which many of the early reliability studies were conducted was viewed as an unsupervised nursery for clinical errors. Fertile soil and proper climatic conditions may be good for orchids, but if they are untended, weeds sprout and flourish as well.

Researchers grouped these errors into two general categories. One group of diagnostic errors occurs because two or more clinicians evaluating the same person accumulate different information about the person and this difference in acquired information may contribute to different diagnostic conclusions. This can happen easily. Clinicians, separately and sequentially interviewing a patient, may ask different questions; receive slightly different responses to similarly worded questions; note, remember, or interpret responses differently; or by style and demeanor elicit different behavior from the patient. Or, in other situations, each clinician may have access to different types, quantities, or quality of information about the patient in addition to that obtained during an interview. For example, they could learn about the patient from family or friends, referral sources, colleagues, or case records.

These various sources of error are called *information variance* by those studying these matters. Clinical judgments may be different because the information obtained is different. Gathering information from different sources in different ways is endemic to clinical practice. The errors encountered are normal in the sense that they are common, understandable and inevitable. Not only are they largely uncontrollable sources of error *in practice*, but indigenous aspects of psychiatric practice indirectly promote them. For example, an important element in psychotherapeutic practice is the use of self in establishing a therapeutic relationship with a patient. An important component of psychodynamic theory and practice rests on the assumption that these idiosyncrasies of the relationship between therapist and client will become a crucial part of the treatment, through transference and countertransference. Thus, information variance is part of the normal and expected character of clinical work. What is welcomed as part of normal practice to clinicians is, to researchers seeking diagnostic consistency, a fertile source of idiosyncratic error.

Another source of diagnostic error, called *criterion variance*, involves how clinicians make diagnostic decisions. Even if information variance can be controlled or eliminated completely, clinicians might still disagree about what pieces of information are relevant, how they should be interpreted, and what diagnostic category the disorder, if any, should be placed in. At clinical case conferences where groups of therapists are presented with the same case information, they frequently reach different diagnostic conclusions. Often in clinical settings, these disagreements allow for the display of subtle clinical acumen in an arena in which different inferences about underlying etiology and diagnosis can be debated. Disagreements about diagnoses in these situations rest on different assumptions about the meaning of and criteria for making particular diagnoses. Criterion variance, like information variance, is the stuff of normal psychiatric practice. It enlivens debate and provides opportunities to examine the meaning, i.e., the validity, of different perspectives on mental disorder. Until the introduction of DSM-III, little in the official diagnostic taxonomy discouraged such tendencies.

These sources of diagnostic disagreement, however, preoccupied those who wished to solve the reliability problem. If the sources of diagnostic error were endemic to clinical practice, and if clinical practice occurred in relatively uncontrolled environments, solutions to the reliability problem would have to involve the control of normal clinical practice. This was a formidable task, one that was not resolvable by developing some new statistical formula.

Not all psychiatric researchers were discouraged by the challenge. Two teams of investigators, who would ride this problem into positions of prominence and influence, began working on ways to control the behavior of freewheeling clinicians. They set out to improve reliability and thereby protect the conceptual integrity of psychiatry by tinkering with the diagnostic discretion of practitioners and then measuring their success with kappa. Within a decade, they announced that victory over diagnostic unreliability was within sight; a few years later, with the introduction of DSM-III, they claimed that victory had largely been achieved. By 1990, few psychiatric researchers argued that unreliability was a central challenge to psychiatry any longer (although privately some would acknowledge it). How this was accomplished is an intriguing chapter in the history of American psychiatry.

The Control of Discretion

The twin strategies for improving reliability required that information variance and criterion variance be greatly reduced, if not eliminated altogether. To do this, first the decision-making of clinicians had to be controlled, and second, the nature and structure of the psychiatric interview had to be changed. Two teams of psychiatric researchers, one at Washington University in St. Louis and the other at the New York State Psychiatric Institute affiliated with Columbia University, set out both separately and through joint activity to confront these challenges.

As psychiatrists, they constituted a small, but very able group. Few psychiatrists devoted themselves to research and among them only a much smaller group was concerned with nosology, diagnostic criteria, and diagnostic reliability. They were a minority among a minority, devoting their professional careers to issues that most mental health professionals did not view as central to their profession; they were on the margins of the profession. They constituted an "invisible college" of neo-Kraepelinians who had personal or intellectual allegiances to each other, who worked on similar research problems, who shared preliminary research findings and methods, and who through citations to each others' publications developed one of the important intellectual networks in contemporary psychiatry (Blashfield, 1982; Guze, 1982; Strauss, 1982; Katz, 1982; Kendell, 1982). The basic beliefs of these neo-Kraepelinians have been described by Klerman (1978) in Table 3.1.

For these teams of researchers, the first task was to develop more specific criteria for determining whether a person should be categorized into one or another subtype of mental disorder. This was no simple task, since the earliest versions of the *Diagnostic and Statistical Manual of Mental Disorders* contained categories with vague definitions that required considerable clinical inference about the nature of the disorder.

For example, in DSM-II the following are the complete descriptions of several disorders:

300.6 *Depersonalization neurosis*: This syndrome is dominated by a feeling of unreality and of estrangement from the self, body, or surroundings. This diagnosis should not be used if the condition is part of some other mental disorder, such as an acute situational reaction. A brief experience of depersonalization is not necessarily a symptom of illness. (p. 41)

Table 3.1.   Neo-Kraepelinian Credo

---

1. Psychiatry is a branch of medicine.
2. Psychiatry should utilize modern scientific methodologies and base its practice on scientific knowledge.
3. Psychiatry treats people who are sick and who require treatment for mental illness.
4. There is a boundary between the normal and the sick.
5. There are discrete mental illnesses. Mental illnesses are not myths. There is not one but many mental illnesses. It is the task of scientific psychiatry, as of other medical specialties, to investigate the causes, diagnosis, and treatment of these mental illnesses.
6. The focus of psychiatric physicians should be particularly on the biological aspects of mental illness.
7. There should be an explicit and intentional concern with diagnosis and classification.
8. Diagnostic criteria should be codified, and a legitimate and valued area of research should be to validate such criteria by various techniques. Further, departments of psychiatry in medical schools should teach these criteria and not depreciate them, as has been the case for many years.
9. In research efforts directed at improving the reliability and validity of diagnosis and classification, statistical techniques should be utilized.

Note: From Klerman, G.L. (1978). The evolution of a scientific nosology. In J.C. Shershow (Ed.), *Schizophrenia: Science and practice*. Cambridge: Harvard University Press. Reprinted with permission.

301.6   *Asthenic personality:*   This behavior pattern is characterized by easy fatigability, low energy level, lack of enthusiasm, marked incapacity for enjoyment, and oversensitivity to physical and emotional stress. This disorder must be differentiated from Neurasthenic neurosis. (p. 43)

308.3   *Runaway reaction of childhood (or adolescence):*   Individuals with this disorder characteristically escape from threatening situations by running away from home for a day or more without permission. Typically they are immature and timid, and feel rejected at home, inadequate, and friendless. They often steal furtively. (p. 50)

295.0   *Schizophrenia, simple type:*   This psychosis is characterized chiefly by a slow and insidious reduction of external attachments and interests and by apathy and indifference leading to impoverishment of interpersonal relations, mental deterioration, and adjustment on a lower level of functioning. In general, the condition is less dramatically psychotic than are the hebephrenic, catatonic, and paranoid types of schizophrenia. Also, it contrasts with schizoid personality, in which there is little or no progression of the disorder. (p. 33)

What precisely were such things as "lack of enthusiasm," "estrangement from the self" or "a slow reduction of external attachments"? No further guidelines were given for making such determinations or any clear indication whether all or some of these ambiguous criteria had to be fulfilled in order to make the diagnosis. It was little wonder that clinicians reached different diagnostic decisions about the same person, if they were given ambiguous descriptions about what constituted a particular disorder. The obvious, technical solution to this cause of unreliability was to develop specific diagnostic criteria for including or excluding disorders from specific categories.

The group of researchers at Washington University in St. Louis addressed this problem directly by developing diagnostic criteria for 15 mental disorders. Their work had an enormous impact on psychiatric research. Their contribution, referred to as the *Feighner criteria* after the senior author (Feighner et al., 1972), was described in an article in 1972 that has since been cited in the literature almost four thousand times, making it one of psychiatry's classics (Spitzer, 1989). Basically, this St. Louis group tried to develop much more specific criteria for determining whether a disorder was present in a person. The contrast between DSM-II descriptions and the Feighner criteria is striking. For example, the Feighner criteria for depression are more elaborate and specific, indicating in much more detail what signs and symptoms must be present to make the diagnosis, than the DSM-II description (see Example 3.1).

The New York group, headed by Robert Spitzer, built on the Feighner criteria by changing some criteria and adding diagnostic categories to produce the *research diagnostic criteria* (Spitzer, Endicott, & Robins, 1978), commonly known as the RDC, also destined to become enormously influential in the development of DSM-III. The article proposing the RDC has also become a "citation classic" with nearly six hundred references to it in the literature (Spitzer, 1989). These two articles (Feighner et al., 1972; Spitzer et al., 1978) and the work on which they were based are among the most influential developments in psychiatry in the last quarter of a century.

A prominent, but often overlooked, feature of both the Feighner and RDC criteria is that both were proposed *explicitly for use in research*. This purpose is made clear in the titles of each article, in the fact that they were published in the leading psychiatric research journal of the American Medical Association, and in that they explicitly addressed the problems that researchers had in designing and comparing results of studies. Neither article proposed that these elaborate diagnostic systems be adopted by clinical psychiatrists. It was only later that these research techniques, spawned in research environments to remedy the narrow problem of criterion variance, would be imposed on clinicians.

The problem of *information variance* was attacked in a similar manner. The general approach was to structure the amount, nature, and sequence of information that a psychiatric diagnostician would gather. Just as criterion variance was approached by limiting a diagnostician's discre-

Example 3.1.   Comparison of DSM-II and Feighner Criteria

From DSM-II for *Depressive Neurosis*
This disorder is manifested by an excessive reaction of depression due to an internal conflict or to an identifiable event such as the loss of a love object or cherished possession. It is to be distinguished from Involutional melancholia and Manic-depressive illness. Reactive depressions or depressive reactions are to be classified here.

From the 1972 Feighner Criteria for *Depressive Disorder*
The following three requirements *must* be met:

1. *Dysphoric mood* characterized by symptoms such as the following: depressed, sad, despondent, hopeless, feeling "down in the dumps," irritable, fearful, worried, or discouraged.
2. *At least 5 of the following 8 criteria:*
    (a) Poor appetite or weight loss of 2 pounds a week or 10 pounds or more a year when not dieting.
    (b) Difficulty in sleeping, including insomnia or hypersomnia.
    (c) Loss of energy, namely fatigability, tiredness.
    (d) Agitation or retardation.
    (e) Loss of interest in usual activities, or decrease in sexual drive.
    (f) Feelings of self-reproach or guilt (either may be delusional).
    (g) Complaints of or actually diminished ability to think or concentrate, such as slow thinking or mixed-up thoughts.
    (h) Recurrent thoughts of death or suicide, including thoughts of wishing to be dead.
(Note: If only 4 of these 8 criteria are found, diagnose as "probable depression" rather than "depression.")
3. *A psychiatric illness lasting at least one month with no preexisting conditions* such as schizophrenia, anxiety neurosis, phobic neurosis, obsessive, compulsive neurosis, hysteria, alcoholism, drug dependency, antisocial personality, homosexuality and other sexual deviations, mental retardation, or organic brain syndrome.
(General Note: Patients with life-threatening or incapacitating medical illness preceding and paralleling the depression do not receive the diagnosis of primary depression.)

Source: From Matarazzo, Joseph D. "The Reliability of psychiatric and psychological diagnoses," *Clinical Psychology Review,* Vol. 3, pp. 103–145. Copyright © 1983. Reprinted with permission.

tion, information variance was controlled by structuring the diagnostician's exposure to clinical information about a case. Since the usual method of acquiring clinical information was through a face-to-face interview, the interviewer's behavior was controlled. Psychiatric interviews, however, are enormously difficult to structure or control. Clients are far from regimented in how they choose to reveal their problems or other sensitive information about themselves. Likewise, clinicians are infinitely diverse in the way they go about gathering information. What questions they ask, how and when they ask them, depend on their purposes in the interview, their training, their individual clinical style, their theoretical orientation, what they already know about a prospective client, and diligence, among other factors. To structure this free-form process required control over what clinicians asked, when they asked it, and how the answers should be recorded. Criterion variance was controlled by structuring decision-making, but information variance was controlled by structuring interviewer behavior with patients.

The development of highly structured interview protocols was the technical solution to the problem of clinicians conducting assessment interviews in their own individual ways and producing diagnostic unreliability. Building on work done earlier on the Present State Examination in Great Britain, the St. Louis and New York research teams developed structured interview schedules that limited the way in which clinicians could elicit information. The New York group developed the Schedule of Affective Disorders and Schizophrenia (SADS) in three versions to measure either current, lifetime, or changed mental state (Endicott & Spitzer, 1978), while the St. Louis group developed the Diagnostic Interview Schedule (DIS) and the Renard Diagnostic Interview (RDI) (Robins, Helzer, Crougham, & Ratcliff, 1981; Helzer, Robins, Crougham, & Wilner, 1981). These were later followed by the Structured Clinical Interview for DSM-III-R (SCID), marketed to clinicians by the APA as one of many costly accessory items.

Interview schedules were not a new methodology. Social and behavioral scientists had been using them for decades in situations where they wanted to gather information from respondents in a consistent and structured way. But they were not the standard practice of mental health workers making diagnostic judgments. These psychiatric interview schedules provided a progression of questions to be asked of patients. The responses to these were then matched with the diagnostic criteria that systematically allocated symptom patterns into specified diagnostic categories. By controlling what information was gathered and how it was used, researchers hoped to prevent research interviewers (and later clinicians) from falling back solely on professional judgment and intuition when making diagnoses. Thus, the interview schedules comprised the second prong of the integrated attack on diagnostic error. (See Example 3.2.)

The problem of diagnostic reliability was transformed into the technical task of controlling clinical behavior and decision-making and then measuring success with the new yardstick, kappa. The St. Louis and New York groups set out to demonstrate that the problem of reliability was solvable. They reasoned that if they (1) limited the information that

Example 3.2. One section of an interview schedule

The next 5 items are screening items to determine the presence of manic-like behavior. If any of the items are judged present, inquire in a general way to determine how he was behaving at that time with such questions as, *When you were this way, what kinds of things were you doing? How did you spend your time?* Do not include behavior which is clearly explainable by alcohol or drug intoxication.

If the subject has only described dysphoric mood, the following questions regarding the manic syndrome should be introduced with a statement such as: *I know you have been feeling (depressed). However, many people have other feelings mixed in or at different times so it is important that I ask you about those feelings also.*

Elevated mood and/or optimistic attitude toward the future which lasted at least 7 hours and was out of proportion to the circumstances.

Have (there been times when) you felt very good or too cheerful or high—not just your normal self?

If unclear: When you felt on top of the world or as if there was nothing you couldn't do?

(Have you felt that everything would work out just the way you wanted?)

If people saw you would they think you were just in a good mood or something more than that?

0   No information
1   Not at all, normal, or depressed
2   Slight, e.g., good spirits, more cheerful than most people in his circumstances, but of only possible clinical significance
3   Mild, e.g., definitely elevated mood and optimistic outlook that is somewhat out of proportion to his circumstances
4   Moderate, e.g., mood and outlook are clearly out of proportion to circumstances
5   Severe, e.g., quality of euphoric mood
6   Extreme, e.g., clearly elated, exalted expression and says "Everything is beautiful, I feel so good"

(What about during the past week?)   PAST WEEK   0 1 2 3 4 5 6

Less need for sleep than usual to feel rested (average for several days when needed less sleep).

Have you needed less sleep than usual to feel rested? (How much sleep do you ordinarily need?) How much when you were [are] high?)

0   No information
1   No change or more sleep needed
2   Up to 1 hour less than usual
3   Up to 2 hours less than usual
4   Up to 3 hours less than usual
5   Up to 4 hours less than usual
6   4 or more hours less than usual

(What about during the past week?)   PAST WEEK   0 1 2 3 4 5 6

54

(*continued*)

Unusually energetic, more active than his usual level without expected fatigue.	0	No information
	1	No different than usual or less energetic
Have you had more energy than usual to do things?	2	Slightly more energetic but of questionable significance
	3	Little change in activity level but less fatigued than usual
(*More than just a return to normal or usual level?*)	4	Somewhat more active than usual with little or no fatigue
(*Did it seem like too much energy?*)	5	Much more active than usual with little or no fatigue
	6	Unusually active all day long with little or no fatigue
(*What about during the past week?*)	PAST WEEK 0 1 2 3 4 5 6	

From Matarazzo (1983), this is part of the SAD probes for screening manic syndrome. Adapted from "A diagnostic interview" by J. Endicott and R.L. Spitzer. (1978), *Archives of General Psychiatry*, 35:839. Reprinted with permission.

clinicians collected, (2) structured the sequence in which it was gathered, (3) guided the manner in which follow-up questions would be asked, and (4) provided explicit instructions about what diagnostic decisions could be reached, they had a chance of greatly reducing disagreement among interviewers. It seemed like a rational approach, and it was in keeping with standard research methodologies. By reducing professional judgment, clinician discretion, and the free unsystematic flow of information, unreliability would be lessened. The development of diagnostic criteria and of structured interview schedules were the expressions of these strategies. The desired end was to supplant clinical diagnostic decision-making as it was routinely practiced with a structured research interview. Since these techniques were primarily addressed to researchers, clinical goals for an interview, such as establishing rapport and a therapeutic relationship with the patient, directing the inquiry into areas suggested by the patient and so forth, were secondary. Instead, primary emphasis was placed on gathering standardized information. Having developed these new technologies, the research teams now needed to show that when they enforced these special instructions and prohibitions, diagnostic reliability would improve. They needed to demonstrate that their solutions worked.

Before they offered their improvements to the psychiatric world, they revisited the reliability problem to emphasize just how bad the situation was. Beck and other earlier reviewers of diagnostic reliability were ambivalent about the interpretation of previous studies. Beck, for example, had not been pleased with the magnitude of diagnostic agreement, but he hedged his assessment by emphasizing the methodological problems that obscured any clear interpretations of the actual state of reliability. It was better to suspend final judgment, he seemed to suggest, than to jump to dire conclusions based on faulty studies. By the mid-1970s, those who were now in the forefront of solving the reliability problem indicated no strategic need for such hesitation.

Interpreting the Past

Progress is often affirmed by denigrating the past and by reinterpreting it to be much less satisfactory than it actually seemed at the time. The new owners of cars with electric power windows quickly wonder why they labored so long with manual ones. Those who recently acquired their first microwave oven talk smugly about the disadvantages of the old way. The cold war now seems anachronistic, a terrible waste of national energy and wealth. Lobotomies, while still performed, are viewed as rather brutal interventions for mania. We boast about our current enlightenment by disparaging yesterday's beliefs.

In 1974, in the midst of the development of what were viewed as the technical solutions to diagnostic reliability, a very influential article (Spitzer & Fleiss, 1974) reported that the early reliability studies were even worse than they had seemed. Written by the leader of the New York group, this reinterpretation takes on added significance. We will examine that paper in some detail. Such attention is justified because, first, the paper played a pivotal role in recasting the past, a recasting that has proved durable for the past two decades. Frequently, reference to this article is the only citation needed when contemporary authors make assertions about psychiatry's poor reliability prior to DSM-III. The paper was pivotal in setting the stage for the introduction of a second wave of reliability studies. Furthermore, it introduced interpretive standards for kappa, although, as we will argue later, these standards were liberalized a few years later when they were used to demonstrate the improved reliability of DSM-III.

Spitzer and a well-known statistician, Fleiss, both of whom had been coauthors of the 1967 paper introducing kappa to a psychiatric audience, reexamined the early reliability studies (Spitzer & Fleiss, 1974). But for the first time, they used kappa as the common metric for the reinterpretation and comparison of the early studies. They minced no words in declaring the significance of reliability for psychiatric nosology, the problem that they were diligently working on. Referring to classification systems, they stated:

A necessary constraint on validity of a system is its reliability. There is no guarantee that a reliable system is valid, but assuredly an unreliable system must be invalid. Studies of the reliability of psychiatric diagnosis provide information on the upper limits of its validity. (p. 341)

Having emphasized the fundamental significance of reliability for psychiatry, they proceeded through familiar territory by describing the limitations of the older measures of agreement that ignored chance agreement and base rates. They offered hypothetical data to illustrate the problems of interpretation created by chance agreement.

The new contribution of the article consisted of the use of kappa to recompute the findings of five earlier published reliability studies (Schmidt & Fonda, 1956; Kreitman, 1961; Beck et al., 1962; Sandifer et al., 1964; Cooper et al., 1972) plus one study of their own, which they described as "in preparation" but which was never subsequently published (R. L. Spitzer, personal communication).

In a summary table, they array kappa values for each study by major diagnostic categories (see Table 3.2). Their interpretations of the data are firm and direct:

There are no diagnostic categories for which reliability is uniformly high. Reliability appears to be *only satisfactory* for three categories: mental deficiency, organic brain syndrome (but not its subtypes), and alcoholism. The level of reliability is *no better than fair* for psychosis and schizophrenia and is *poor* for the remaining categories. (p. 344, emphasis added)

They follow this bleak review by reminding the reader that in most of these studies the diagnosticians were of similar background and training, and that special efforts were made in some studies to have the participants come to some agreement on diagnostic principles prior to the beginning of the study. In case these implications were missed by the reader, they draw the conclusion explicitly:

One can only assume, therefore, that agreement between heterogeneous diagnosticians of different orientations and backgrounds, as they act in routine clinical settings, is even poorer than is indicated [in their table]. Further, there appears to have been no essential change in diagnostic reliability over time . . . The reliability of psychiatric diagnosis as it has been practised since at least the late 1950s is *not good*. It is likely that the reasons for diagnostic unreliability are the same now as when Beck et al. (1965) studied them. (pp. 344–345, emphasis added)

They conclude by referring to the work of the New York and St. Louis groups as working on "two major innovations which may provide solu-

Table 3.2. Kappa Coefficients of Agreement on Broad and Specific Diagnostic Categories from Six Studies

| | | | | | \multicolumn{2}{c}{*Study*} | | |
Category	*I*	*II*	*III*	*IV*	*V* NY	*V* London	*VI*	*Mean*
Mental deficiency				.72				.72
Organic brain syndrome	.82	.90					.59	.77
Acute brain syndrome				.44				.44
Chronic brain syndrome				.64				.64
Alcoholism					.74	.68		.71
Psychosis	.73	.62		.56	.42	.43	.43	.55
Schizophrenia	.77		.42	.68	.32	.60	.65	.57
Affective disorder					.19	.44	.59	.41
Neurotic depression			.47		.20	.10		.26
Psychotic depression				.19	.24	.30		.24
Manic-depression				.33				.33
Involutional depression			.38	.21				.30
Personality disorder or neurosis	.63			.51	.24	.36		.44
Personality disorder			.33	.56	.19	.33	.29	.32
Sociopathic			.53					.53
Neurosis		.52		.42	.26	.30	.48	.40
Anxiety reaction			.45					.45
Psychophysiological reaction				.38				.38

Note: From R.L. Spitzer & J. Fleiss "A re-analysis of the reliability of psychiatric diagnosis," *British Journal of Psychiatry, 125,* 341–347. Copyright © 1974. Reprinted with permisssion.

tions to these problems" (p. 345). These innovations were, of course, structured interview schedules and explicit diagnostic criteria. They end their important article with this bold statement, which links problems of validity with their confident prediction that they are on the road to solving the reliability problem:

> These two approaches, structuring the interview and specifying all diagnostic criteria, are being merged in a series of collaborative studies on the psychobiology of the depressive disorders sponsored by the N.I.M.H. Clinical Research Branch. We are confident that this merging will result not only in improved reliability but in improved validity which is, after all our ultimate goal. (p. 346)

This article carefully and dramatically sets the stage for DSM-III. It reinterprets and denigrates the past, refers to innovations being currently developed by the authors and others, and predicts success in the future.

As important, the article was the first one explicitly to offer interpretive standards for kappa, something that Spitzer and his colleagues had avoided in prior articles. In telling the tale of poor reliability in the past, the article links specific kappa scores with interpretive language (p. 344, as cited above). Since these links were largely obscured a few years later when DSM-III was being promoted, it will be useful to examine them carefully.

Five interpretive standards were proffered in the text: *uniformly high, only satisfactory, no better than fair,* and *poor*; the general state of reliability was described incidentally as *not good*. In their table, kappa scores were provided from each study within similar diagnostic categories. By examining the kappas in their table and matching them to their interpretive language and the categories they mention, we can identify their interpretive standards (see Figure 3.1).

Their interpretations of these data are central to the analysis in this book. First, each level of interpretation contained a broad range of scores, from a 31- to 54-point spread. Each level contained broadly overlapping kappa scores. For example, a kappa score of .60 in one study could have been included in any of the interpretive categories from poor to only satisfactory. Second, the interpretations are all *phrased negatively* and, third they use different interpretive referents. These last two points require some attention.

The negative wording is important. Starting at the top, by stating that no categories have reliability that is *uniformly* high, they accomplish two rhetorical goals. First, they are leaving the top rating vacant, without an occupant or even a close challenger. Second, by claiming that none are high, they are able to make the blanket judgment about all reliability studies that reliability as it had been practiced for decades was "not good" (p. 345).

Good in their scheme apparently occupies a rhetorical position above *only satisfactory.* The interpretation of *only satisfactory* is damning by faint praise. Labeling something as only satisfactory offers grudging acknowledgment to an attempt that achieves minimal success.

No better than fair is a clear put-down. Who can accept an achievement that is no better than fair? No better than fair is worse than fair. Try describing your partner's driving, cooking, looks, or intelligence as no better than fair and his or her reaction will quickly help you realize the not so subtle nature of your assessment. *No better than fair* implies that even when one is being charitable and giving something the benefit of the doubt, it is, at best, fair, and probably considerably worse.

Poor, in their scheme, is everything that is less good, satisfactory, or

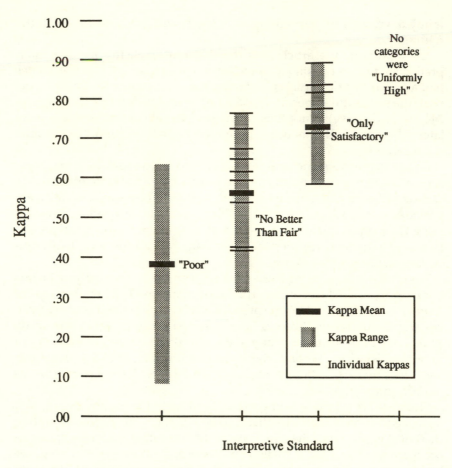

Figure 3.1. Interpretations of kappa in the reanalysis of six earlier studies (Spitzer & Fleiss, 1974).

acceptable than all the rest. At the bottom of the bottom is where they consign the reliability of most diagnostic categories. Using kappa as the hammer, the poor reliability of psychiatric diagnosis was soundly nailed home.

There was nothing inherent in the kappa values that suggested the interpretive labels that they used. The interpretation of kappa coefficients had not been standardized in any scientific manner. As was true of many other statistical measures, kappa came with no predetermined evaluative meaning for scores between chance agreement (assumed to be bad) and perfect agreement (obviously good). There was no normal or expected level of kappa for any study.

Thus, the interpretation of kappa falls within an area of enormous scientific discretion. Despite the appearance of precision in behavioral and psychological research, there are few set standards for interpreting the substantive meaning of many statistics, beyond making some broad probabilistic statement about the likelihood of their occurrence given certain assumptions (usually referred to as testing for statistical significance). One well-respected psychometrician (Nunnally, 1978) has argued that with regard to measures of reliability, however, standards for research purposes can be considerably lower than the reliability standards for measures that will be used to make decisions about people in applied settings. In the latter, where individuals will be seriously affected by the measurement, e.g., classroom placement based on IQ score or treatment for a patient, he argues that practically no reliability error should be tolerated in measures. These are crucial points: that interpretations of reliability depend on the purpose and consequences of the measure and that research purposes may permit greater unreliability than clinical purposes in some circumstances.

Since the originators of kappa had enormous discretion, these data from the early studies could have been grouped differently and the categories could have been described quite differently. The authors were restrained by no prior interpretive standards. The field for interpretation was unmarked and, consequently, the lines they chose to draw on it have rhetorical significance. Had their purposes been to promote optimism in psychiatry, they could have described the state of reliability as quite good, but needing to get better. In fact, one commentator, a psychologist trying to persuade other psychologists to accept psychiatric diagnosis as a useful tool, has made this kind of optimistic interpretations of the same reports (Matarazzo, 1983). They could have stressed that in the early studies every single diagnostic category in every study achieved psychiatric agreement that was considerably better than chance! This absolutely factual observation could have been described as a diagnostic achievement of psychiatry that had been earlier obscured, but now was revealed by the advent of kappa.

Many other interpretive approaches were possible. They could have used different sets of descriptors. For example, they could have employed *very high, high, medium, low.* Or *very satisfactory, satisfactory, somewhat satisfactory, unsatisfactory.* Or *very good, good, not so good, bad.* And, more importantly, having the comparative freedom of originators, they could have placed the findings of the early studies into any of these categories, either inflating or deflating their acceptability. For example, they could have described all the findings as falling into the categories of moderately high and high and celebrated the value of current psychiatric practices. Instead, they emphasized negative descriptors to argue that the findings were in some way marginal or worse. Their interpretations struck forcefully at the vulnerability of the field.

This 1974 article contained no new methodological or statistical information, no new theory, no new findings, with the exception of reference to data from a study by the senior author that was never published. What may have prompted the appearance of this review of the early studies in 1974, when it could have been included in the 1967 article announcing and promoting kappa? The 1974 reinterpretation is a logical extension and illustration of kappa. In addition, the illustration shows how comparisons can be made across actual studies and suggests interpretive guidelines for kappa. Showing the uses of the new kappa by reinterpreting the early studies would have made the 1967 article more straightforward and powerful and less mystifying.

Although these articles are closely related, they had very different purposes. In 1967, psychiatry was under assault from many directions. Introducing new scientific technology, like kappa, could be viewed as supportive of current psychiatry, a sign of scientific progress in a beleaguered profession. If the introduction of kappa had been accompanied by an assault on diagnostic reliability, kappa might have been viewed as a new weapon that was being used against the profession. Kappa's promise might then have been permanently damaged by being associated with the antipsychiatry movement. It was much safer to talk about the intricacies of weighted kappa and Fortran programs in 1967 than about more controversial matters such as the sorry state of reliability.

A systematic approach to the reliability problem had not been developed by 1967. The nature of the problem itself was still being identified. However, by 1974 both the St. Louis and New York groups were completing a variety of studies that were to report better reliability under conditions where discretion was controlled. Thus, by 1974, belittling the state of reliability in the past became an effective way of preparing for diagnostic criteria and structured interview schedules.

A normal part of "problem-making" is to emphasize the negative, the potential threat of some putative condition (Spector & Kitsuse, 1987). The current state of affairs must be presented as grossly unacceptable to those who are being called on to take action to remedy the problem. If diagnostic unreliability is unacceptably low, and that implies that diagnoses are invalid, then surely something must be done or the mental health enterprise is gravely threatened. Making a condition a problem implies that the condition can be otherwise, that a solution is possible. Problem-making often advances a particular approach to a solution (Spector & Kitsuse, 1987).

By 1974, the Task Force to Develop DSM-III (hereafter DSM-III Task

Force) was being formed. Robert Spitzer, the coauthor of the paper introducing kappa to a psychiatric audience in 1967 and the leader of the New York group developing structured interviews and diagnostic criteria, was also the senior author of the 1974 paper offering a scathing reinterpretation of the past reliability studies. At the same historical moment, he was appointed as the head of the DSM-III Task Force, one of the most important committee assignments in psychiatry in the twentieth century. He and others certainly were not ignorant of the new interviewing and decision-making technologies that were in the final stages of development or of the enormity of the task that lay ahead in revising the diagnostic manual to reflect this new technology. A renewed and escalated attack on the weaknesses of DSM-II, and indirectly on the state of American psychiatry, gave these researchers extra leverage in the struggle to define what the diagnostic problems were and to propose how to renovate psychiatric nosology. The 1974 paper reinterpreting the past had very different political consequences than it would have had in 1967, before the appointment of the DSM-III Task Force. Why make the state of American psychiatry appear even worse in 1967 if you had little to offer to make it better? The 1974 article served as a dramatic pronouncement about the reliability problems of the past, while it set the stage for the proposed solution.

The Second Wave: Announcing Initial Success

Both the St. Louis and New York groups worked on developing diagnostic criteria and structured interviews. Beyond developing technical materials, they also worked on selling the importance of those twin strategies to an audience of clinicians. Many of these researchers' publications in the major psychiatric journals took the form of communications addressed not to each other or to other researchers who already constituted the converted, but to clinical practitioners who could be expected to be resistant to attempts to control clinical judgment. For example, in 1975, the *American Journal of Psychiatry* published an article coauthored by researchers from New York and St. Louis (Spitzer, Endicott, & Robins, 1975) in which unreliability was deplored, blame was heaped on DSM-II for allowing so many sources of clinician discretion and error, diagnostic criteria were touted, and it was suggested that DSM-III—which was then in development—would solve these problems. The article concludes, as many others do in the mid- and late 1970s, on a new optimistic note:

We believe that the major potential beneficial effect of including specified diagnostic criteria in DSM-III would be to improve the reliability and validity of routine psychiatric diagnosis. This in turn should improve the value of the standard nomenclature for all of its many uses—clinical, research, and administrative. (p. 1191)

By the mid-1970s the psychiatric journals were alive with pronouncements about structured interviews and appeals for diagnostic criteria. We will refer to these articles as the second wave of reliability studies, since they followed the gloomy earlier reports. To appreciate their significance fully, we need to examine them in some detail.

The Helzer Report

In the mid-1970s, while the DSM-III Task Force was at work, the St. Louis and New York groups were actively publishing articles that they clearly expected to play a critical role in solving the reliability problem and influencing the nature of DSM-III and, therefore, of psychiatric nosology in general. From St. Louis, Helzer et al. (1977a, 1977b) contributed an influential paper during this crucial period, which has since been referred to as a "classic" (Matarazzo, 1983:112). In a two-part article, "Reliability of Psychiatric Diagnosis," published back-to-back in one issue of the *Archives of General Psychiatry*, the authors review the methodological issues of prior reliability studies, the uses of kappa, and some reliability data from a study that used diagnostic criteria and structured interviews.

The first part contains little that was new. It presents what had by then become the conventional wisdom about the incomparability of prior studies, their methodological shortcomings, the sorry state of diagnostic agreement, the benefits of kappa, and the need to do better. It ends by reporting that of all the sources of inconsistency in diagnosis, only 5% is due to inconsistency in patients' reports, about 30% is due to inconsistency among clinicians, and over 60% is due to inadequacies of the nosological system itself. Thus, blame is strategically shifted away from clinicians and placed instead on the then current diagnostic manual. By identifying DSM-II (the nosological system) as the major culprit, they set the stage for DSM-III, its footsteps already faintly discernible coming down the hall, ready to make an appearance as the hero who solves the reliability conundrum.

The second part of the Helzer classic was a report of a new reliability study. This article is a fine example of advocacy in science. It was a frontal assault on those who might not believe in the importance of the

Feighner diagnostic criteria or the potential merits of structured interviews. The paper made reference to the close links between these issues and DSM-III, which was in active development. The article even optimistically claimed that DSM-III was "scheduled to go into effect in 1978" (p. 136), actually two years earlier than its publication date. The authors, however, wanted to link their work in St. Louis with DSM-III.

The study is simple. Three clinicians interviewed separately 101 patients shortly after they were admitted to Renard Hospital. Two of the three clinicians interviewed each patient, usually 24 hours apart. The three senior authors of the article conducted the research interviews. In the article, they reported their level of diagnostic agreement, compared it with the 1974 reanalysis of the early reliability studies, and offered some interpretations.

First, let us look at what they report in terms of the level of their diagnostic consistency (see Table 3.3, adapted from their Table 2), as measured by kappa. As can be seen in Table 3.3, the kappa coefficients range from .19 to .85, with a mean of .66.

Next (see Table 3.4), the authors compared their results with those of the earlier studies reported in Spitzer and Fleiss (1974). They did this by

Table 3.3. Reliability Levels Reported by Helzer et al. (1977)

Diagnosis	Kappa
Depression	.55
Mania	.82
Anxiety neurosis	.76
Schizophrenia	.58
Antisocial personality	.81
Alcoholism	.74
Drug dependence	.84
Hysteria	.72
Obsessional illness	.78
Homosexuality	.85
Organic brain syndrome	.29
Undiagnosed psychiatric illness	.19
Average (mean)	.66

Source: From Helzer, J.E., Clayton, P.J., Pambatian, R., Woodruff, R.A., & Reveley, M.A. Reliability of psychiatric diagnosis: II The test/retest reliability of diagnostic classification. *Archives of General Psychiatry, 34,* 136–141. Copyright © 1977, American Medical Association. Reprinted with permission.

Table 3.4. Comparison of Spitzer & Fleiss with Helzer et al.

Spitzer & Fleiss (1974)		Helzer et al. (1977)	
Diagnostic Category	Kappa	Kappa	Diagnostic Category
Affective disorder	.41	.55	Depression
Manic depressive	.33	.82	Mania
Sociopathy	.53	.81	Antisocial personality
Anxiety reaction	.45	.76	Anxiety neurosis
Alcoholism	.71	.74	Alcoholism
Schizophrenia	.57	.58	Schizophrenia
Organic brain syndrome	.77	.29	Organic brain syndrome
Kappa range	(.33–.77)	(.29–.82)	
Kappa mean	3.77/7 = .54	4.55/7 = .65)	

Source: From Helzer, J.E., Clayton, P.J., Pambatian, R., Woodruff, R.A., & Reveley, M.A. Reliability of psychiatric diagnosis: II The test/retest reliability of diagnostic classification. *Archives of General Psychiatry, 34*, 136–141. Copyright © 1977, American Medical Association. Reprinted with permission.

averaging the kappas across the different studies and attempting to match the earlier diagnostic categories with their own. The resulting comparison in Table 3.4, as the authors recognize, is cumbersome. One of the enduring problems in making comparisons across reliability studies is the fact that many studies use different diagnostic categories. Even if studies used similar methodologies, which they do not, the constantly changing diagnostic nomenclature ensures that these comparisons are flawed. Thus, the very process of constantly revising the diagnostic system makes it difficult to accumulate adequate comparative data about it. More will be said about this in Chapter 8.

What did Helzer et al. make of these numbers? They concluded that "in every category except organic brain syndrome, the kappas from the present study are higher" (p. 138). That appeared to be an accurate summary of the data presented. The mean kappa in their study was .65, higher than the .54 reported by Spitzer and Fleiss. (Remember that, for Helzer et al., the results were obtained among research psychiatrists with considerable experience developing and using diagnostic procedures and structured interviews.) For our purposes, however, we want to know what their interpretation is of those higher kappas. Several pages later, they say that their results "represent some improvement over previous reports" (p. 139). That statement is ambiguous and does not help the reader know what might constitute meaningful improvement. For example, a kappa rising to .58 from .57 for schizophrenia could be considered improvement, but we are still left wondering whether an improvement of .01 is meaningful (no one believes it is) and, more importantly, whether both .57 and .58 should be viewed as poor or good reliability.

In their text they offer a few clues to interpretation. They describe the organic brain syndrome by referring to a "low k" (kappa) and "low reliability" (p. 140). They review several reliability studies of medical diagnosis where kappas of .70, .43, and .47 are reported. With regard to this latter figure from a study of agreement among radiologists, they inform us that the original authors found the .47 "unacceptable." Helzer et al. then concluded:

> Thus, by comparison to previous studies of psychiatric diagnosis and to reliability of medical judgments, the results reported in the present investigation seem *good*. . . . Of the major psychiatric diagnoses, affective disorder and schizophrenia are on the *low* end of the reliability scale at .55 and .58 respectively. (p. 140, emphasis added)

By the very next paragraph, however, these modest conclusions were inflated: "Probably a major contributory factor to the *high* inter-rater reliability obtained in this study was the use of operational criteria" (p. 141, emphasis added).

They ended their article with a rousing defense of the importance of operational criteria as the way out of the confusion that had confronted American psychiatry. Their conclusion was a spirited display of what became the standard formula: the seriousness of the reliability problem, if it was not solved; the reasonableness of a technical approach to its solution; and the presentation of original data to claim that the proposed solution actually worked.

Figure 3.2 presents the interpretive standards that appear to be operative in this article, recognizing that even within the article there is some inconsistency. This inconsistency will be examined in greater detail in Chapter 6.

The Research Diagnostic Criteria Report

Perhaps no single report captures the spirit of the mid-1970s as well as a lengthy article published in 1978 titled simply "Research Diagnostic Criteria: Rationale and Reliability" (Spitzer et al., 1978). Historically, it was sandwiched between the common complaints about the sorry state of psychiatric diagnosis and the publication of DSM-III. It was authored by individuals in both the New York and St. Louis groups, who were all heavily involved in the development of DSM-III. Like the Helzer et al.

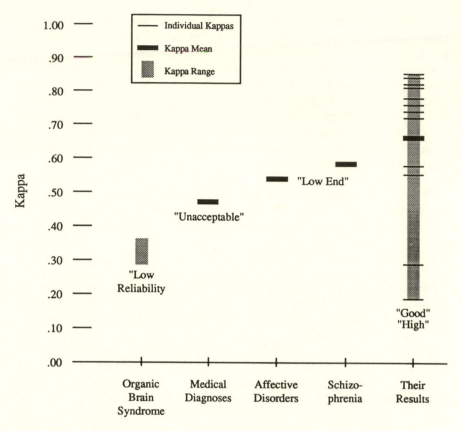

Figure 3.2. Interpretive standards of the Feighner diagnostic criteria by Helzer et al. (1977).

article, it attempted to demonstrate that the way to achieve diagnostic consistency was to control discretion. The authors' task was to show that if discretion could be controlled, reliability would improve. In their article, they accomplished these objectives using the familiar formula: denigrate the state of reliability from earlier studies and promote the most positive interpretation of the new diagnostic procedures.

The opening and final sentences in the article's abstract told the story of the success of the RDC:

> A crucial problem in psychiatry, affecting clinical work as well as research, is the generally low reliability of current psychiatric diagnostic procedures. . . . The data presented here indicate *high reliability* for diagnostic judgments made using these (RDC) criteria. (p. 773, emphasis added)

The article covered the following outline: (1) it blamed reliability problems on the lack of specific diagnostic criteria; (2) it reviewed the development of the RDC, how it grew out of the work of the St. Louis group and was being considered for use by those developing DSM-III (without mentioning that all the coauthors were, of course, the senior actors in both developments); (3) it described the nature of the RDC and the various diagnostic categories that it included; and (4) it reported reliabilities from three related studies that used the RDC.

The authors were clearly conscious of the pivotal position of this report. They explicitly connected it to the "crucial" reliability problems of the past and to the concurrent work going on in developing DSM-III, which was nearing completion and would be published in final form two years later.

They were also careful to emphasize that "a major purpose of the RDC is to enable investigators" to determine diagnoses more precisely and that "special attention was given to reliability" (p. 774). They reported using the SADS, a structured interview protocol. As research psychiatrists, they were on much firmer ground promoting the RDC and the SADS as technical, research tools rather than clinically useful instruments. Note that they labeled their instrument the research diagnostic criteria (as opposed to simply the diagnostic criteria). They had not demonstrated the clinical advantages of RDC or the SADS, but they felt that they could document the research advantages.

In their article, several pages were used to present reliability data from three related studies that they refer to as Study A, Study B, and the Test-Retest study. The latter two used both a structured interview protocol (the SADS) as well as the RDC. The studies were conducted by the New York and St. Louis groups as well as by investigators at two other important psychiatric research centers in Iowa and at Harvard. In five tables and accompanying text they presented their results using kappa.

As an example of how subtle "technical" research decisions may appear insignificant, but can greatly affect the findings, consider one small footnote to their tables. In it the authors indicate that in making diagnoses, a rating of "probable or definite was counted as present" in computing reliability scores (see Table 3.5). Clinicians were apparently asked to express their diagnostic judgments in terms of how confident they were about the presence or absence of a disorder in the cases. If only clinicians' judgments of definite were used to indicate the presence of a disorder, reliabilities would have been lower. But by combining those judgments about which the clinicians were definite with those in which the clinicians thought that there was a probable disorder, a more ambiguous range of opinion was collapsed into present or absent. Since the authors never revealed the kappas using only definite judgments,

Table 3.5. Kappa Coefficients of Agreement* for Major Diagnostic Categories Using the Research Diagnostic Criteria

	Joint Interviews		Test-Retest (N = 60)
	Study A (N = 68)	Study B (N = 150)	
Present episode only			
Schizophrenia	.80	**	.65
Schizo-affective disorder			
Manic type			.79
Depressed type	.86	.85	.73
Manic disorder	.82	.98	.82
Major depressive disorder	.88	.90	.90
Minor depressive disorder		.81	
Alcoholism	.86	.97	1.00
Drug abuse	.76	.95	.92
Lifetime diagnosis			
Schizophrenia	.75	.91	.73
Schizo-affective disorder			
Manic type			
Depressed type	.94	.87	.70
Manic disorder	.89	.93	.77
Hypomanic disorder	.85		.56
Major depressive disorder	.97	.91	.71
Minor depressive disorder		.68	
Alcoholism	.88	.98	.95
Drug abuse	.89	1.00	.73
Obsessive compulsive disorder		1.00	
Briquet's disorder	.79	.95	
Labile personality			.70
Bipolar I	.93	.95	.40
Bipolar II	.79	.85	
Recurrent unipolar	.81	.83	.80
Intermittent depressive disorder		.85	.57

 * Rating of probable or definite was counted as present.
** Less than 5% frequency by either rater.
Source: From Spitzer, R.L., Endicott, J. & Robins, E. Research Diagnostic Criteria. *Archives of General Psychiatry,* 35, 773–782. Copyright © 1978, American Medical Association. Reprinted with permission.

we cannot know to what extent this definitional liberalism increased the kappa scores reported. And since this maneuver was mentioned in a footnote to a table, it is unlikely that readers would pay much attention anyway. There is nothing obviously wrong with how the data were handled or reported. Nothing about this technical decision is uncommon to research reports. It is simply an example of how subtle decisions about the management and analysis of data can shape the results that are reported, but in a way that is beyond the ready comprehension of nonresearchers.

How did they interpret the data presented in the article? Their summary interpretations of their findings were as follows (see Figure 3.3): "The results of these three studies indicate that the reliability of the RDC categories is very high, even under the test-retest conditions where a much lower reliability is expected" (p. 779, emphasis added). They dismissed the importance of a few low kappas on the basis that there was a small number of cases in those diagnostic categories. (The occurrence of a small number of cases in a diagnostic category is another technical matter that is handled inconsistently throughout the reliability literature. For example, in the presentation of data about DSM-III, as we shall review later, high kappas are not dismissed when they are based on small numbers.) They emphasized that their findings, based on the New York RDC, are even higher than those shown by the St. Louis–based studies of the Feighner criteria.

When they examined the kappas for the subtypes of major depression, they concluded that they "are quite satisfactory for research use, and much higher than generally reported" (p. 780). They also reported

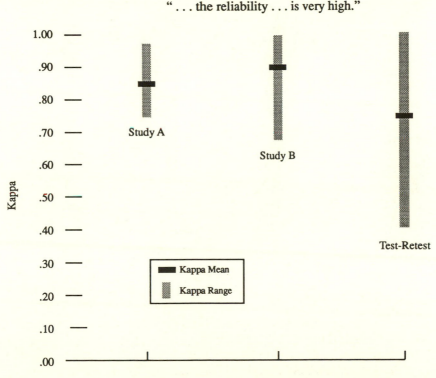

Figure 3.3. Interpretation of the RDC (Spitzer et al., 1978).

on a study using the RDC and SADS (lifetime version) with relatives of patients. They described those results as "amazingly high" (p. 781). Beyond these comments, they made few definitive statements that tied the data directly to its assessment. Using their own language, the interpretive standards used in this key article are given in Figure 3.4.

At the end of their article, they left no doubt about their appraisal of their own efforts: "The use of operational criteria for psychiatric diagnosis is an idea whose time has come!" (p. 781) they boasted. To them, their success was so impressive that they concluded, "It is amazing that this approach was not widely used before the 1960s since the problems of the unreliability of standard clinical diagnostic practice have been known for decades" (p. 781). In a rather curious inclusion for a scientific article, they then proudly quoted an authority on medical nosology who praised their efforts to include diagnostic criteria in DSM-III as a breakthrough of fundamental importance to psychiatry, comparable to demanding "that obstetricians and surgeons wash their hands before operating on the human body" (p. 781). They left little doubt about the value of what they defined as major accomplishments.

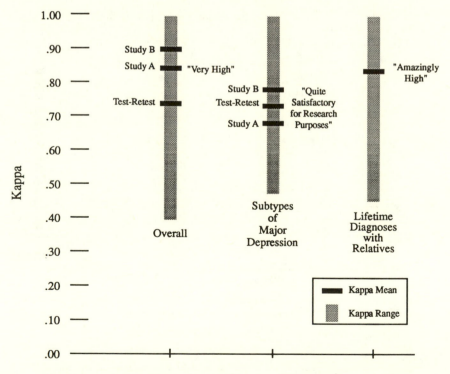

Figure 3.4.   Interpretive standards for the RDC (Spitzer et al, 1978).

They then argued that the only alternative to the RDC was to limit clinicians "to collecting and recording diagnostic data and then having a computer apply an algorithm to yield one or more diagnoses" (p. 782). They mentioned that they have developed such computer programs but they were somewhat impractical (at least they were before the era of microcomputers). They preferred the RDC, they wryly noted, which "does not, of course, eliminate clinical judgment" (p. 782). Thus, while advocating for a method of achieving greater reliability that clearly would limit clinical discretion, they presented themselves as backing away from computerized decision-making systems because they "eliminate clinical judgment." Rhetorically, this is important. While in the process of advocating for the adoption of a research protocol and decision criteria for clinical practice, they presented themselves as sensitive to and protective of clinical practice. Appearing to reject computer programs had this effect.

In their final sentence, they claimed that a large number of studies were under way using the RDC and that results would appear very soon. Like the Helzer article the previous year, they took a strong advocacy position for a particular type of solution to an important problem that they helped to define.

Their enthusiasm for their approach was not temporary. A decade later, it had not dampened. In a brief note in *Current Contents*, in which the RDC report was selected as a citation classic, Spitzer, reflecting on his earlier work, asserted that,

> The true historical significance of our article was that it heralded the way for the inclusion of specified diagnostic criteria for virtually all of the over 200 specific mental disorders included in the third revision of the DSM (DSM-III), published in 1980. (1989:20)

There are several noteworthy aspects of the Spitzer et al. (1978) RDC article. First, the language is all positive. Even in the text where they acknowledged some low kappas, the authors quickly obscured them in the tide of good news. Second, as in the earlier reports, there was a tendency to use summary evaluative terms for kappas that fall within a very broad band. Third, the positive statement "quite satisfactory for research purposes" encompassed the entire range of what in the reanalysis of the early studies report was described negatively as "only satisfactory." While both phrases used the term *satisfactory*, each biased the interpretation of the data in opposite directions. In the first "quite satisfactory," they connote acceptance and modest achievement. The findings are welcomed into the research family, without ever specifying whether "research purposes" implies more or less stringent criteria. In

the second "only satisfactory," they convey begrudging and bare tolera-
tion, as if allowing in an unwelcome relative. These differences in rhetorical presentation for essentially similar data nicely illustrate the effect
of context, intent, and language on scientific interpretation.

These points about the rhetoric of interpretation, however, should not
obscure the fact that in the RDC article the overall means and the top
end ranges are generally higher than in the previous studies. Despite
the inconsistency in the use of the terms *very high, quite satisfactory,* and
amazingly high to describe results that fall in similar ranges and have
similar means, the fact is that these ranges and means themselves are
higher than those in the earlier studies, although perhaps not as much
higher as the inflated language might suggest. The data they presented
in 1978 appeared to signal some moderate success in raising kappa levels
in controlled research settings and, hence, to buttress their case for
technical solutions to the reliability problem (see Figure 3.5).

The 1978 article, while promoting the use of the RDC and structured

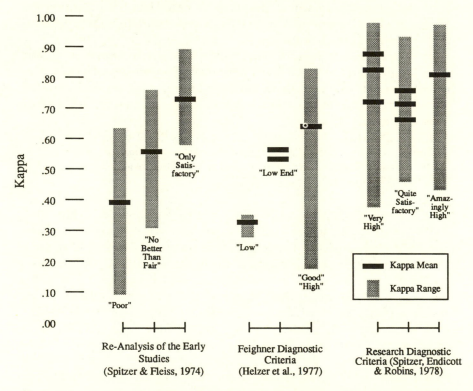

Figure 3.5. Summary of three articles and their interpretation of kappa. (The
kappa ranges are of the reported reliability coefficients.)

interviews, did present reliability levels that are considered achievable and, by any implicit standard used up to then, good. One of the major purposes of the paper was in fact to signal that the way had been found to solve the reliability problem. Describing kappas as very or amazingly high is a way of announcing success and setting the standards for what could be achieved and what should be expected. The interpretive language of the review of early studies and the RDC article set the standards within which the authors forecast that the reliability problem would be solved by DSM-III.

By the late 1970s, the development of diagnostic criteria to control diagnostic decision-making and structured interview schedules to limit information variance had claimed center stage in the reliability drama. The mystery would be solved by superior techniques, rigorous control, and the right leadership. Moreover, the development of DSM-III had been earmarked as the theater in which this play whose themes were now being rehearsed would be produced. The executive producer and most of the supporting cast had been selected.

It was through the development of a new psychiatric manual that research psychiatrists, by emphasizing the sorry state of diagnostic reliability and its significance and, further, by claiming that they could do better, positioned themselves near the center of American psychiatry. With their claims of initial success in solving reliability problems, they forecast to one and all that if given the chance, they could carry their success to a larger stage. The house was DSM-III and the script was a new psychiatric nosology.

4

MAKING A MANUAL

> Finally, interest in the development of this manual is due to awareness that DSM-III reflects an increased commitment in our field to reliance on data as the basis for understanding mental disorders.
>
> Robert L. Spitzer, *Introduction to DSM-III*

There is great irony in the story of how the new manual was developed. Once the work started, questions of reliability and other scientific issues took a back seat to political struggles about the appropriate place of various diagnoses such as homosexuality, neurosis, and post–traumatic stress disorder. The committee appointed to revise DSM-III was controlled by Robert Spitzer and his colleagues in the New York and St. Louis groups, who had pioneered the use of explicit diagnostic criteria and structured interviews. On the basis of their earlier work they devised an "atheoretical" diagnostic system that emphasized specific descriptions of directly observable behaviors. Their approach was a radical departure for American psychiatry, which had accepted as a first axiom that its task was to identify and treat causes, not symptoms. This oft-repeated homily led Freud and his followers to discount symptoms or to interpret them as symbolic clues to underlying psychological processes, which could be understood principally in terms of psychoanalytic theories. By pursuing an atheoretical approach, Spitzer inevitably ran afoul of many psychoanalytically oriented psychiatrists.

The controversies that arose from this conflict consumed the attention of the new manual's architects. It compelled them to use political tactics and to engage in strategic compromises that were not based on empirical data. In this political struggle, questions of reliability and other more-or-less data-related issues were overshadowed by the politics of diagnosis.

His work on reliability established Spitzer's scientific credentials to oversee the process of revising the new manual, but it was his ability to resolve an embarrassing dispute over the diagnosis of homosexuality that demonstrated his political usefulness to newly emerging leadership of the APA. This chapter reviews some of the major controversies that developed just prior to and during the development of DSM-III. This will not be a thorough examination of the revision of the manual, or a complete description of any of the individual controversies. The purpose is to identify the limited role of research and empirical data in key controversies that arose as the new manual was formulated. The first of the conflicts that we will describe, a confrontation over the diagnosis of homosexuality, occurred just prior to the time when the revision of the manual began. We will explain some of the details of this struggle, particularly the intricate process that was used to settle the conflict, to illustrate how diagnostic controversies were conceptualized and debated. This introduction to the Byzantine committee structure of the APA may seem elaborate, but these details are necessary to understand the process that psychiatrists use to decide about official changes in the diagnostic manual. To resolve the dispute over homosexuality, ad hoc procedures were developed that became a model for negotiating compromises during the later efforts to revise the manual. More significantly, this controversy also provided the opportunity for Robert Spitzer to demonstrate his extraordinary ability to handle the enormously complex task of revamping DSM. The conflict over homosexuality was resolved with little regard for questions of reliability, and in the final analysis, it had little to do with empirical issues. The pattern that was established during this controversy carried over to events that occurred during the following six years when DSM-III was created.

Early Planning for the Third Edition of DSM

There are many reasons why the APA decided to revise DSM-II. No doubt, the demands that homosexuality be eliminated from the manual caused great discomfort, particularly after gay activists staged protests at the annual APA conventions, starting in 1970. Furthermore, many researchers, including some who were highly respected within the profession, criticized both the theoretical foundations of the diagnostic system and the reliability of diagnostic practices. There were many other pressures that have been less publicized. The needs of the drug industry for a reliable, standardized nomenclature for the diagnosis of participants in government-required drug trials is one that is seldom mentioned (Sartorius, 1990).

Third-party support for psychotherapy grew rapidly during the 1970s and this led to an unprecedented expansion of outpatient treatment. Insurance companies and other third-party payers often required diagnoses and they pushed for a closer relationship between diagnosis and treatment (Chu & Trotter, 1974). This focused more attention on diagnosis, and, as a result, the deficits in the existing diagnostic system, DSM-II, became more evident.

Public protests, disturbing research, third-party financing, and clinician dissatisfaction all played some part in the mounting pressure on the APA. The pressures were not necessarily consistent or well focused, nor was it certain that more tinkering with the diagnostic manual was the solution to many of these concerns. Although the decision to revise the manual was made within five years after the publication of DSM-II, what the APA hoped to achieve is unclear. In a memo dated March 20, 1973, Walter Barton, the chief executive of the APA, described some of the first steps that had been taken to initiate DSM-III. The memo was addressed to the chairman of the APA Council on Research and Development, one of the many committees in the chain of command between the APA governing board and the group that would actually revise the manual. The council was directed to "appoint a task force to revise DSM-II and prepare DSM-III within the next two years." The type of change contemplated by the board was:

> that the revision be related to problem-oriented records, and that in the new terminology an attempt be made to determine the functional disabilities that accompany any given diagnostic condition so that it can be subjected to quantitative revision.

Although it is not entirely clear, the thrust of the recommendation seemed to be to develop a system that would be useful in various administrative and forensic settings, so that it would be possible, for instance, to use the diagnostic system to accurately assess the amount of a disability award, or to provide the participants in a lawsuit with an accurate measure of damages.

Barton also reported some other concerns of the board:

> The Trustees noted that while the new terminology should relate to ICD-9 [International Classifications of Diseases, 9th ed. (WHO, 1977)], national concerns should be overriding; that classification of the aged, children and mental retardation are more important; that the quantitication (*sic*) of the degree of disability is most important.

Although some of the recommendations were incorporated into DSM-III, many of the barely formed ideas of the board of trustees were ignored as DSM-III took shape. As the board recommended, national concerns, particularly about children, were given much greater emphasis than an attempt to coordinate the new revision of the manual with the next edition of ICD, which was the medical classification system devised by the United Nations for reporting medical disorders. The principal reason for publishing DSM-II was to create a manual that would mesh with ICD, which the United States was required, by international treaty, to use for statistics-keeping purposes, but this objective was given very low priority for DSM-III.

However, the recommendation of the board that the new revision be problem oriented and that the degree of disability be subject to quantification quickly fell by the wayside as the agenda of those who actually developed the manual superseded the concerns of the Board and its committees.

The board also made another recommendation that never came to fruition. Barton reported that:

> At this time also, the Trustees recommended the formation of a Task Force to Define Mental Illness and What Is a Psychiatrist. The Reference Committee has assigned this to the Council on Emerging Issues. It was the Trustees wish that the definitions that this task force develops be used as a preamble to the new DSM-III.

The definition of mental illness became one of the major controversies that developed as DSM-III was formulated. But the Task Force to Define Mental Illness would have no apparent role in the controversy. In hindsight, the idea that the makers of the manual would let this important issue escape their control is ironic.

As an aside, Barton passed along a recommendation for membership on the new task force to revise DSM. The candidate was not a full-fledged psychiatrist; he was a:

> Member in Training. . . . An older man [who] was in the general practice of medicine for many years; his psychiatric training was in a GP program. . . . He has had experience in a community mental health center and as an inspector of psychiatric hospitals for the JCAH [Joint Committee on the Accreditation of Hospitals]. He's "gung-ho" on problem-oriented records and . . . knows quite a bit about them.

In retrospect, this suggestion is also amusing, because the candidate falls so far short of the type of member the DSM-III Task Force would have: aggressive, research-oriented, technically sophisticated psychiatrists who were at the cutting edge of new developments in nosology, a far cry from the good old boy approach that Barton suggested. But then, neither he nor the other APA leaders had any idea of how important DSM-III would become for the association, and how significant would be the selection of members of the drafting group.

In the next few years, several developments converged that led to changes. A new generation of psychiatrists who referred to themselves as Young Turks came to power in the APA. They were less bound by psychiatric tradition than their predecessors (although this has to be understood in context, since they were not on the cutting edge of social change). Although the majority of psychiatrists identified themselves as Freudians up until the 1980s, many younger psychiatrists were not as wedded to Freudian orthodoxies as the older members of the profession. Some of this disaffection occurred because psychoanalysis had not proved to be as useful as earlier practitioners had believed it would be. Psychoanalysis in the United States was used as an intensive, long-term treatment. The psychotherapy market was flooded with newer treatments such as Transactional Analysis and Gestalt therapy that claimed to do as much as psychoanalysis, but to do it much faster. For inpatients, even when psychoanalysts were available, long-term analysis was not a viable treatment because hospital stays were greatly shortened after the introduction of psychotropic medication. Added to these clinical challenges were researchers' reports that psychoanalysis showed no higher cure rates than other treatment approaches and that patients in psychotherapeutic treatment did no better than those who remained on the waiting list for the same length of time.

There were other differences among the psychiatrists who were now coming to power within the APA. Many were influenced by the social activism of the 1960s. A prominent publication of the new medical director, Melvin Sabshin, who replaced Barton in 1974, was "Dimensions of Institutional Racism," which appeared in the *American Journal of Psychiatry* a few years before he was appointed to head the association (Sabshin, Diesenhaus, & Wilkerson, 1970). The article called for a regular section of the journal to be devoted to issues of racism (a proposal that was short-lived).

DSM and Homosexuality: A Cautionary Tale

Although changing leadership of the APA did not propel the organization into the forefront of social activism in the United States, it reflected a greater responsiveness to the social problems from which psychiatrists had traditionally insulated themselves. This change was evident in the dramatic events surrounding the controversy over the diagnosis of homosexuality, which occurred just as plans for DSM-III were being formulated. This controversy illustrates both the sensitivity of the APA to public opinion and its organizational difficulties in dealing with internal dissension or external critics. These dual vulnerabilities allowed an enterprising and able nosologist, Robert Spitzer, to step into the breach. His eagerness to do so and his tenuous success at managing the controversy placed him at the political heart of psychiatric diagnosis and foreshadowed his subsequent efforts to develop DSM-III.

The principal source of information about the DSM controversy over homosexuality is Spitzer. Bayer's (1981) book length description of these events was heavily dependent on material provided by Spitzer. This is evident not only from reading his account, but also because he collaborated with Spitzer (Bayer & Spitzer, 1982) on an edited report of the correspondence of the principals. Bayer and Spitzer (1985) also coauthored an account of another closely related episode, the attempt to extirpate neurosis and other Freudian aspects of DSM.

Despite these limitations, Bayer and Spitzer reveal a good deal of information, some of it critical of Spitzer. On the other hand, claiming to provide information on "both sides," or more accurately on all sides of the debate, the story that is presented could be incomplete. If key elements are missing, they are hard to identify. This is a problem that pervades the entire history of the development and revisions of the manual. Nevertheless, the recounting of this key episode illustrates some of the politics of psychiatric diagnosis that existed just as the campaign to transform DSM was about to begin.

At stake was a minor modification of DSM-II. At the 1970 annual convention of the APA in San Francisco and at subsequent psychiatric meetings, gay activists picketed and disrupted conference events in order to draw attention to their demand that homosexuality be dropped as a psychiatric category. In addition to disrupting the presentations by psychoanalysts who were well known for their views that homosexuality was a form of pathology, gay activists forced the APA to schedule panels at the annual meetings where the protesters presented an alternative view of homosexuality as a normal variation of sexual activity. This pattern of protest persisted for several years and at the 1972 meeting a masked and cloaked psychiatrist, "Dr. Anonymous," joined the panel and declared that he was a homosexual as were more than two hundred of his associates, some of them members of the Gay Psychiatric Association, which met socially but secretly during the annual APA meetings.

A standoff persisted until late in 1972 between the protesters and psychoanalysts such as Irving Bieber and Charles Socarides who insisted that the "scientific evidence," principally derived from studies that they had conducted, demonstrated that homosexuality was a pathological condition, and that a positive response to gay demands would constitute an unjustified political accommodation. Enmeshed in the controversy was a challenge to psychoanalytic orthodoxy.

The man who took control was Robert Spitzer. Although he was a member of the Committee on Nomenclature and Statistics, which produced DSM-II, he had not been assigned to resolve the conflict. As the story has been told, he was at a meeting in October 1972, when more than a hundred gay activists protested antihomosexual bias. This was his first contact with gays protesting against psychiatric mistreatment and he stayed afterwards to talk with one leader of the protest, Ron Gold. As Spitzer has described the encounter:

> I went to this conference on behavioral modification which the gay lib group broke up. I found myself talking to a very angry young man. At that time I was convinced that homosexuality was a disorder and that it belonged in the classification, I told him so. (Spector, 1977:54)

Gold also described the exchange:

> He said he believed in the illness theory. I said, all right, who do you believe? And he hadn't read any of it. . . . But he happened to know Socarides and thought he was a nut. Whom do you believe? Bieber? I don't know. Have you read it? No. But they all believed it. (p. 54)

The result of this encounter was that Spitzer agreed to arrange a meeting with the Committee on Nomenclature and to schedule a panel at the next meeting of the APA in May 1973 in Honolulu.

Although this chance encounter has been reported in several different accounts of the controversy of the diagnosis of homosexuality, the story leaves much to be explained. Spitzer, by all accounts, was unfamiliar with the literature and had little, if any, clinical experience with homosexuals. Nevertheless, as a result of an unanticipated discussion, he agreed to undertake a major role in this struggle.

Spitzer had spent much of his professional career devoted to psychiatric diagnosis and the development of DSM. He knew that during the next year a decision would be made about who would head the effort to revise the manual. And here with Ron Gold, without hesitation or explanation, he walked into the middle of the biggest public battle then confronting the APA. One can only speculate that he must have considered how this would affect his opportunity to be selected as head of the task force to revise DSM, a fitting capstone for his entire previous professional career. As it turned out, he demonstrated that he was the man for the job. He ended the embarrassing public controversy, without capitulating to either the psychoanalytic faction or the gay activists, and he did it on his own initiative. If there was a question about who should head the upcoming effort, his performance in the controversy added to his credibility. Furthermore, when later disputes emerged in the development of DSM-III, the way that he handled this controversy demonstrated that he was to be deferred to as a master of the professional politics involved in developing an acceptable nosology.

Spitzer conveyed the request to meet with the Committee on Nomenclature and Statistics to its chairman, Henry Brill, who agreed. Spitzer's explanation for the decision: "We couldn't think of any good reason not to meet them" (Spector, 1977:54). Perhaps not, but there were many good reasons for the members of the committee to proceed in a different manner than they did. When they met with gay spokesmen in February 1973, they did not invite the established psychiatrists who vehemently opposed dropping homosexuality from the manual. And they made their deliberations public. The following day there was an article in *The New York Times* about the meeting, and Brill was quoted as saying that some change was indicated.

Actually, as early as 1971 Brill had reported that there was strong sentiment within the Committee on Nomenclature and Statistics to recognize "that homosexual behavior was not necessarily a sign of psychiatric disorder; and that the diagnostic manual should reflect that understanding" (Brill to Barton in Bayer, 1981:113). But the story in *The New York Times* was different because these private sentiments were now a part of the public record. Furthermore, Brill indicated that the committee hoped to have a resolution prepared within two months, in time for the APA annual meeting. This deadline was not met despite the apparent enthusiasm of the Committee on Nomenclature and Statistics and its chairman, because Spitzer balked and would not agree to incorporate a recommendation to declassify homosexuality in a position paper he was asked to coauthor for the committee.

Although the May 1973 convention was not punctuated by the dramatic disruptions that had occurred in prior years, there were several events that had a major impact on the conflict over the diagnosis of homosexuality. First of all, as he had promised, Spitzer arranged for a panel that included leading psychiatrists on both sides of the controversy, as well as a gay speaker. This program was unlike the previous year's panel, which had consisted of gay activists and their psychiatrist supporters. The whole atmosphere had changed dramatically in the three years since protestors first disrupted a panel on "Issues of Homosexuality" and created so much pandemonium that some conventioneers demanded a refund of their airfares, and at least one physician asked that police shoot the protesters (Bayer, 1981:103). By contrast, the panel at the 1973 convention was very well attended by almost a thousand people, and there was a positive response to those who criticized the view that homosexuality was a pathological condition. The media made optimistic predictions that homosexuality would be dropped soon from DSM.

Another event at the conference had a profound effect on Spitzer, who was still undecided about homosexuality. Spitzer, who, we are told, had never knowingly met a gay psychiatrist, was invited to attend a social meeting of the Gay Psychiatric Association. Although participants were upset by Spitzer's unannounced appearance, many were persuaded to explain how they felt. "Spitzer heard homosexual psychiatrists declaring that 'their lives had been changed by what they had heard at the panel discussion'" (Bayer, 1981:126). They confirmed Spitzer's belief that many homosexuals (among them psychiatric colleagues) functioned at a high level. His encounter gave Spitzer such "an emotional jolt" that he prepared a proposal within a month for the deletion of homosexuality from DSM.

Actually, Spitzer's position paper, "Homosexuality as an Irregular Form of Sexual Development and Sexual Orientation Disturbance as a Psychiatric Disorder," did not recommend the entire elimination of homosexuality from the manual. Although homosexuality per se was not enough to warrant a diagnosis, those who were troubled should be given a new diagnosis of Sexual Orientation Disturbance. Spitzer did not accept the position of gay activists that homosexuality was a normal variant of sexual behavior. He proposed a middle ground between their position and the assertion that homosexuality was pathological.

Spitzer's reasoning was as follows. In order to answer the question of whether homosexuality was an illness, he felt that it was necessary first to define mental disorder as a behavior that was accompanied by subjective distress or a general impairment in social effectiveness or functioning. Since some gays, such as those he met at the APA meeting, did not suffer from subjective distress because of their sexual orientation and were obviously high functioning, they could not be considered mentally ill.

On the other hand, he did not want to give them the stamp of normalcy. He decided that homosexuality was a form of irregular sexual behavior. But, if psychiatry was to broaden its diagnostic system to include "suboptimal" behaviors as mental disorders, he reasoned, it would have to recognize celibacy, religious fanaticism, racism, vegetarianism, and male chauvinism as diagnostic categories (Spitzer, 1973:1215). The choice of examples, obviously meant by Spitzer to be humorous, reveals what was likely to persuade his audience composed primarily of white males who understood the distinctions between racism, sexism, and the disorders they diagnosed and treated.

Bayer offered an admiring evaluation of the proposal:

> The position paper as well as the proposed new diagnostic category thus attempted to provide a common ground for those who had been locked in combat for the past three years. To homosexual activists it granted the removal of homosexuality from the Diagnostic Manual, allowing them to claim a stunning victory. To psychoanalytically oriented psychiatrists, it stated that their own view of homosexuality as suboptimal was not being challenged but rather was not central to the restricted concept of psychiatric disorder. To those seeking an end to the pattern of disruptions that had beset psychiatric meetings, the new classification provided a formula that could remove the APA from the center of controversy. Finally for psychiatrists concerned with the extent to which the psychiatric nosology had become a tool in the hands of government officials attempting to deprive homosexuals of their rights, the proposed shift promised to put an end to such unwanted collaboration. That all this could take the form of a theoretical refinement rather than a political accommodation made the proposal more attractive to those willing to yield polar positions defined in the course of conflict. (1981:129)

However, few of the participants in this controversy viewed Spitzer's handiwork in this way. The Committee on Nomenclature and Statistics refused to adopt his proposal. The chairman, Brill, seemed to back away from his earlier position that the committee should do something about the diagnosis of homosexuality. Instead, he suggested a survey of APA members to determine whether Spitzer's proposals would elicit a strong reaction. Spitzer's proposal, without committee approval, was bucked upstairs to the Council on Research and Development. The chair of the council rejected Brill's suggested survey as "ridiculous," saying, "You don't devise a nomenclature through a vote" (p. 130).

The Committee on Nomenclature and Statistics was not the only group that refused to accept Spitzer's compromise. Ron Gold objected to Spitzer's proposal, particularly the new diagnosis, Sexual Orientation Disturbance, which would be used only for homosexuals. Gold urged the council to limit its action to deletion of Homosexuality from DSM. Judd Marmor, a highly respected psychiatrist, also objected because of Spitzer's description of homosexuality as "irregular," rather than as "a variant form of sexual development" (Spector, 1977:54). Despite reservations by many of its members, the council voted unanimously to adopt Spitzer's proposal. The reasoning of the council was that they should not override the recommendation of a committee they had appointed to evaluate a scientific issue. Their logic was questionable, since the proposal was not recommended to them by the Committee on Nomenclature and Statistics; it was solely Spitzer's work.

Next to review the proposal was the Assembly of District Branches, and it was overwhelmingly approved. However the assembly called upon the Council on Research and Development to reword the proposal to eliminate pejorative phrasing such as the reference to homosexuality as an irregular form of sexual behavior.

Finally, in December 1973, the matter was considered by the board of trustees. After listening politely to the objections of opponents, the board voted unanimously to delete homosexuality and to replace it with the diagnosis of Sexual Orientation Disturbance. The final text made a distinction between homosexuality per se and Sexual Orientation Disturbance. "This diagnostic category is distinguished from homosexuality which by itself does not necessarily constitute a psychiatric disorder" (APA press release cited in Bayer, 1981:137).

The meeting was followed by a press conference attended by the president of the APA, gay activists, and Robert Spitzer. Major newspapers across the country carried stories announcing the revision. Many reports missed the nuances of the compromise. For example, the *Washington Post* reported "Doctors Rule Homosexuals Not Abnormal" (December 12, 1973, p. 1). Their headline ignored the careful denials of the APA president and Spitzer that the board had not declared that homosexuality was normal. Spitzer's statement infuriated gays, but it made little difference in the public perception of what had happened.

Spitzer's comments were a tip-off that he was not done tinkering with the problem. But it was a while before he had an opportunity to deal with these issues again. Other participants had scores to settle. Charles Socarides forced the board to submit its decision to a referendum of the APA membership. Many people ridiculed the idea that a scientific issue should be settled by a plebiscite. Ironically, Socarides and Bieber, who had complained that scientific decisions were being subjected to political pressures by gays, now justified the use of a political device to reverse the decision.

The reputation of the organization was not the only thing at risk. Individual careers were deeply affected. Not long after the decision, Judd Marmor replaced Bieber as the author of a chapter on homosexuality in one of the leading psychiatric textbooks. A new group of experts, many with views more sympathetic to gays and lesbians, was called on to express their opinions about issues related to homosexuality in court proceedings, in the popular media, and in professional publications.

Spitzer was among those most directly affected. Although he expressed "severe discomfort" (Bayer, 1981:143) over the idea of a referendum, he and gay activists drafted a letter that was signed by all of the candidates in an upcoming election for president and vice president of the APA. The letter was sent to the entire APA membership, paid for by funds raised by gay groups, although their participation was concealed. This was a risky strategy, but he felt that the stakes were very high. Spitzer's career was directly linked to the outcome of the vote, since he had just been appointed to oversee the publication of DSM-III. Later he acknowledged how important these factors were in his decision to help draft the letter:

> We knew the other side would be angry with what we did. Frankly I was very worried by the referendum. . . . We were very apprehensive and we didn't win by much. . . . If we had lost I would probably have been asked to resign and just after becoming Chairman at that. (Spector, 1977:55)

The vote was not close although it was described this way in later accounts: 58% were in favor of deleting homosexuality from DSM, while only 37% voted against the proposal. Those familiar with voting patterns among large groups of people would characterize this as a landslide, but describing the vote as close served other purposes in subsequent conflicts over the diagnosis of homosexuality.

Before describing the sequelae to this debate, four aspects of the controversy deserve to be highlighted, since they recurred repeatedly in the conflicts over the revisions of DSM. One is the claim of the proponents on every side that they were being scientific and their opponents were not. Even though they had done little research and had very little hard data to support their position, psychiatrists who wanted to change the diagnostic system claimed that they were making informed, scientific decisions. A fallback position was that the scientific evidence presented by their opponents was invalid and should be discounted, which was easy enough to show by looking at it in terms of basic scientific standards. Few of the psychiatrists involved in the controversy had done studies that could pass muster as credible research, but before a decision could be made each side had to couch its arguments in the terms of science. The presentations by gay activists were very important in this respect, because they were careful to mobilize whatever scientific reports were available to support the declassification of homosexuality. The earlier disruptions by gay rights groups were crucial, but a scientific rationale was also needed before the APA and its committees could act. Science was a rallying cry; politics a term of denigration.

A second factor involves the strategy of presenting issues as though they came from a position of organizational authority. For example, even when Spitzer did not have the support of the Committee on Nomenclature and Statistics, his proposal was seen as its recommendation. Perhaps the best illustration of this strategy was in the final referendum. In addition to the circulation of the letter signed by the leaders of the organization, the strategy was reflected in the way that the referendum was worded. Members were asked to vote whether they were in favor of the decision of the board of trustees or whether they opposed it. In this way the proposal was persuasive to both liberals who wanted to declassify homosexuality and to some conservatives who wanted to maintain the status quo and to reestablish traditional authority of the organization.

A third very important phenomenon that will reappear in the struggles about DSM-III was the sense that someone took control in a stalemated situation and resolved it; without active intervention the more conservative membership of the APA would not have acted. In addition to Spitzer, leadership was provided by Judd Marmor, who had greater popular support. Marmor, who had been forthright about his position that homosexuality was not pathological, was elected president of the APA within months after the board declassified homosexuality and the referendum was defeated.

Furthermore, a more liberal proposal of the Massachusetts Psychiatric Association to declassify homosexuality appeared to have a good chance of being adopted when it was withdrawn in deference to Spitzer's efforts. Although the story has generally emphasized his ability to get things done, there is an additional way of looking at it, namely to see the controversy as an opportunity that he used to advance his own interests.

The final consideration about this episode is how important it was symbolically, but how *unimportant* its consequences were. Although Spitzer insisted that Sexual Orientation Disturbance should be limited to homosexuals, the impact of this formulation was inconsequential. Lawrence Hartmann, who headed the initiative of the Massachusetts Psychiatric Association to declassify homosexuality, told an interviewer:

> [Hartmann] If you're seeing a homosexual patient and had to fill out an insurance form, I would still . . . not use the word homosexual. I think it is such a damaging word.
>
> [Interviewer] What is the most convenient one?
>
> [Hartmann] Depression is easy, anxiety neurosis is easy, adjustment reaction of adulthood or adolescence. Usually a patient has quite a few worries. I write as brief notes as I can. I use as vague and general categories as I think are compatible with the truth. Insurance companies realize that they are getting watered down diagnostic labels in order not to harm the patient. (Spector, 1977:56)

The gay activists clearly realized the symbolic significance of the decision about the diagnosis. Although they were angry with Spitzer for the way that he had formulated the diagnosis of Sexual Orientation Disorder and for his continued unwillingness to recognize that homosexuality was a normal variation of sexual activity, they pushed for the APA press conference which announced the change in the nomenclature.

Following the 1974 referendum, Spitzer went back to the drawing board. He was dissatisfied with the definition of mental disorder that he had used to justify revising the diagnosis of homosexuality (Bayer, 1981:167–68). He came up with a new definition of mental disorder, which in his mind necessitated a further revision of the diagnosis. The revised diagnosis was first called homodysphilia and then dyshomophilia; it finally appeared in the next edition of DSM as Ego-Dystonic Homosexuality, a diagnosis for those who are troubled about their homosexual impulses (Spitzer, 1981a:210–15). This effort was not the result of any significant pressure by Bieber, Socarides, or their allies who gave up the fight to retain homosexuality in the manual. The major impetus came from Spitzer.

There was a protracted exchange of letters with some of the gay activists and their supporters who opposed Spitzer's initiative, but eventually he prevailed. Gay activists decided against another public battle that they might lose as the APA began to shift back to a more conservative orientation. By not publicizing the insertion of Ego-Dystonic Homosexuality, they felt that there would continue to be a public perception that the APA had abandoned homosexuality as a pathological condition. Even with the revision, this was technically true, although less so than was generally believed.

The wisdom of their decision was confirmed in 1987 when Ego-Dystonic Homosexuality was quietly eliminated from the next revision of the manual, DSM-III-R. The principal justifications offered for deletion from DSM-III-R were that Ego-Dystonic Homosexuality was used infrequently in clinical practice and that very few articles had been written about it in the scientific literature. This reasoning was far different than the scientific justifications that were used in the 1974 battle over the diagnosis of homosexuality. Gay rights leaders had used the opportunity presented by another embarrassing public battle (this time between the APA and feminists over controversial new diagnoses that Spitzer had proposed for disorders that principally affect women) to successfully press for the elimination of Ego-Dystonic Homosexuality.

Architect, Critic, and Defender of DSM

The controversy over homosexuality was a prelude to many of the issues that emerged in the development of DSM-III and provides some lessons about the way that the APA dealt with them. As is by now evident, Spitzer's role cannot be ignored in any discussion about the evolution of modern psychiatric diagnosis. His presence and his method of handling controversy were an intimate part of the development of the manual. Allen Frances, the psychiatrist in charge of the publication of DSM-IV, has described him as a man whose entire life, private and public, personal and professional, is occupied with diagnosis and particularly with DSM (Frances, 1990a, 1990b).

Spitzer was trained as a physician, psychiatrist, and psychoanalyst. Not long after completing his training he became a prominent figure among the small group of psychiatrists who were interested in psychiatric nomenclature in the 1960s. He has been employed by the New York State Psychiatric Institute, a major research facility affiliated with Columbia University, throughout his career, which has been devoted principally to research, an unusual career pattern for psychiatrists.

He was a major participant in the development of DSM-II, but his role deserves attention because he did not unequivocally support its formulations. DSM-II opened with an acknowledgment, signed by Spitzer and two other psychiatrists, who "served as consultants to the APA Medical Director, and approved the final form of the manual before publication" (APA, 1968:iv). Spitzer was at once an apologist for the manual and for psychiatric diagnosis in general, and at the same time a major critic. Some examples will illustrate how he managed this dual role. After DSM-II was published, an explanatory chapter was added, "A Guide to the New Nomenclature," coauthored by Spitzer and Paul Wilson (1968). They stated that their purpose was to "facilitate the transition" from DSM-I to DSM-II "by explaining how the new manual differs from the old one and how in many ways it is improved" (p. 130). Much of the chapter was devoted to a comparison between DSM-I and DSM-II and an explanation of the changes in the new manual. The chapter concluded with an interesting prediction:

> With the adoption of DSM-II, American psychiatrists for the first time in history will be using diagnostic categories that are part of an international classification of diseases. While this is an important first step it is only an agreement to use the same sets of categories for classifying disorders. For many disorders it is clear that clinicians in different countries will still define these categories in different ways. (p. 134)

They observed that "the next step must be to establish a common set of definitions for these categories," and that the World Health Organization had already started this process. Anticipating Spitzer's agenda for DSM-III they observed: "Even this is not an end in itself. The ultimate purpose of this work is the improvement in treatment and prevention that will evolve with better communication among psychiatrists of all nations" P. 134).

Spitzer's dual role as defender and critic of DSM-II is even more pronounced in an article, "DSM-II Revisited" (Spitzer & Wilson, 1969), that he and Wilson published a year later. The occasion for their reevaluation was a symposium on DSM-II in which various international experts participated. First, they responded to the complaints of Karl Menninger, the most famous psychiatrist in America at that time. They dismissed Menninger's criticism that diagnoses are used improperly:

> Because psychiatric diagnoses are sometimes misused to the detriment of patients does not seem to us an adequate reason for denying the profession a classification system by which they can communicate with each other regarding the conditions for which they have professional responsibility. (p. 422)

This complaint about the misuse of psychiatric diagnosis was increasingly voiced in both professional literature and in popular works of the period such as Kesey's *One Flew Over the Cuckoo Nest*. Spitzer and Wilson did not express concern that a diagnostic system such as DSM-II should develop procedures to protect against the misuse of diagnoses. They also dismissed the criticism that clinicians in different settings often used the same diagnostic terms in different ways. This was one aspect of the reliability problem that Spitzer was already attempting to solve, but no mention was made of his work. In general they did not acknowledge a number of problems that would be of major concern to Spitzer when he began developing DSM-III.

The most interesting part of the article, however, was that it revealed the blueprint that Spitzer would use in the development of DSM-III. Answering the self-imposed question, What have we learned that can be useful in preparing DSM-III? their first recommendation was that "the small committee in charge of producing DSM-III be supplemented by subcommittees of experts in the various psychiatric disorders" (p. 425). And, indeed, one of the hallmarks of DSM-III was the involvement of hundreds of experts in 14 committees that advised the main DSM-III Task Force. The names of the participants in these advisory committees are displayed prominently at the beginning of DSM-III, offering an unmistakable look at a massive effort to obtain professional consensus.

Spitzer and Wilson's second recommendation was that "a draft version of any subsequent manual be given an adequate clinical trial" (p. 425). Here too, they were prophetic, since the clinical trials for DSM-III were a linchpin in selling the manual, and some of the results of the trials, about which we shall have much to say, were included in the 1980 revision.

Spitzer and his colleague also recommended a multidimensional system, which, renamed the multiaxial system, was later publicized as one of the major new features of DSM-III. They even identified two of the added dimensions or axes that would be incorporated in DSM-III. Subjective distress would become one aspect of Axis IV (Psychosocial Stressors) and social and occupational role functioning were evaluated on Axis V (Highest Level of Adaptive Functioning) in DSM-III.

This article was not only remarkable because it so precisely forecast major steps in the development of DSM-III, but also because it appeared within a year of the publication of DSM-II. Although few members of the APA were considering the next edition, it was clear that Spitzer was giving the matter considerable thought. These plans came to fruition five years later, when he was appointed to head the Committee on Nomenclature and Statistics.

There is another episode that illustrated the way that Spitzer played a dual role as defender of psychiatric diagnosis and, at the same time, as an effective critic. The occasion was a symposium to evaluate David Rosenhan's "On Being Sane in Insane Places" (1973), which was published in the highly respected journal *Science*. In the article Rosenhan described an experiment in which eight "pseudopatients" gained admission to 12 hospitals by falsely reporting a single symptom. They each claimed that they heard an unclear voice that seemed to say "empty," "hollow," and "thud." These "existential symptoms" had never been associated in the literature with schizophrenia, but 11 of the 12 admissions were made with this diagnosis. The one exception was diagnosed as manic depressive. The pseudopatients exhibited no other pathological behavior, and reported all other events of their lives accurately, with the exception of identifying information such as their names and, in the cases of a psychiatrist and other mental health workers, of hiding their profession to avoid special attention. Once they were in the hospital they acted normally and stopped pretending to hear voices. They engaged in one unusual behavior, which was to take extensive notes, but this apparently did not make the staff suspicious. The only ones who recognized that they were faking were other patients. The pseudopatients remained in the hospital from 7 to 52 days, with an average of 19 days.

When they were released, each was given a diagnosis of "schizophrenia in remission." Rosenhan used the results to substantiate some principles of labeling theory, particularly that a psychiatric diagnosis will continue to be applied to the patient even if it is no longer warranted. This simple experiment was widely publicized, and, even today, it is often discussed in introductory college courses in psychology and sociology. Along with the earlier work of Szasz and Scheff, and the publicity from the quarrel over homosexuality, Rosenhan's experiment provided some of the most powerful arguments against the value of psychiatric diagnosis.

Not long afterwards, as Spitzer was starting to revise DSM-II, he submitted a critique of Rosenhan's work (Spitzer, 1975). The DSM-III assignment placed him in the awkward, but by now familiar role of being an official defender of psychiatric diagnosis while he undertook to reconstruct it. He obviously took Rosenhan's work very seriously; it constituted a frontal assault on psychiatric diagnosis. In many respects, Spitzer's critique was forceful and quite clever. He characterized Rosenhan's experiment with pseudopatients as "pseudoscience." He countered Rosenhan's reports about diagnosis of schizophrenia in remission by observing that his examination of Rosenhan's methods, results, and conclusions led him to a diagnosis of "logic in remission." Some of Spitzer's criticisms of the design of the study were warranted, although his zeal to discredit Rosenhan sometimes led him simply to disregard or distort basic observations. For instance, he conjectured that staff may have spent too little time with patients to assess them accurately. Spitzer speculated that the pseudopatients note-taking may have been overlooked, and therefore the staff developed no suspicion that the pseudopatients had simulated illness to gain entry into the hospital. Actually, Rosenhan reported that in at least four cases staff members commented on note-taking, but they attributed it to pathological causes, as in the case of a nurse who observed in her records that a pseudopatient was engaging in "note-taking behavior" or another case when a psychiatrist assured a pseudopatient that he did not have to write down the name of the medication he was receiving, because the doctor would remember it for him.

There are other instances in which Spitzer distorted what Rosenhan said in order to defend psychiatric diagnosis. For instance he asked, "But where did Rosenhan get the idea that psychiatry is the only medical speciality plagued by inaccurate diagnosis?" (p. 450). He then cited data that indicated that there is often misdiagnosis of pulmonary disorders, unreliability in the interpretation of electrodiagrams and of X-rays, and inaccuracies in the certification of the causes of death. The problem with his defense of psychiatry is that Rosenhan did not argue that physicians in other branches of medicine diagnose without error. In fact, Rosenhan observed:

> Failure to detect sanity during the course of hospitalization may be due to the fact that physicians operate with a strong bias toward what statisticians call the type 2 error. This is to say that physicians are more likely to call a healthy person sick (a false positive, type 2) than a sick person healthy (a false negative, type 1). The reasons for this are not hard to find:

it is clearly better to err on the side of caution, to suspect illness even among the healthy.

But what holds for medicine does not hold equally for psychiatry. Medical illnesses, while unfortunate, are not commonly pejorative. Psychiatric diagnoses, on the contrary, carry with them personal, legal and social stigmas. (1973:252)

Rosenhan not only acknowledged unreliability in medical diagnosis, but offered a reasonable explanation to account for it. The principal problem he was concerned with was not unreliability, but the consequences of incorrect diagnosis.

The importance of Spitzer's comments are not what they tell us about Rosenhan's study but what they tell us about Spitzer's new enterprise, the making of DSM-III. First, he had to invalidate Rosenhan's basic point, which was to criticize diagnostic practices of psychiatrists because they could not distinguish those who were sane from those who were mentally ill.

Spitzer argued that: "A correct interpretation of [Rosenhan's] own data contradicts his own conclusions. In the setting of a psychiatric hospital psychiatrists are remarkably able to distinguish the 'sane' from the 'insane'" (1975:451).

In order to support this remarkable reinterpretation, Spitzer took the unusual step of gathering his own data on discharges of patients from hospitals where there were no (known) pseudopatients. He reported that, in his hospitals, patients were almost never diagnosed as being "in remission" at the time they were discharged. They were almost always found to be still suffering from the disorder. Since all of Rosenhan's pseudopatients were considered to be in remission, it was obvious, at least to Spitzer, that the doctors of these pseudopatients could detect that they were not insane and so they gave them an in remission diagnosis. It appears that Spitzer concluded that schizophrenia in remission was the equivalent of sanity in disguise.

Spitzer had a second objective, which was at least as important as the task of defending psychiatric diagnostic practices. As discussed in Chapter 3, he also used the article to redefine the problems in psychiatric diagnosis:

If psychiatric diagnosis is not quite as bad as Rosenhan would have us believe, that does not mean that it is all that good. What is the reliability of psychiatric diagnosis? A review of the major studies of the reliability of psychiatric diagnosis prior to 1972 (Spitzer & Fleiss, 1974) revealed that "reliability is only satisfactory for three categories . . . reliability is no better than fair for psychosis and schizophrenia and is poor for the remaining categories." (p. 450)

Citing himself as authority, he pinpointed the problem of psychiatric diagnosis as one of unreliability.

If reliability of psychiatric diagnosis was the problem, there was also a solution. Once again citing his own work, he used the opportunity to reiterate that the problem of unreliability in psychiatric diagnosis can be solved by establishing criteria for each of the diagnostic categories:

> Recognition of the serious problems of psychiatric diagnosis has resulted in a new approach to psychiatric diagnosis, the use of specific inclusion and exclusion criteria, as contrasted with the usually vague and ill-defined general descriptions found in the psychiatric literature and in the psychiatric glossary of the American Psychiatric Association. (p. 451)

He gave credit to Guze and his colleagues from St. Louis for initiating this new approach which "has been further developed by Spitzer, Endicott and Robins (1974)." He then discussed how the RDC that he and his associates developed had improved the reliability of psychiatric diagnosis, and he cited himself for a third time as the principal author of the study demonstrating that there was a dramatic improvement of reliability that resulted from the use of the RDC. Although he did not mention it, he was already engaged in incorporating specific criteria into DSM-III, one of the new manual's principal innovations.

He acknowledged other problems. He noted that it had been difficult to define mental disorder and cited himself once again as the principal author of a new definition, which he prophetically admitted might not be adopted. He also observed, with little elaboration, that there were serious problems of validity of many of the traditional categories, including some of the subtypes of schizophrenia. Because of validity problems, he observed, these categories had not been "useful for prognosis or treatment" (p. 451). He acknowledged the limited value of traditional psychiatric categories for outpatients, but he did not articulate any solution to the problem of validity. He ended his discussion of problems by recognizing that psychiatric diagnoses have been misused to hurt patients rather than to help them. But he concluded, without providing any citations: "However, whatever the solution to that problem, the misuse of psychiatric diagnostic labels is not a sufficient reason to abandon their use because they have been shown to be of value when properly used" (p. 451).

Spitzer's rebuttal to Rosenhan's critique revealed a great deal about the instrumental way that he furthered his plans to rewrite psychiatric diagnosis in America. As in his 1969 assessment of DSM-II, he first rejected the attack on the psychiatric enterprise of diagnosis. He then acknowledged criticism, but only after redefining it in a way that furthered his efforts. In 1969, he spelled out the process by which he intended to revise DSM through the use of a multitude of experts in a large number of committees, and by testing the manual through large-scale field trials. He also suggested some of the substantive ways that he wanted to change the manual, principally through the adoption of a multidimensional system. In the 1975 article he subtly introduced more about his approach. He dismissed a concern about the misuse of psychiatric diagnosis once again and refocused the problem as a question of reliability, how to obtain consistent agreement among diagnosticians. He then spelled out his solution to the problem, the adoption of diagnostic criteria he had pioneered, and the testing of the criteria using statistical measurements he had helped to develop, principally relying on the use of the kappa statistic, which he discussed in his Rosenhan rebuttal.

The Palace Revolt and Invisible Colleges

In several essays, Theodore Millon (e.g., 1983, 1986) has provided an insider's account of the early stages of revision of the manual. Millon, a prominent psychologist, played a very special role in the evolution of DSM-III and defended the new manual against repeated attacks by his fellow psychologists. Millon had two other qualities that were important for the development of the DSM-III: He was a friend and colleague of the new chief executive of the APA, Melvin Sabshin, and he was an authority on personality disorders, which were given special prominence in DSM-III.

As a colleague at Northwestern University, Millon complained to Sabshin for many years about DSM-II. Encouraged by Sabshin's interest, in 1971 Millon prepared a memo for him in his capacity as chairman of the APA's Council on Research and Development, the group that had responsibility for the Task Force on Nomenclature and Statistics, which was responsible for the revision of DSM- II. (Earlier this was referred to as the Committee on Nomenclature and Statistics, but it is the same group. The discrepancy is due to the fact that participants at the time and in their later writing gave the committee various names.) He criticized "the total lack of creative innovation" (Millon, 1986:37) in DSM-II, and he urged the establishment of a group to review new research and theoretical proposals that could improve DSM. Although an ad hoc committee was established for this purpose, its work was spurned by the Task Force on Nomenclature and Statistics. According to Millon, the DSM-III Task Force appeared to be starting the same unimaginative process of revision that it had gone through in the previous edition, DSM-II.

As part of the palace revolution by the Young Turks within the APA, Sabshin accepted the post as medical director in January 1974, to become effective the following June. In April, Sabshin held an all-day meeting with Millon and Spitzer devoted to the future of DSM-III. According to Millon:

> Spitzer, a member of the DSM-II Task Force, noted that substantive advances would not be likely if those who then comprised that committee were asked to extend their responsibilities to the development of DSM-III. With an essentially new membership however, one composed of active researchers and innovative theoreticians who could study and debate ideas with the view of constructing an empirically grounded and functional classification system, . . . a scientifically sound and clinically useful instrument might be developed. (p. 29)

The result of this meeting was a recommendation to the Council on Research and Development and the incoming president of the APA to reconstitute the Task Force on Nomenclature and Statistics and to appoint Spitzer as its chairman. These recommendations were approved at the May 1974 APA annual conference the following month.

Having secured the prize he sought for many years, Spitzer acted quickly. By September, he had selected the new task force, which consisted of five psychiatrists. There were also two psychologists and an epidemiologist who were committee consultants. Contrary to the strategy for revision of the manual that Spitzer had advocated publicly in his 1969 critique of DSM-II, the actual decision-making group that completed the initial plan for the new manual was very small. Furthermore, it did not represent a diversity of opinion, but a rather narrow range of interests. Two of the psychiatrists, Andreasen and Woodruff were associated with the St. Louis group that had pioneered the development of behaviorally oriented, diagnostic criteria. Klein, a colleague of Spitzer's at Columbia University, is a leading spokesperson for a biologically oriented approach to diagnosis and to psychiatry as a whole, and Saslow also had a long-term interest in a behavioral approach to diagnosis (Kanfer & Saslow, 1965). Spitzer, of course, had already committed himself to the criteria-based approach pioneered by the St. Louis group. Thus among the five original psychiatrists on the task force, there was a remarkable congruence of interest. More importantly, there were no major divergent viewpoints, and the primary, psychodynamic perspective in psychiatry, had no representative at the table. Blashfield (1982) has described the participants in the task force as members of an invisible college, and Klerman has identified them as neo-Kraepelinians. Although Spitzer steadfastly refused to be identified as a neo-

Kraepelinian, his approach is far closer to this early pioneer than it is to Freud and the psychodynamic school.

Within a year, the DSM-III Task Force produced the first draft of the new manual, which incorporated all of the major innovations that were eventually included in DSM-III. Although another five years passed before the manual was published, the essential decisions about its approach, structure, and contents were made quickly by Spitzer and this small group. Millon substantiates this view, although he claims that the initial DSM-III Task Force had more theoretical diversity than it is possible to identify from their published work. Millon observed about the initial DSM-III Task Force and its progress:

> Most were well recognized contributors to the research and theoretical literature; as a committee, they formed an unusual alliance, possessing a significant array of professional interests combined with a substantial diversity in theoretical orientations. New members were added in later years to further broaden the Task Force's perspectives and expertise, but the original nucleus worked intensely and productively as a single, unified committee for over a year, meeting frequently, debating issues vigorously, and establishing a firm foundation and structural framework. . . . Important modifications continued to evolve of course, but the basic conceptual schema and its distinctive features were set well in place by the end of its first full year of deliberation. (Millon, 1986:38)

When the DSM-III Task Force completed its work in 1980, the membership of the committee had expanded to 15 psychiatrists and 4 consultants, but neo-Kraepelinians continued to dominate its deliberations. Some of the later appointees were not identified with the neo-Kraepelinian approach and were added for other reasons, but all of the members were recruited with an expectation that they would be in basic agreement about the committee's approach. For instance, John Frosch was asked to join the committee in 1977 specifically because he was a psychoanalyst, and Spitzer hoped that his participation would stem the growing tide of opposition to the manual among his psychoanalytic colleagues. But he was not a typical psychoanalyst. According to an account by Bayer and Spitzer:

> John Frosch, a senior figure, with an interest in the epistemological and conceptual problems of diagnosis was a perfect choice from Spitzer's perspective. Although committed to psychoanalysis, he had made clear his belief that psychiatry had suffered in the past from its failure to distinguish between etiological, dynamic and descriptive levels of analysis. (1985:1990)

In spite of Spitzer's hopes, Frosch later resigned from the committee because of disagreements over the treatment of psychoanalytic concepts.

Spitzer also invited William Frosch, another psychoanalyst who was John's nephew, to join the committee for the same reasons. William Frosch had already shown that he could participate in the work of the DSM-III Task Force in a way that satisfied Spitzer. He had

> demonstrated his capacity to work within the Task Force perspective by contributing to its work on substance abuse disorders. Sympathetic to what he believed were the needs of the research community, he accepted the descriptive criteria-based approach to diagnosis. (p. 190)

When Spitzer was criticized for not including prominent psychoanalysts among those who participated in the development of the manual, he protested indignantly that he had attempted to recruit many, but they were not interested, since the manual was not very important to them before the publication of DSM-III (Spitzer, 1984). But he protested too much, since he also did his best to discourage participation by antagonistic psychiatrists, not only on the main DSM-III Task Force but also on the many subcommittees that were formed to deal with specific topics. These were the groups that he had earlier said he would use to encourage widespread, diverse participation in the development of the manual.

On January 20, 1975, he reported to the chairman of the Council on Research and Development,

> I do have some good news. There are two members of the Child Subcommittee that should be removed from the list because they have other duties that prevent them from attending future meetings. They are Drs. Dane Prugh and Irving Berlin. (letter from Spitzer to Schwab, January 20, 1975)

It was not that Berlin and Prugh were simply too busy to attend meetings. They had major disagreements with Spitzer, as his letter hinted. On December 10, 1975, Berlin, in his role as president of the American Academy of Child Psychiatry wrote to Judd Marmor, president of the APA, to complain:

> Our concern as an organization is that the variety of clinical concerns relevant to the development of a new diagnostic nomenclature for children's disorders requires a much broader representation than is currently available. The three or four members of the Academy, who have acted as consultants of this committee and have been at one or another meeting

feel equally strongly that there is not as great an involvement of a sample of clinicians as there should be. Thus, I am asking you as President of the American Psychiatric Association to both clarify with Dr. Spitzer our concern, and to ask him to work closely with a committee which is already in existence and which I have just enlarged called the Committee on Diagnostic Categories. This committee of the Academy is chaired by Dane Prugh who was the principal author of the GAP [Group for the Advancement of Psychiatry] Diagnostic Categories for Children's Disorders and who has been very much involved in psychosocial diagnosis. (letter from Berlin to Marmor, December 10, 1975)

It is worth noting that GAP was an organization of reform-minded psychiatrists; and when DSM-III was published, the developers went out of their way to assert the superiority of the scientific status, i.e., reliability, of the new manual's section on children's disorders over the GAP nosology. Although Spitzer may have claimed that he was encouraging widespread participation, he was selective in who should participate and how they should be involved. The two participants he struck from the lists so eagerly were major figures in the field of child psychiatry. Their struggle is particularly important because children's disorders was one of the areas where there was the largest increase in diagnostic categories in DSM-III. Although Prugh had a substantial amount of experience with diagnostic issues, his approach was not of sufficient value to encourage his participation.

Psychoanalytically oriented child psychiatrists were not the only group who felt that their concerns were not represented. Spitzer dismissed questions about the adequacy of representation by minorities and women. In his January 20, 1975, letter to the chairman of the Council on Research and Development, Spitzer replied to these complaints:

As far as the concern in the Council and the Reference Committee about the relative absence of minority members on the task force, I believe that no further action is necessary. There are two members of the central committee that are women (Dr. Jean Endicott, a psychologist and Dr. Nancy Andreasen, a psychiatrist, and a woman psychiatrist Dr. Diane Settlage is a member of the subcommittee on sex). In addition, Dr. Richard Green a member of the subcommittee on sex, is also a member of the Task Force on Women's Issues, so that any nosological issues relevant to the status of women can be dealt with. (letter from Spitzer to Schwab, January 20, 1975)

The facility with which women's issues and the concerns of gay men are compressed speaks for itself. (Dr. Green figured prominently as a spokesman for gay protesters in the struggle over the diagnosis of homosexuality.)

As for racial minorities, none were members of the DSM-III Task Force in 1975 or at any later time. When a committee of black psychiatrists later recommended that racism be included as a mental disorder, Spitzer rejected the recommendation, as well as their request for minority representation on the task force. In a letter to them, he responded:

> As you know, we are still struggling with the problem of defining what is a mental disorder. With our current working definition racism would not meet the criteria for a mental disorder since it is only in certain environments that it is associated with distress. We would regard it as a good example of a condition which should be regarded as a vulnerability in that in certain environments patients with this condition will evidence subjective distress. In your report you give good examples of the special environments in which racists will become symptomatic. The same logic would apply to other conditions such as male chauvinism and religious fanaticism.
>
> I would expect that in DSM-III in the discussion of what is a mental disorder we would list racism as a good example of a condition representing a non-optimal psychological functioning which renders a person vulnerable in certain environments to manifesting signs of disorder. (letter from Spitzer to Committee of Black Psychiatrists, December 29, 1975).

When DSM-III was finally published, not even this condescending suggestion was included, that racism would be described as an example of nonoptimal psychological functioning.

Spitzer added insult to injury by rejecting a request for minority representation:

> In suggesting individuals for membership in the Task Force on Nomenclature and Statistics, the criteria were special expertise in problems of classification of mental disorders. I applied what I regarded as the principles of affirmative action in considering minority group members who had such expertise. In so doing several women are members or consultants to the Task Force. Although there is no black psychiatrist on the Task Force we would be glad to meet with representatives of your group to further discuss this or any other matter relevant to DSM-III.

Once again, Spitzer not only lumped together women and minorities, but he compounded the affront by suggesting that there was no black psychiatrist among the 18 thousand members of the APA with adequate expertise to meet his criteria for membership on the DSM-III Task Force.

These examples of the exclusion from the DSM-III Task Force and its subcommittees of psychoanalysts, minorities, and other potential participants who may have added diverse views to the development of DSM-III support the claim that there was an invisible college, and provide a filter through which to view the claim of massive participation in the development of the manual. Although hundreds of names are listed in DSM-III as participants in its creation, their carefully structured participation colored (or left lily white) the final product.

Throughout the subsequent development of DSM-III during the next five years, particularly as the realization grew that something of great importance was occurring, individuals and groups with a variety of interests attempted to participate in the process of shaping the manual. Some appealed directly to Spitzer, and others attempted to go over his head and force him to respond to higher authorities within the APA. Among the many factions, psychoanalysts, sensing that they had the most to lose, were among the most persistent. But Spitzer was able to rebuff many of their efforts, and even when he made concessions, he never lost control over the process. There were several reasons for this: One was his ability to mobilize support and to maneuver effectively in the arcane political structures that governed psychiatrists and other professionals in the field of mental health. Another reason that Spitzer and his allies succeeded is that none of his opponents could articulate a full-scale alternative. After the first year of work, when the basic structure of the new manual was developed, there was no competing design for the assessment of mental disorders that was offered as a challenge.

Ratifying DSM-III

As Millon described it, the actual creation of DSM-III took less than a year, but this was followed by a long tortuous process of refining the manual and seeking official approval of it. There were many who had to be convinced. First of all (and last) there was a formal procedure for approval. Many of the steps in this process had been established during the production of earlier editions of DSM, and in the controversy over homosexuality. The formal procedure required that the manual be approved by a hierarchy of APA committees, progressing from the Task Force on Nomenclature and Statistics, to the Council on Research and Development, then to the Assembly of District Branches, the Reference Committee, and finally to the board of trustees. Along the way other groups were formed on an ad hoc basis to deal with DSM-III. In 1976, the assembly appointed an Assembly Liaison Committee to the DSM-III Task Force, which had many members who were antagonistic toward the manual that was emerging, but had to be placated, if not convinced, to allow the manual to proceed up the organizational hierarchy. Even the board of trustees, which balked at adopting the manual at the eleventh hour, appointed a special Ad Hoc Committee on DSM-III in 1979, to undertake another review before final approval (APA, 1980:3–4). In addition to these groups, the Committee on Confidentiality, the Task Force on Women's Issues, the Task Force on the Problem Oriented Medical Record, the Committee of Black Psychiatrists, the Council on Mental Health Services, the Council on Medical Education and Career Development, The Commission on Standards of Practice and Third Party Payment and other groups within APA were involved in one aspect or another of the development of the manual.

True to the promise he made in his 1969 article, Spitzer also created a series of specialized advisory committees to review recommendations about specific diagnoses that appeared in the drafts produced by the Task Force on Nomenclature and Statistics. Of course, these committees were not empowered to make final decisions; they acted as sounding boards and offered opinions to the DSM-III Task Force. Furthermore, the scope of their activity was severely limited. Spitzer set the agenda and arranged for the appointments of more than one hundred participants to the 14 advisory committees. He was also a member of 11 of the committees.

In addition to these standing committees, subcommittees, and ad hoc committees of the APA, a variety of organizations within the psychiatric profession and in other mental health disciplines also participated. Among the psychiatric groups, DSM-III lists some with specialized concerns that established "liaison committees" with the DSM-III Task Force. They included the Academy of Psychiatry and the Law, the American Academy of Child Psychiatry, the American Association of Chairmen of Departments of Psychiatry, and the American Academy of Psychoanalysis. This does not give a full picture of all of the psychiatric organizations that demanded to be heard. For instance, in the community of psychoanalysts there are many organizations, such as the Baltimore–District of Columbia Society for Psychoanalysis, whose leaders exerted substantial political effort to have their recommendations adopted (letter from Boyd L. Burris, president, to Spitzer, January 22, 1979). The international psychiatric community, and in fact the entire medical establishment, also had a substantial role to play, particularly in the coordination of DSM-III with the publication of the *International Classification of Diseases, 9th Edition* (ICD-9). This required interaction with the United Nations World Health Organization, as well as many other professional medical groups within the United States that were concerned about the impending publication of ICD-9 in 1977.

Professional organizations that were not composed exclusively of psychiatrists or physicians also entered the melee. The American Psychological Association, whose membership was substantially larger than that of the APA, objected vigorously when Spitzer and a colleague proposed that psychiatric disorder was a subset of medical disorder. As a result of their protests, psychologists forced a modification of that position. Nonprofessional groups also were involved. A notable example was the Vietnam Veterans Working Group, which waged a successful campaign to include post–traumatic stress disorder in the manual (Scott, 1990). In many of these controversies, the APA mobilized resources to transform perceptions about psychiatric diagnosis by arguing that DSM-III was now a scientific enterprise and no longer simply an arbitrary stigma-producing exercise in labeling.

The Unveiling

The APA had many resources at its disposal, and it used all of them. Starting in 1975, Spitzer and his DSM-III Task Force made presentations about DSM-III at each annual meeting of the APA, where sessions are devoted to discussions of scientific advances in the field. Some of the presentations were later reprinted in the prestigious periodical, the *American Journal of Psychiatry*, published by the APA. Other APA publications also contributed. Its monthly newsletter, *Psychiatric News*, carried drafts of the manual and other relevant information. *Hospital and Community Psychiatry*, a popular mental health journal also published by the APA, carried news about DSM-III, including a regular column, "Questions and Answers about DSM-III," written by Janet B. W. Williams, the text editor of the manual. Other scientific publications were also enlisted, including the American Medical Association's *Archives of General Psychiatry*. As Spitzer has pointed out, prior to the advent of DSM-III, articles about psychiatric diagnosis were infrequent in professional journals; all of this changed dramatically when the revision was initiated. In one sense this can be seen as a revival of scholarly interest, but in another it can be interpreted as an enormous publicity campaign to raise concerns about the scientific status of diagnosis and to encourage support for the revised manual. Whichever interpretation one chooses to believe, it is clear that the manual received an unprecedented amount of attention in the publications and meetings of the association.

The first public presentation of the new manual came at the 1975 annual meeting of the APA (Spitzer et al., 1975). This was a major test. One commentator reported the following:

> At the 1975 meeting of the American Psychiatric Association, members got
> their first look at a draft of DSM-III. Spitzer fielded an onslaught of objec-

tions with genial flexibility. A number of times he accepted suggestions of critics on the spot, promising changes with comments such as, "That's a good idea. We hadn't thought of that." Spitzer's political style is one of accommodation. Rather than turn his dissenters into enemies he prefers to join them.

A number of examples were offered to demonstrate how Spitzer's "genial flexibility" and accommodating style led to alterations. Because of complaints about sex bias, changes were made in the description of Gender Identity Disorder of Childhood to make it clearer that a tomboy would not be considered as mentally disordered. Another category, Sexual Sadism, was rewritten after the Committee on Women complained that it could be used to provide a psychiatric defense by murderers and rapists.

Although Spitzer may have attempted to operate flexibly, in a spirit of accommodation, it was within ground rules that he and the Task Force on Nomenclature and Statistics had established. Criteria could be modified and rewritten, descriptions changed, and even, in some instances, categories of disorders could be added or deleted. But a change in criteria did not change the frame of reference that led to criteria-based diagnoses or to the other basic assumptions about the newly developed manual.

A Place On the Platform

A bigger test for the new manual occurred a year later in St. Louis. A two-day conference, "DSM-III in Midstream," cosponsored by the APA and the Missouri Institute of Psychiatry, was attended by over one hundred experts on diagnostic issues and others with special interests in the field. This conference was a major milestone in the campaign for the manual. A year later, *Psychiatric News* (March 18, 1977) reported that:

> According to Spitzer, the single most significant gathering in the development of DSM-III to date was a conference held last summer at the University of Missouri at St. Louis. Out of that conference came substantially stronger emphasis on disorders of adolescence, a commitment to the multiaxial approach (it has been tossed around for some time before) and a host of other changes. Spitzer said that none of the changes, then or now, is political in nature. "We have strongly and successfully resisted any changes in the draft DSM-III not based on good sound knowledge. We have welcomed all input, but we weigh it by that measure." (p. 26)

The Introduction to DSM-III summarized the results of the meeting: "As a result of discussions at this conference, additional diagnostic categories were added, some were deleted, and a decision was made to proceed with the development of the multiaxial system" (p. 4).

Some of the discussion took the form of professional give-and-take suggested by this description, although not all of the changes were the result of scientific considerations. For instance, Sexual Assault Disorder was dropped after the American Academy of Psychiatry and the Law protested that it would provide a defense for rapists in criminal trials (Halpern, 1986). As this example illustrates, the committee responded to other concerns besides scientific or clinical problems, but it was part of a tempered, well-controlled process of development.

However, not everyone was so moderate or focused in dissent. The growing frustration and anger of many APA members was manifested in the person of Howard Berk, M.D., representative from the Queens District Branch of the APA, who was present in his capacity as chairman of the newly organized Assembly Liaison Committee to the DSM-III Task Force. The liaison committee had been established less than a month earlier, after assembly delegates complained that the DSM-III Task Force was operating with relative autonomy and that assembly members wanted an opportunity for greater input and review. After the St. Louis conference, Berk expressed his concerns in a statement that he sent to Spitzer (letter from Berk to Spitzer, June 29, 1976). His approach was reflected in the cover letter that accompanied his comments:

> At the plenary on June 11, 1976, I took my place on the platform as I had on the previous day. I had not expected to be on the platform or to be called on to speak at the first plenary session, so I had spent some time prior to the last session writing down some of the observations of Dr. Jaso [another committee member] and myself in order to better contribute to the final session.
>
> However, omitting no other person on the platform, the member of the Task Force presiding at the final session did not call upon me to speak. Unfortunately, at the time I did not feel well, did not call the attention of the presiding member to the omission, and I did not speak.
>
> Afterwards in reviewing my notes I realized that my failure to speak had denied the Conference views to which it was entitled.

In order to remedy this failure, Berk requested that his revised and extended comments be distributed with "the remarks of the other platform speakers at the final session." Furthermore, Berk sent a copy of his statement to all of the conference participants.

His comments consisted of an eight-page statement (Berk & Jaso, 1976), which reviewed the development of successive editions of DSM and the relationship of DSM-III to ICD-9. In it, he complained that:

In the process of simplification and restriction we see that the proposed nomenclature displays a generous measure of linguistic and conceptual sterility. DSM-III gets rid of the castle of neurosis and replaces it with a diagnostic Levittown. (p. 3)

He objected that:

The elimination of the past by the DSM-III Task Force in the face of the considered judgement of many that it continues to have a high degree of validity and probable usefulness can be compared to the director of a national museum destroying his Rembrandts, Goyas, Utrillos, van Goghs, etc. because he believes his collection of Comic-Strip Type Warhol's (or what have you) has greater relevance. (p. 7)

Although he was obviously agitated about the structure of DSM-III and the way it was being developed, he did not offer a very clear idea of how to remedy the problem.

The APA leadership quickly responded to this revolt in the ranks. Shortly after Berk's comments were circulated, Bernard Glueck (memo, July 6, 1976), a highly respected senior psychiatrist who had been involved in the preparation of DSM-II, sent a memorandum to the APA's Council on Research and Development, to inform them about the St. Louis meeting. He reported that the meeting was "energetic" and "a great deal was accomplished in the interchange of viewpoints." The discussion "while at times heated, was generally friendly." However, he observed:

There were several important exceptions to the above statement, the most serious being the attitude as demonstrated in the attached critique [Berk's statement], both verbally expressed and, throughout the two days, non-verbally demonstrated by Dr. Berk. I do not know how representative of the attitudes in the Assembly Dr. Berk's comments may be, but I am hopeful that he would represent a rather tiny minority. As such, I am wondering whether he should continue as Chairman of the Liaison Committee to work with the Task Force.

I have discussed this problem at some length with Bob Spitzer, who will be talking to Mel Sabshin and Irwin Perr. I think the Council, however, needs to consider very seriously what actions it should take in terms of dealing with the type of attitude expressed in Berk's comments.

Berk continued to direct hostile fire at the DSM-III Task Force, but the APA leadership quickly mobilized a counterattack. Spitzer, outwardly at least, maintained a spirit of accommodation. He sent a letter to Berk stating:

It seems to me that it would be extremely useful for your Committee and for our Task Force if I met with your Committee prior to your preparing your report to the Assembly in October. At such a meeting, it would be possible for me to fill you in on the latest details of decisions regarding DSM-III, and to answer any questions you might have. In addition I would very much appreciate the opportunity of listening to your Committee regarding some of its concerns. It is possible that some of these concerns are based on misunderstandings which I would be able to hopefully clarify. (letter from Spitzer to Berk, August 3, 1976)

Spitzer offered to make the arrangements for the meeting wherever Berk wished and to pay for the travel expenses.

By October 15, 1976, Spitzer was able to send the APA leadership the report from Berk's committee that was to be presented later in the month to the APA assembly. In an accompanying memorandum (October 15, 1976) to DSM-III Task Force members and other APA officials, Spitzer commented that "You will note that the tone of the report is considerably changed from the initial document produced by the committee." The document was more moderate, balanced and focused than Berk's post–St. Louis comments. In instances where there was a specific criticism of DSM-III, the report acknowledged that Spitzer and the DSM-III Task Force had taken steps to incorporate suggestions made by Berk's committee. For instance, Berk's complaint that disorders of adolescence had been underemphasized was acknowledged by the DSM-III task force. The Berk committee report noted that:

Since the June, 1976 meeting there has been a considerable expansion in the number of terms available to diagnose adolescents. This will be a considerable advance over the classification available for adolescents in DSM-II or ICD-9. One of our members says that there has been considerable agreement in the Childhood and Adolescent Subcommittee to include as an appendix or possibly as an axis the Symptom List of GAP Report 62, Psychopathological Disorders in Children. This would be a more general classification and symptoms from the list would be added to characterize the primary diagnosis. However there has been no written announcement of this at the time of this writing. (Assembly Liaison Committee, 1976:8)

When DSM-III was finally published in 1980 the report of the reform-minded Group for the Advancement of Psychiatry (GAP) was not included, and in fact GAP was mentioned only once in the manual, in disparaging terms (p. 469). But the promise to consider the GAP report did help to subdue the mounting criticism of the DSM-III Task Force in 1976.

Some changes were adopted as a result of the objections of Berk and the assembly committee. In his interview with *Psychiatric News* (March 18, 1977) quoted above, Spitzer denied that accommodations were political, but this was because of the way that political pressures were translated into "scientific" concerns. Spitzer had demonstrated his mastery of this ability to reformulate these issues in the earlier fight over homosexuality. He could honestly say that the accommodations were based on scientific considerations, although there is no record of new scientific knowledge that was brought to bear before changes were made in response to the assembly's objections. Spitzer's formal reply, which accompanied the committee's report, began "I am extremely appreciative of the work of the Assembly Liaison Committee on DSM-III. It has provided valuable input to our committee which has and will continue to help guide our work." Spitzer was even able to use the Berk committee's criticisms to support his plan for field tests for DSM-III.

The potential revolt in the ranks had been neutralized, but Berk was not satisfied for long. In February 1977, Spitzer made an interim report to the APA Executive Committee. *Psychiatric News* (March 18, 1977) reported that:

> Howard Berk, M.D., chairperson of the Assembly Liaison Committee to the APA Task Force, speaking apparently for himself, criticized the draft DSM-III charging a bias toward biological etiology, a charge which Spitzer hotly disputed. Berk also charged that the task force is circumventing assembly scrutiny of the draft DSM-III, but Spitzer countered that the assembly had been kept informed on all points of the draft. Speaker Irwin Perr [chairman of the assembly] stated that he felt that there is concern in the assembly about DSM-III, but Speaker-elect Daniel Grabski said that he did not perceive any dissatisfaction. The Executive Committee took no action other than referring Berk's objections to the assembly Executive Committee, asking it to determine whether the objection represents an official position of a constituent group or is an individual's opinion. In general, however Trustees voiced praise for Spitzer's work.

In an angry letter to the editor of *Psychiatric News* Berk (1977a) objected to the news account of this meeting. He attempted to establish his own legitimacy as a spokesman by claiming that he was there along with Spitzer to discuss the October 1976 report of his committee to the assembly. He complained that the issue of Spitzer's biological bias was not the major dispute. The substance of his objection was that Spitzer had imposed a February 15, 1977, deadline on all changes in nomenclature and coding in DSM-III. Berk also complained because Spitzer had submitted the current DSM-III draft to be incorporated into the upcoming revision of the ICD. Berk claimed that this circumvented the approval process in

APA, since DSM-III was not scheduled for formal approval by the APA assembly and Board of trustees until the following year, 1978.

Spitzer's rationale for imposing a deadline was that anything that was to be incorporated into ICD-9 had to be submitted by July 1977. Since ICD was the official manual for reporting medical and psychiatric disorders, and was used by insurance companies for reimbursement and for other crucial record-keeping purposes, Spitzer argued that it was important to coordinate the work of DSM-III with that of ICD-9, so that there could be sufficient correspondence between the two manuals. Failure to coordinate the work could result in nonrecognition of DSM-III or in some of the diagnostic categories in DSM-III. As a result, it was necessary to impose a deadline on additions and major changes to DSM-III that was no later than the ICD-9 deadline.

Spitzer went back to the assembly to explain his actions, and at their May 1977 meeting, they approved his decisions. Shortly thereafter, Howard Jaso replaced Berk as chairman of the liaison committee. Berk continued to object to DSM-III and to APA's process for approval. At the October 1977 meeting of the assembly, he criticized Spitzer, the board of trustees, *Psychiatric News*, and others, but this time he added a new target, the Assembly Liaison Committee to the DSM-III Task Force. He was now clearly speaking for himself. Complaining that the process for approval was "a closed system," he added that:

> The present assembly DSM-III Task Force [referring to the Assembly Liaison Committee to the DSM-III Task Force, not the DSM-III Task Force headed by Spitzer] provides no exception to this, because it has given up considering alternatives and has committed itself to accepting the current draft without fundamental objection. (Berk, 1977b:8)

Opposition from within the APA would surface again and Berk's dissatisfaction was shared at the highest levels of the organization. But every time it took shape in an organized manner, it was defeated or deflected.

The Medical Model Under Siege

It was not as easy to stem the flow of criticism outside the organization, although the developers of DSM-III eventually succeeded here as well. To do this, they made some accommodations, but none of the compromises resulted in significant changes to the integrity of the new manual itself. The major professional challenge came from the American Psychological Association, and it took the form of a dispute over the definition of mental disorder. The conflict had little to do with the most important innovations that had been introduced.

The dispute arose from an attempt by Spitzer to develop a definition of mental disorder. In May 1975, soon after initiating its deliberations, the DSM-III Task Force began trying to define mental disorder. This was contrary to the earlier plan of the board of directors to establish a separate committee to develop this definition and append it to the manual. However, the debate over homosexuality hinged on the definition of mental disorder, and it seemed logical that the effort to identify specific disorders was dependent on the general definition. Spitzer was dissatisfied with the definition that he had developed in order to resolve the homosexuality controversy; furthermore, he intended to revive the diagnosis of homosexuality in a somewhat modified manner (Bayer, 1981:170).

Spitzer and Jean Endicott, a psychologist, drafted a new definition of mental disorder for consideration by the DSM-III Task Force, and they also used this as a basis for a paper presented at the 1976 annual meeting of the APA (Spitzer & Endicott, 1976). Many mental health professionals objected to the definition, and agitation mounted after it was published the following year. Psychologists disagreed with one assertion in particular: "mental disorders are a subset of medical disorders" (Spitzer & Endicott, 1977:4).

On August 8, 1977, Theodore Blau, president of the American Psychological Association, wrote to the president of the APA to register a formal complaint. He stated that his board of directors had received information that the DSM-III Task Force "proposes—and is confident that it will succeed—to append to DSM-III the'Proposed Definition of Medical and Psychiatric Disorders for DSM-III.'" Declaring that the two documents—the manual and the proposed definition—were "immiscible," Blau specifically objected to the offending statement that mental disorders are a subset of medical disorders. "Of the 17 major diagnostic classes," Blau asserted, "at least 10 have no known organic etiology." He then went on to discuss a number of disorders that were "obviously acquired though learning experiences," and to discredit the idea that they were medical disorders.

Millon, the psychologist on the DSM-III Task Force, offered an account that differs from Blau's interpretation of the actions of the task force. According to Millon, the adoption of a definition of mental disorders was first mentioned at a meeting of the DSM-III Task Force in May 1975, and the group decided to consider proposals drafted by their members. Spitzer and Endicott later presented their statement, but "it was discussed only cursorily and assuredly not given official status as a formal statement by the task force" (Millon, 1983:805). When Spitzer and his colleague published their proposal, despite their repeated assertions that it represented their personal view, many assumed—incorrectly, but with good reasons—that it was the official statement of the DSM-III Task Force. Millon observed that:

> In the end, the uproar proved to be a tempest in a teapot. At no time would the task force have jeopardized acceptance of the substantive advances they had wrought in the DSM-III by including a statement so obviously provocative to one of the major mental health professions. Perhaps two or three task force members might have seen the fight as worth pursuing, but it would have been a pyrrhic victory at best. With the support of . . . a special liaison committee of the American Psychological Association to the DSM-III Task Force, when the concept was put to the test of a vote in February 1978, it was soundly and wisely defeated. (p. 806)

Millon's account of the deliberations of the DSM-III Task Force may be accurate, but Spitzer and the leadership of the APA were willing to include a statement that was obviously provocative to one of the major mental health professions. In fact, they were spoiling for a fight. When the APA received the American Psychology Association's protest, Spitzer was asked to draft a reply. He forwarded his draft for the APA president's consideration along with a cover letter in which he observed about the psychologists, "these guys have some chutzpah." He also suggested that the exchange be publicized in *Psychiatric News*, and noted that a reporter from a Pittsburgh paper had already contacted him. In his draft, which Spitzer characterized as "perhaps too combative," he refused to abandon the idea that mental disorder was a subset of medical disorder. Spitzer felt that there was a secondary benefit to publicizing the controversy:

> I personally would enjoy having this [exchange of letters between the two associations] made public to our membership, as it would be another way of demonstrating our conviction that psychiatry is a speciality within medicine. It would also make it clear to our profession that DSM-III helps psychiatry move closer to the rest of medicine. (letter from Spitzer to Sabshin, October 26, 1977)

The APA president, Jack Weinberg, included Spitzer's language in his reply to the American Psychological Association, and he retained the combative tone. Weinberg observed that it was unlikely that the new manual would incorporate Spitzer's paper, "The Proposed Definition of Medical and Psychiatric Disorders for DSM-III," but this did not settle the matter. Using Spitzer's wording, Weinberg asserted that:

whether or not the paper is included in DSM-III is not the issue, since there will certainly be a statement in DSM-III indicating that the DSM-III classification of mental disorders is a subset of medical disorders. It is apparently this concept, rather than the particular definition of mental disorder contained in Dr. Spitzer's paper, to which your association is objecting.

I would hope that you will be able to appreciate that as far as we are concerned we have always regarded mental disorders as a subset of medical disorders. The only difference is that in DSM-III this will be explicitly stated. (letter from Weinberg to Blau, November 3, 1977, p. 2)

In an effort to soften the impact of Spitzer's formulation of mental disorder, Weinberg proposed that DSM-III might include the following disclaimer that had been drafted by Spitzer in consultation with the American Psychological Association's liaison committee:

Although DSM-III is conceptualized here within the medical model, it should be noted that while psychiatry is a speciality of medicine, it is also one of the mental health professions, which includes clinical psychology, psychiatric social work and psychiatric nursing. For this reason, issues regarding the role of members of these professions in dealing with a specific disorder or group of disorders are to be considered within the framework of applicable legal statutes and regulations, as a function of the training and the competence of members of these professions. (p. 4)

Weinberg's (and Spitzer's) view was that this disclaimer might be useful in resolving the conflict, but the offer to include the disclaimer was provisional. "Obviously [the disclaimer] requires further study by us." To add insult to injury, Weinberg did not continue in this conciliatory manner for long. He concluded his letter with a challenge:

Where are we to go from here? You can continue to try to convince us that most mental disorders in the DSM-III classification are not medical disorders. You will not only fail to convince us, but we believe that it is inappropriate for you to attempt to tell us how we should conceptualize our area of professional responsibility. You can try to convince us that even if we believe that mental disorders are medical disorders, we should not explicitly say so in DSM-III. You will not convince us of this either. We believe that it is essential that we clarify to anyone who may be in doubt, that we regard psychiatry as a specialty of medicine. (p. 4)

Blau responded to the challenge in Weinberg's letter by observing (letter from Blau to Weinberg, December 6, 1977) that "Using the concepts of 'mental' and 'medical' synonymously or inclusively may exclude or deny the promising independent research and service" by other mental health professionals besides psychiatrists. He complained that the APA formulation "suggests disdain" for these professionals. He did acknowledge that the proposed disclaimer may be helpful. "At a minimum," he warned, " we look forward to its inclusion in the form that we discussed, in the next draft of DSM-III.'

However, this solution did not mollify the psychologists. Blau continued, "Candidly DSM-III, as we have seen it in its last draft, is more of a political position paper for the American Psychiatric Association than a scientifically-based classification system." Warming to the subject, Blau complained, "To continue to promulgate a classification system that does not meet the needs of emotionally troubled persons is not in the best interest of society or of either of our professions." Furthermore Blau felt, "It would be irresponsible to produce a diagnostic system without an empirical scientific data base after so much scientific input by our many colleagues in both professions over the past thirty years.'

To remedy the problem, Blau announced that the American Psychological Association had decided "to embark on a truly empirical venture in classification of behavioral disorders." They intended for the proposed classification system to be an interdisciplinary venture.

As Millon observed, in the end, none of the threats or counterthreats were realized. DSM-III did not include the offending statement or the disclaimer. His assertion may have been technically correct that "At no time would the *task force* [emphasis added] have jeopardized acceptance of the substantive advances . . . in the DSM-III" by including the provocative statement. However, the leaders of the APA were willing to include the provocative statement. At no time did the DSM-III Task Force have the final authority over what was included in the manual. In fact, Millon documents the fact that the definition of mental disorder finally approved by the DSM-III Task Force was altered by the APA before it was published in DSM-III.

More to the point, it is quite clear from the correspondence that the chairman of the DSM-III Task Force and the leaders of the APA were not only willing to include the offending statement, but they wanted to encourage open conflict over it to promote greater commitment among psychiatrists to the medical model.

The conflict was never over scientific data. When the president of the American Psychological Association offered evidence that there were mental disorders that were not medical disorders, this line of reasoning was summarily dismissed by the president of the APA. Repeating Spitzer's words, Weinberg informed Blau that he would not convince psychiatrists and that it was inappropriate to try. The debate had nothing to do with science or the examination of data. The claim that DSM-III was based on empirical information did not extend to the basic definition of mental disorder.

The American Psychological Association did not publish its own classification system, but it was not because of compromises over DSM-III. The association found that it did not have the resources or the sustained organizational interest to produce an alternative manual. Its threat to develop an alternative system was revived again in the mid-1980s, when there was renewed conflict between the two organizations over a subsequent revision of DSM-III.

Even if one accepts Millon's interpretation, the offending definition of mental disorders was dropped for reasons unrelated to empirical data. The DSM-III Task Force had other more important goals according to Millon, and it did not want to jeopardize them. Furthermore, Spitzer, Sabshin, and Weinberg had achieved important objectives, especially moving the psychiatric profession closer to a medical approach, simply by airing the controversy, even though they eventually deleted the contested phrase from the definition of mental disorder that appeared in DSM-III.

There were many other controversies that engrossed Spitzer and the DSM-III Task Force during the revision process but, like the fight over the definition of mental disorders, empirical data were seldom the basis for resolving them. Chief among the disputes was an astonishing quarrel over a word—neurosis (Bayer & Spitzer, 1985). Psychoanalysts, alarmed at their loss of influence over the theory and practice of psychiatry eventually focused their attention on the deletion of the term *neurosis* from the manual, although many neurotic disorders were renamed and retained. The dispute involved countless meetings and communications over several years, and it almost resulted in the rejection of the manual prepared by Spitzer and the DSM-III Task Force. Throughout this entire period, 1977–1979, Spitzer and his colleagues were conducting extensive studies of successive drafts of the manual, although this research seemed to have had little influence on the acrimonious debate.

The Final Product: DSM-III

When all was said and done, the board approved DSM-III because there was too much "bureaucratic momentum" (Bayer & Spitzer, 1985:193) behind the new manual. After six years of preparation, a substantial financial expenditure, and the promotion of the manual in many of their journals and in the popular press, it would have been hard to reject the new product. It is informative to compare it with DSM-II.

DSM-II was a small, spiral-bound notebook, less than 150 pages long, that clinicians could purchase for $3.50. DSM-II opened with a list of the ten members of the Committee on Nomenclature and Statistics who developed the manual, and all of the 30 other members who had served on the committee in the previous 20 years. The certification of the manual by Spitzer and two other consultants followed. There was a foreword by the committee chairman, Ernest Gruenberg and an introduction, which was entitled "The Historical Background of ICD-8," by Morton Kramer of the National Institute of Mental Health. This was followed by seven sections. The first was an introduction that provided instructions for the use of the manual. A second listed the disorders. The most important part of the manual was the third section, which consisted of short descriptions of all the diagnoses. A fourth section entitled "Statistical Tabulations" was a brief discussion about statistical reporting of mental disorders. There was a fifth section that compared DSM-I and DSM-II. Another section provided a detailed list of the major disease categories in the ICD-8. The concluding section, added to later printings, was the "Guide to the New Nomenclature," by Spitzer and a colleague.

The heart of the manual was a brief section that listed the mental disorders and their code numbers, followed by a section that contained the definitions for 182 specific disorders grouped into 10 classes in less than 40 pages. The one-paragraph description of schizophrenia—the pivotal disorder from which modern psychiatric classifications have evolved—illustrates the brevity of these definitions. Even the more extended discussion of subtypes of schizophrenia was less than a page.

By contrast, DSM-III devoted a dozen pages to Schizophrenic Disorders. DSM-III was an oversized volume, five hundred pages long, that sold for more than ten times the price of its predecessor. Everything about it was bigger, swollen in length and in importance. Starting in the first-page acknowledgments by Spitzer, there was the first of several lists of names of people who had participated in the creation of the manual, in this case those in the APA hierarchy. This was followed by several pages that listed the 19 members of the Task Force on Nomenclature and Statistics (the DSM-III Task Force) and more than a hundred names of members of the 14 task force subcommittees and various APA liaison committees. Before one read a single word of text, one already had a sense of a massive undertaking with great participation and widespread approval.

This long list was followed by the introduction, signed by Spitzer. This was no ordinary statement. As many struggles had been waged over the content of the introduction as over any other aspect of the manual, and Spitzer had been able to keep control of it, despite the attempts by some of the most powerful groups in the mental health field to wrest it from him. The dispute over the definition of mental disorder was only one of many battles that had been fought over the contents and authorship of the introduction. The introduction as published was more like a carefully worded preamble to a legal document than a scientific report. In addition to a recitation of the story of the development of DSM, there was an account of the field trials, which set the tone for future discussions about reliability. "Perhaps the most important part of the study was the evaluation of diagnostic reliability" (p. 5), the introduction stated, thus establishing from the outset the importance of reliability and the field trials.

The other notable aspect of the introduction is the disclaimers, which give it a legalistic quality. In a section of the introduction entitled "Cautions" readers are advised, "The use of the manual for nonclinical purposes such as determination of legal responsibility, competency or insanity, or justification for third party payment must be critically examined in each instance within the appropriate institutional context" (p. 12). Of course, the architects of the manual could not help but know that these were the concerns that were of great importance to most of its users.

The text of the manual included elaborate instructions for its use, which were particularly important since many features were new to most mental health professionals. The new manual included a multiaxial system. Instead of limiting a diagnosis to a single word or phrase clinicians were asked to evaluate five dimensions or "axes" of human behavior. Axis One, entitled Clinical Syndromes, included descriptive words like *schizophrenia, agoraphobia,* or *pyromania* that we usually associate with psychiatric diagnosis. Two groups of diagnoses, Personality Disorders and Specific Developmental Disorders of Childhood and Adolescence, were listed on Axis Two. Medical conditions related to the patient's mental disorder were to be reported on Axis Three. Axis Four and Axis Five were both eight-point scales. Axis Four assessed psychosocial stressors and Axis Five rated the highest level of adaptive functions during the previous year. These numerical scales added to the sense of scientific precision the new manual conveyed, although they were not required to complete an "official" diagnosis.

The bulk of the new manual was once again devoted to description of the specific disorders. There were now 265, a third more than appeared in DSM-II. Some, such as Post–Traumatic Stress Disorder, appeared for the first time, and there were many that had been deleted. For instance, neurasthenia, the most popular diagnosis throughout the rest of the world, was dropped from DSM-III. The greatest expansion had occurred among the children's disorders, oddly, and probably unwittingly, following the initial dictate of the APA board of trustees.

The entry for each specific disorder was far more elaborate than the simple one-paragraph description in DSM-II. The principal change was a list of criteria that had to be satisfied for each diagnosis. In order to make a diagnosis the clinician had to identify specific symptoms, which were listed as the criteria. Only if a certain number of symptoms had been manifested were the criteria met. In addition to the listing of essential and associated features, the entry for disorders contained information about the age of onset, course, impairment, complications, predisposing factors, prevalence, sex ratio, and familial pattern. There was also a discussion in each entry about the differential diagnosis, that is, the way that the disorder differed from other illnesses with which it might be confused. There was additional information in the manual's appendices that attempted to help differentiate various disorders, and implicitly to reduce the risk of error in diagnosis.

There were five appendices to the manual. Appendix A was a series of Decision Trees for Differential Diagnosis. These algorithms were a new feature and increased the look of scientific accuracy about the diagnostic enterprise. Appendix B was a glossary of technical terms, also a new feature, which attempted to standardize the definitions of many of the descriptive terms such as delusion, hallucination, and loosening of associations, that were used to characterize disorders. There was another appendix that compared the listing of diagnoses in DSM-II and DSM-III and that discussed the relationship of DSM-III to ICD-9. Another curious appendix listed sleep disturbances—a compromise that set a precedent. It was included as an appendix because the manual's architects were reluctant to incorporate it in the text. They promoted sleep disturbances to full-fledged mental illnesses in the next addition, DSM-III-R, and included other disputed new diagnoses about women's disorders in a new appendix.

Finally, Appendix F was the report of the reliability data from the field trials. This 14-page report consisted of a brief, two-page description of the field trials, three tables and an eight-and-one-half-page list of the names, degrees, and institutional affiliations of more than six hundred field trial participants. In the end, as at the beginning, the manual clearly signaled the massive effort that had been made to produce a document that included the contributions of an army of professional and scientific workers who had helped to create the best document that science could produce.

5

A CAREFUL LOOK AT
THE FIELD TRIALS

The field trials were not research conducted for the purpose of testing and comparing the efficacy of the completed manual in relation to the efficacy of other systems of diagnosis. The field studies were primarily concerned with debugging the new classification system: Could clinicians understand how to use the manual, were the instructions clear, were the descriptions of disorders adequate, and should the criteria be changed or clarified? The project did not stress careful, uncontaminated data gathering among random samples of clinicians or patients. Nor were the field trials attempts to test the construct validity of the categories rigorously.

The tasks of innovation require fluidity and flexibility—the work of product development and marketing. The field testing was a method of gauging how user-friendly the new product was and how much resistance might be encountered; it was not a final or comprehensive assessment of the scientific credibility of the instrument. The distinction is important because some of the results, particularly the data from the reliability tests, were presented as though they represented a definitive assessment of the manual. The kind of field studies that were performed are a necessary part of the scientific process, but different from the rigorous psychometric testing of a new scientific instrument. However, the field trials, which played no important role in the initial development of the manual nor in the controversies that surrounded it, were used when the manual was published as evidence of the scientific respectability of the enterprise. The architects of the manual repeatedly claimed that the reliability tests showed that DSM-III was so much better than expected and better than DSM-II. Although they repeated this claim a number of times, they actually did not have any new data that systematically compared the overall reliability of DSM-III with previous versions. Although a comparative study would have been easy to do, the reliability tests were not designed to produce information about the relative reliability of different systems or different approaches to diagnosis.

Shortly after the 1976 St. Louis conference, "DSM-III in Midstream," Spitzer began to organize field trials. Preliminary studies were conducted at eight different sites in the early months of 1977, and findings were reported at a special session at the annual APA meeting in May. Diverse sites were used, including a college mental health facility, an outpatient clinic for severely disturbed patients in a poverty area, a marriage counseling program that concentrated on sexual dysfunctions, a psychiatric consultation service in a hospital, and a program for children and adolescents. According to the APA,

> the purpose of this pilot field trial . . . was to test the feasibility of field trials, identify major problem areas in the classification and develop a simple reporting system that would preserve confidentiality and at the same time provide data which would enable the Task Force to further develop DSM-III. (APA, 1977:1)

Many of the on-site coordinators in the early tests of DSM-III were very involved in the development of the manual. In one report presented at the 1977 APA special session, Robert Arnstein (1977:2) confessed, "I would hesitate to say that the trial was a Simon-pure, Mr. Clean test of DSM-III for a variety of reasons." He explained how he became involved:

> About a year ago Bob [Spitzer] came to Yale to lecture on the subject of *DSM-III*, and at the time he passed out a draft list of the then projected *DSM-III* classifications. Although I had arrived at his lecture with indifference, approaching dissociation, the indifference changed rapidly to alarm when I saw the draft list, which seemed to me to have eliminated every diagnosis that I would be likely to choose for a college student. As a result I talked with some people at the American College Health Association [ACHA], who talked with Bob and the upshot was that Bob invited the ACHA to send a representative to the June planning meeting in St. Louis, and I was it. From that point on I became involved in developing relevant classifications and have been working quite closely with Bob and the Childhood and Adolescence Subcommittee ever since, as well as a committee of college mental health workers appointed by ACHA. (pp. 2–3)

Arnstein not only acted as a liaison from the ACHA, but he eventually became a full member of the DSM-III Task Force. His participation in the field trials was a logical extension of his involvement in the creation of the classification system. "When Bob suggested that a college health service be included in the field trial, I felt it only appropriate to participate" (p. 3).

He was not the only person who ran field trials who was so actively involved in the development of the manual. Michael Sheehy was another DSM-III Task Force member who reported at the 1977 APA session on his study, "DSM-III Field Trial in an Outpatient Service." His clinic was located in the same institution where Spitzer was employed. Among the others who reported at the 1977 special session were Dennis Cantwell, another DSM-III Task Force member, and Harold Lief, who was an active participant in the DSM-III Advisory Committee on Psychosexual Disorders.

Although the issue of reliability became a matter of primary concern in the reports of subsequent field trial research, most of the initial studies did not concentrate on this subject. Cantwell's project, "A reliability study of the Childhood and Adolescent Section of DSM-III," was an exception, and the results were not promising for DSM-III. When Cantwell and his associates used DSM-II and a draft of DSM-III, the reliability scores for mental disorders of children were slightly better for the old manual, although the differences were not statistically significant (Cantwell et al., 1979).

The preliminary trials were fluid and informal. The draft of DSM-III used to make diagnoses was not complete. Arnstein observed:

> The initial draft of the classification write-up that we received had some rather large gaps so that some of the diagnoses were unquestionably applied on the basis of what someone thought the title ought to cover, rather than because he or she had a clear cut list of operational criteria to check against. From time to time a packet would arrive from Bob Spitzer's office, filling this gap or that. (1977:2)

Furthermore, changes were often made on the basis of informal feedback from the field sites, without waiting for a final analysis of the data from the projects. In their report at the APA session, Clancy and Noyes (1977) described the process. Commenting on problems in the draft manual, they noted:

> In the trial these problems were noted and referred to the Task Force for discussion and resolution. In some instances this resulted in changes or rewrites of the offending portion of *DSM-III*. The committee's opinion was then relayed to the field trial coordinator. Constant feedback was a feature of the relationship between the Task Force Committee and the coordinators of the field trial. (p. 6)

Spitzer reported that well over 80% of the suggestions submitted by the participating clinicians "were either accepted outright, or provided the stimulus for some modification." (APA, 1978:7)

The initial projects were also used to devise some of the instruments that were employed in the major study done by the DSM-III Task Force, which has generally been referred to as the NIMH Field Trials. Even before the preliminary trials had started, on October 7, 1976, the APA contacted the head of the National Institute of Mental Health to ask for support for field testing. He agreed that careful field testing was needed, and assigned staff to work out the details. The project was eventually funded by NIMH and Spitzer served as the principal investigator. The project ran for two years, from September 1977 to September 1979.

The APA used a variety of settings to field test the manual. There were both public and private hospitals, including those run by the Veterans Administration, universities, and state governments. In addition, the APA used outpatient settings in community mental health facilities and private offices, as well as emergency facilities. They tried to ensure that most participants were not involved in the previous development of DSM-III, although some DSM-III Task Force members and some of those who participated in the preliminary trials continued to take part in the tests. They also tried to select clinicians who would provide a wide distribution of cases that included children, adolescents, adults, and geriatric patients over 65. However, they were careful to note that:

> no attempt will be made to insure that the types of facilities and patients be statistically representative in this country. . . . the major purpose of the study is to identify and solve potential problems with the DSM-III draft. . . . The purpose of this study is not to conduct a scientifically designed epidemiological study of the distribution of mental disorders in the population or according to different types of services. (APA, 1977:2)

The researchers wanted participants who had an unusual level of commitment:

> Our experience with the initial *DSM-III* field trials has convinced us that few facilities have more than two to four clinicians with sufficient motivation to provide us with the kind of quality data that is required. Merely coercing a clinician to use the *DSM-III* form and make a *DSM-III* diagnosis does not elicit the identification of problem areas which is the major purpose of the study. (p. 3)

They recruited candidates by placing a notice in the APA periodical, *Psychiatric News*, and other journals, and they directly solicited volunteers from some specific organizations such as the Veterans Administration where they felt that representation in the project was particularly important and by letters sent to the membership of the American Academy of Child Psychiatry. All groups of clinicians who applied were accepted as participants in the reliability study. Participants were from all parts of the country, and most were involved in the evaluation and care of patients. There were also many clinicians at other institutions who participated in the field trials but were not considered part of the formal NIMH trials. There were more than six hundred participants in the field trials that took place in this final period, 1977–1979, but only one fourth of them were considered to be part of the official NIMH tests of reliability. As an incentive, all of the volunteers were offered continuing medical education (CME) credits, which physicians must accumulate.

There were two phases of the project. The goal of the first phase was to gather information about a draft published on January 15, 1978. Information from Phase One was analyzed, and then, for Phase Two, the manual was revised, and a new draft was distributed and retested, repeating many of the same procedures that had been used in Phase One.

During Phase One, each participating clinician received drafts of the manual, instructions, and forms. Everyone was expected to complete 20 initial diagnostic evaluations, on consecutive admissions to the facility or on a catch-as-catch-can basis as the clinician was available, but they were not to select cases on the basis of patient characteristics such as cooperativeness. The clinicians were asked to complete a form called DIRE that asked for the DSM-III diagnosis and the corresponding DSM-II diagnosis. They were also asked to identify potential problems from a checklist on the form and to rate the difficulty of making the diagnosis using a scale the researchers had prepared.

As was true in the preliminary field tests, the NIMH Field Trials stressed interchange between the clinicians and the research staff. In order to facilitate this, clinicians were encouraged to include suggestions about problems that they had identified. They were assured that there would be a prompt response, as had occurred in the preliminary trials.

The field tests consisted of four subparts: a diagnostic study, a case summary study, a reliability study, and a debugging study. The 20 diagnoses completed in Phase One on the Dire forms along with the critiques of each diagnosis provided data for the diagnostic study and the debugging study.

In addition, for the reliability study, two or four of the cases were to be selected after at least 15 diagnoses had been completed. One article (Spitzer, Forman, & Nee, 1979:815) indicated that participants were each asked to evaluate at least two patients, but in the manual itself and in a 1982 article, the researchers stated that participants were asked to make at least four evaluations (APA, 1980:467; Hyler, Williams, & Spitzer, 1982). Whatever the specific number requested, these assessments were to be done only after each clinician had already used the DSM-III draft in evaluating at least 15 patients. Clinicians were to monitor their own compliance with this request. Patients were selected either as

> consecutive admissions or on a catch-as-catch-can basis. . . . Each individual was evaluated on each of the five axes.
> The two clinicians could either be present at the same evaluation interview or arrange to do separate evaluations as close together in time as possible. (APA, 1980:467–468)

The researchers cautioned participants "not to choose cases specifically because they presented no differential diagnostic problems and not to discuss a case before each clinician's independent completion of the diagnostic forms" (Spitzer et al., 1979:815). Clinicians were allowed to have access to the same information on patients and case records and to share other information "while at the same time avoiding communication of [their] diagnostic impression" (p. 816).

Of the 365 volunteers participating in group settings who saw adult patients, only 274 participated in the first phase of the reliability study (p. 816). No information was given about the attrition of 25% of the participants. Who were they? Why after volunteering did they not participate? Did they participate in a later phase? Did they begin to participate in the reliability study, but simply failed to send their data in? Did they send results in, but these results, for whatever reasons, were not used in this report?

Since these pairs of clinicians had to have access to the same patient and were from the same institution, private practitioners did not participate in the reliability study. The interviewers were asked to share all information about the case, but not their diagnosis. After seeing the patient they each filled out a diagnostic (DIRE) form, then compared diagnoses and completed a second form (Reliaform), which asked them to identify the reasons for any disagreement. They were asked whether disagreements were due to information variance, differences in the interpretation of clinical data, differences in the interpretation of diagnostic criteria, or other problems. When the two evaluations and the reliability forms were completed, they were sent to the researchers.

There are several aspects about the field trials that are confusing. In the various reports of the reliability study, the researchers presented different sets of data. The field trials were in two parts (Phase One and Phase Two) and focused on adults, children, and adolescents. At times, information was reported on Phase One and at other times for both phases. This may explain some of the inconsistencies. For example, in reporting on Phase One for adults in 1979, the researchers stated that "slightly more than half of the evaluations were done jointly" (both clinicians were present at the evaluation interview), but the next year they reported just the opposite:

> In Phase One, approximately 60% of adult as well as child and adolescent diagnostic assessments were done in separate evaluations, and in Phase Two about two-thirds of all evaluations were done separately. (APA, 1980:468)

There is also a discrepancy in the reports of how many adult patients were evaluated in Phase One. In the 1979 report they indicate that 281 adult patients were evaluated by 274 clinicians, but in 1980 the figure reported was 339 adult patients. This 20% discrepancy in adult patients was never explained. Such discrepancies as these (and there are others) may not be serious, but they make it difficult to know precisely how the field trials were conducted. Scientific reports should adequately describe research procedures and selection (and attrition) of samples, since these can skew the data and their interpretation. While all this information does not have to appear in every report from a single study, it impedes a full analysis of the field trials since no full, comprehensive report with methodological details was ever made available. Discrepancies about simple matters such as the number of participants in the study illustrate some of the difficulty that even informed researchers would encounter in understanding exactly what was done in the field trials.

The separate case summary study called for each of the clinicians to provide a synopsis of the data on at least one of the cases that had been used in the reliability study. Participants were also asked to complete case summaries for patients who had an unusual, rarely seen diagnosis. These two- to four-page summaries were to be prepared in a traditional, standard format that included information about the chief complaint, history of present illness, developmental history, psychiatric and medical history, mental status examination, and so forth. No mention of a specific psychiatric diagnosis or any information about the family history of the mental disorder was to be made in the summary.

The clinicians submitted 150 summaries, 70 of which were on patients who had also been evaluated as part of the reliability study using live interviews. Forty-six of the 70 summaries, prepared by 41 different clinicians, were selected by the researchers for a separate inquiry. Each of the same 41 clinicians was sent five of the 46 case summaries, but no clinician was sent a case that he or she or another clinician at the same facility had prepared. The participants were asked to record a DSM-III multi-

axial evaluation of each case. In all, 192 (of a possible 205) case summaries were diagnosed. The results of this part of the field trials were
reported in 1982 and will be discussed in Chapter 6.

The case summary study yielded another important by-product.
Many of the case summaries were compiled into *The DSM-III Casebook*, a
learning guide for the manual that has become a best-seller, second only
to DSM-III in popularity among the myriad of publications about psychiatric diagnosis. The *Casebook* consists of a series of vignettes, usually a
few paragraphs long, which illustrate one or another diagnosis. In most
cases the information clearly portrays some diagnosis in an obvious way.

Much less is known about Phase Two of the field trials. In the 1979
article about Phase One the authors promised:

> In future reports we will present the reliability of the individual diagnostic
> categories and the results of phase two of the field trial, which involves
> reliability interviews to assess the effects of changes made in the DSM-III
> classifications and in the diagnostic criteria. (Spitzer et al., 1979:817)

However, no such reports appeared in the literature, except for a brief
appendix in the final DSM-III. And nowhere is there a complete report
of the individual diagnostic categories.

The second phase of the field trials involved the completion of another
series of diagnoses, similar to the first. Although the data from Phase
Two represented the culmination of the effort to obtain information
about the new diagnostic system, there is only one, incomplete report of
these efforts in an Appendix to DSM-III. Phase Two of the trials took
place during the early months of 1979. New revisions of the manual
were circulated, and the participants were asked to make diagnoses on a
revised form, DIRE-2. New questions on this form attempted to elicit
information about the treatment that the diagnostician felt was suitable
for the patient, although this information has never been published.
Once again clinicians were asked to select two cases for a reliability test
after they had practiced on an adequate number of other patients. Diagnostic forms were returned to the researchers and reliability scores were
computed from the paired diagnoses.

In a 1980 article, the researchers indicated that the field trials "used
several versions of the completed draft" and that "as a result of these
trials, continued revisions were made" (Spitzer et al., 1980:152), but in a
1985 article, the coordinator of the field trials, stated that the version of
DSM-III used in Phase One "was virtually identical to the final versions"
(Williams, 1985:181). The DSM-III manual noted that Phase Two used the
earlier draft of Phase One "supplemented by a set of revised criteria" (p.
467).

In the final manual, one can find data that indicated that Phase Two involved the psychiatric evaluation of 331 adults and 55 children (APA, 1980:467, 470, 471). It is difficult to infer from these partial reports exactly how many clinicians were involved in Phase Two, the extent to which they were different from the clinicians in Phase One, or how they were selected. Omissions of this sort usually do not survive normal editorial review, particularly when the findings are purported to address a serious national issue and are being published by the leading journal of the APA. In summary then, there are surprising inconsistencies and gaps in information available about these highly touted field trials.

In addition to these activities, participants in the NIMH Field Trials were sent inquiries about selected subjects. After having completed the first round of studies, the researchers belatedly decided to find out who had participated. They asked participants to identify their profession (psychiatrist, psychologist, social worker, etc.), their practice setting, and their therapeutic orientation (psychoanalytic, behavioral, somatic, etc.). They also asked how much time each respondent had spent on reading the new manual—including the time they had spent consulting it while diagnosing the 20 patients they were asked to examine for the study. Interestingly, 65% of the respondents had spent ten hours or less consulting the complex, voluminous document, which had entirely new, intricate instructions for more than two hundred diagnoses, many of them appearing in the manual for the first time. Even more noteworthy, 38% of these volunteers—who had been characterized as a select group of "clinicians with sufficient motivation to provide us with the kind of quality data that is required"—spent five hours or less reading the manual during the first field trial (APA, 1978b).

There were questions about how often diagnoses were made without satisfying all of the diagnostic criteria, and the majority of participants acknowledged that they made diagnoses without meeting all the criteria at least occasionally. There were questions about various other innovations, including the multiaxial system, and the decision-making algorithms. (Some of the findings were reported in Spitzer & Forman, 1979.)

A number of queries related to the participants' opinions about the manual, and particularly to questions about the deletion of neurosis and other psychodynamic aspects of DSM-II. These data—never published—were used in the battle with Freudians to demonstrate that even psychoanalysts who had used the manual supported the changes. In a showdown meeting with psychoanalysts, "Spitzer and his supporters . . . argued that a sample survey of those engaged in the DSM-III field trials indicated that even among those who identified themselves as psychodynamically oriented, the new approach to diagnosis met with widespread approval" (Bayer & Spitzer, 1985:191). It was true that this nonrandom survey of volunteers who had invested a substantial amount of time and effort to participate in the field trials preferred DSM-III to DSM-II. But the data about the issues in dispute were far from clear. On one question, 65% of those with a psychoanalytic orientation agreed with the DSM-III approach and rejected the proposal that psychodynamic formulations should be included. Responses were more mixed to another query about the deletion of the category Neurotic Depression, which was a major point of contention among opponents to DSM-III. Only 52% of the psychodynamically oriented clinicians agreed with this. Furthermore, in response to another question, only 46% of the psychodynamically oriented respondents agreed to the recommendations to delete the neurotic subtypes, which became the focal point of the dispute with the analysts. Thirty percent rejected the proposal and the rest did not respond. The developers were free to claim that support was widespread because there was no published information about the field trials that could contradict them.

All told, the number of published reports that resulted from the field trials was surprisingly small. Only four short publications appeared that were primary reports of empirical data, and their purpose was to promote the manual. This started early, as illustrated by an April 1979 memo, "Our Travails Never Seem to End," from Spitzer to the DSM-III Task Force. This memo described the 11th-hour efforts of psychoanalysts to block publication of the manual, and the widespread dissatisfaction with DSM-III among the APA board of trustees. Spitzer described a meeting of the board that occurred just two months before the final decision on DSM-III was scheduled to be made: "A straw vote was then taken as to whether or not DSM-III in its current form was preferable to DSM-II. Only one member, Dr. Alan Stone, voted in favor of DSM-III!" The board decided to set up a committee to review the manual and report back in a month at its May 17 meeting.

In the memo, Spitzer described his strategy for obtaining final approval of the manual. The field trials are mentioned twice. Spitzer reported that he was invited to make a presentation to an ad hoc committee of the board, which was appointed to review complaints about the manual. In preparation for the meeting Spitzer stated, "I will be sending them the results of the Field Trial, fan letters we have received, etc. "

The second mention of the field trials was in reference to a subsequent meeting of the full board of trustees, which was scheduled to evaluate the report of the ad hoc committee and to make a final decision about DSM-III. He told his DSM-III Task Force, "I have asked Dick Finn, long-time field Trial Participant to talk about his experience with DSM-III. Janet [Williams, the Field Coordinator] will present the more uplifting data from the Field Trial." Even though work on the field trials had not ended, data were to be presented as part of the sales package to persuade the board to adopt the manual.

Reliability, which had been the ticket of admission for Spitzer to justify a radical revision of the diagnostic manual, was of so little importance during the final stages of the struggle because it was overshadowed by other controversies, principally those with psychoanalysts, over specific diagnoses. Although reliability was substantially less useful as a problem during the process of developing DSM-III, in the end as in the beginning, it played a very meaningful symbolic role. As we shall describe in the next two chapters, it was prominently used in the final sale of the manual to the professional community.

6

RELIABILITY AND THE
REMARKABLE ACHIEVEMENT

> In principle, the problem of reliability has been solved.
>
> Gerald L. Klerman, *Contemporary Directions in Psychopathology*

> Science is rooted in creative interpretation. Numbers suggest, constrain, and refute; they do not, by themselves, specify the content of scientific theories. Theories are built upon the interpretation of numbers, and interpreters are often trapped by their own rhetoric. They believe in their own objectivity, and fail to discern the prejudice that leads them to one interpretation among many consistent with their numbers.
>
> Stephen Jay Gould, *The Mismeasure of Man*

By the time DSM-III appeared, its authors and indirectly the entire DSM-III Task Force claimed to have generated a substantial amount of data about DSM-III, which they offered in support. Both these data and the field trials in which they were gathered were heralded as among the distinguishing features of DSM-III that set it apart from earlier versions of the manual. The problem of diagnostic reliability, submerged by the political controversies generated in the process of transforming the manual, temporarily reemerged as a focal point, this time appearing as the problem that had been substantially remedied by DSM-III.

By design, the field trials played a key role in the development of DSM-III and, as Spitzer et al. (1979:815) stressed as work on DSM-III drew to a close, "one of the most important purposes of the major field trial . . . has been to determine interrater diagnostic reliability." Data from the field trials became pivotal evidence for the claim that diagnostic reliability was no longer a serious problem for American psychiatry. Although it was apparent that unreliability continued to plague certain diagnostic categories, it was argued, nevertheless, that the new system was still much better than the old one. That the psychiatric community did not seriously dispute these claims was a remarkable achievement.

The claims made about the reliability of DSM-III will be examined in some detail in this chapter and the next. We have already reviewed the methodological quality of the field trials themselves. Now, we will review the claims that were made about the reliability of DSM-III based on the results of the field trials and the extent to which these claims appear to have been accepted. Then, using the interpretive standards suggested by the developers of DSM-III, we will review the original interpretations of these data that were offered. Finally, we will examine other reliability studies that appeared in the professional literature shortly after the appearance of DSM-III to evaluate the extent to which they supported the developers' sanguine interpretations of the reliability of DSM-III.

Claiming Success with the DSM-III Field Trials

The introduction to DSM-III stated that the manual's development included a series of field trials in which "12,667 patients were evaluated by approximately 550 clinicians, 474 of whom were in 212 different facilities" (APA, 1980:5). The developers described the reliability tests as the "most important part of the study" and offered the bold conclusion that the results "generally indicate *far greater* reliability than had previously been obtained with DSM-II" (APA, 1980:5, emphasis added). These are enormously important claims. They appeared prominently in the introduction to the revolutionary, long-awaited, new diagnostic manual. They purported to be based not merely on the hopes of the developers, but on a massive scientific study. And, finally, they proclaimed that the problem of diagnostic reliability, for decades an embarrassment to psychiatry, was now greatly ameliorated; reliability was "far greater" than before. The introduction to DSM-III clearly conveyed the good news that, as promised, the reliability problem was substantially diminished.

These claims were made repeatedly. In the first publication appearing about the field trials (Spitzer et al., 1979)—an article that we will examine in more detail in the next chapter—the developers stated that:

> for most of the [diagnostic] classes, the reliability . . . is quite good and, in general, is higher than that previously achieved using DSM-I and DSM-II. These results were so much better than we had expected. . . . It is particularly encouraging that the reliability for such categories as schizophrenia and major affective disorders is so high. (p. 817)

They attribute their success to the improvements contained in DSM-III. In several other articles, interviews, and presentations that were orchestrated to appear just prior to or immediately after the publication of the new manual, they made similar statements. For example, a long interview with Spitzer was published in *Hospital and Community Psychiatry* (Talbott, 1980) for the purpose of introducing the journal's readership to DSM-III. In the interview, Spitzer described many aspects of the new DSM. One brief part of the interview asked about reliability:

> *Interviewer:* Maybe you could tell us a little about the reliability of DSM-III compared with DSM-II or DSM-I.
> *Spitzer:* With the exception of only a few conditions about which it was always pretty easy to get clinicians to agree—organic brain syndrome, mental retardation, and alcoholism—the reliability of psychiatric diagnoses based on DSM-I and II has been fair, at best, or poor. . . . *The reliabilities are much higher for DSM-III* [he cites several categories]. . . . The reliability is not as good for the childhood categories, although again it is far better than it was for DSM-II.
> *Interviewer:* So DSM-III is clearly much more reliable?
> *Spitzer:* Reliability is *much higher.* (p. 27, emphasis added)

On the eve of the publication of DSM-III, another lengthy promotional article for the new manual appeared in the APA's major journal, the *American Journal of Psychiatry* (Spitzer, Williams, & Skodal, 1980). In it, the authors describe themselves as "battle-weary at the time of this writing and in the final throes of reviewing galleys and page proofs" of DSM-III. Nevertheless they wanted to share with the reader their "major achievements and an overview" of the soon-to-be-released DSM-III.

Interestingly, in this lengthy article the issue of reliability merited only one paragraph. This is it, in its entirety:

> The need for reliability, that is, agreement among clinicians on assigning diagnoses to patients, is universally acknowledged. Studies of the reliability of psychiatric diagnosis using DSM-I and DSM-II indicated generally poor or only fair reliability for most of the major diagnostic categories. In the DSM-III field trials over 450 clinicians participated in the largest reliability study ever done, involving independent evaluations of nearly 800 patients—adults, adolescents, and children. For most of the diagnostic classes the reliability was quite good, and in general it was much higher than that previously achieved with DSM-I and DSM-II. (p. 154)

And, in the introduction to DSM-III itself, they reiterate these same claims (APA, 1980:5).

Although progressively less space was used to discuss reliability after the publication of DSM-III than before, it is not because its importance had changed. Rather, the perception of *reliability as a problem* had changed dramatically. For example, two years later at a debate on DSM-

III at the annual conference of the APA in 1982, a principal proponent of DSM-III asserted that the new diagnostic system's reliability was among the five features that contributed to its success (Klerman, 1984). After applauding the APA's decision to promulgate DSM-III as a "significant reaffirmation" of psychiatry's "medical identity and its commitment to scientific medicine," Klerman acknowledged the "serious problems related to unreliability" that had confronted psychiatrists in the 1950s and 1960s, proudly reviewed the development of new "technologies" (such as kappa, diagnostic criteria, and standardized interviews), and stated that all these developments coalesced with Spitzer's appointment to the DSM-III Task Force to provide "the final pathway for funneling these trends into DSM-III" (pp. 539–541). The result, he stated, was that the reliability problem had been "solved" (p. 541). At this important discussion of DSM-III (reprinted in the *American Journal of Psychiatry* in 1984), none of the other distinguished participants, neither those supporting nor those criticizing DSM-III, questioned these assertions about reliability. Four years later, Klerman (1986) reiterated his bold claim: "In principle, the problem of reliability has been solved" (p. 25). Even critics of DSM-III—and there were many who disliked at least some aspect of it—readily accepted the claims that reliability was no longer problematic (Vaillant, 1984; Michels, 1984a, 1984b). The only concern they expressed was that the achievement of high reliability may have been at the expense of diagnostic validity.

This kind of begrudging acknowledgment of greatly improved reliability has continued for a decade. For example, in a special issue of the *Journal of Abnormal Psychology* devoted to the forthcoming DSM-IV, Carson (1991) conceded that DSM-III "fixed [the problem of unreliability] once and (possibly) for all" by draconian measures to restrict professional diagnostic judgments (p. 304). He then belittled the achievement by arguing that construct validity has been given insufficient concern while reliability had been given excessive emphasis. Although the issue of achieving high reliability at the expense of validity is an important one, the noteworthy achievement in selling DSM-III was that by 1982 neither the reliability problem-solvers nor their critics were publicly agonizing anymore about *un*reliability.

The Unmaking of the Reliability Problem

The problem of diagnostic reliability, which had been effectively defined as a serious threat to psychiatry for three decades, had by 1982 begun to recede from public attention. Gone were the frequent laments in the journals about the embarrassingly low level of diagnostic agreement or how unreliability called the scientific status of psychiatry into question. In their place, an occasional warning would appear about validity being sacrificed or about unexpectedly disappointing reliability results from a particular structured interview schedule or for a particular diagnostic category studied at a specific facility. Expectations now were to find reliable, not unreliable, results among diagnosticians.

Some researchers, of course, kept grappling with reliability on a study-by-study basis, as all scientists do to establish the scientific credibility of any measurement instrument. So the fact that psychiatric researchers continued to attend to reliability issues did not necessarily mean that these were problems around which they tried to mobilize the broader professional community or even that they would have been successful in doing so had they tried. A condition that is viewed as a significant problem for a few investigators, may carry little significance for other investigators or for the larger professional community. The intriguing aspect of diagnostic unreliability is that a routine research problem was used as a focal point to reform the psychiatric classification system.

Perhaps, not surprisingly, those from the New York and St. Louis groups who had been the most vociferous in making reliability a crucial problem that demanded attention were among those who were quick to announce that it was no longer a fundamental problem for psychiatry. It is understandable that they were the first to raise the flag of victory, since they had assumed responsibility and leadership in the battle, first by transforming the problem into one that only a few could fully comprehend and, second, by claiming that they possessed the technical innovations that would lead to a resolution. It was their problem to make and unmake.

Problems of diagnostic agreement evolved into something distant, technical, and complex, best entrusted to the specialists. DSM-III and the claims made about the field trials provided welcome relief from the harsh criticism to which psychiatry was routinely subjected. DSM-III promised greater scientific respectability. It was as if a miasma that had once caused distress had been eradicated by specialists whose methods and claims one accepted gratefully, if uncritically.

After the publication of DSM-III and the proud announcements made at its christening, diagnostic reliability as a problem for psychiatry exited from the stage on which it had been so dramatically introduced 15 years before. No longer were strident calls made to alert members of the profession to the serious weaknesses in the reliability of the nosology. No longer did the St. Louis and New York groups hammer away in the professional journals at the perilousness of allowing reliability problems to go unaddressed. No longer were bold promises offered. Reliability as a problem lost its luster.

While studies of reliability continued to appear in the professional literature (some of these will be reviewed below), they no longer possessed the prominence they enjoyed previously. For the most part, they became mere footnotes in a settled controversy, addressed to questions that most believed were satisfactorily answered. The reliability studies that appeared after DSM-III was published focused on specific disorders or specific populations, not on the reliability of the diagnostic system itself. Their objective was to identify and repair minor flaws in the classification system, rather than to raise questions about the nosology itself. These more recent studies represent the puzzle-solving activities that Kuhn (1970) refers to as "normal science," where, after a paradigmatic shift has occurred in a field, researchers look for ways to extend and support, rather than to question it. For a decade after the field trials in 1978, there were no further calls for comprehensive studies of the reliability of the diagnostic manual as a whole.

Diagnostic agreement was the Achilles heel of psychiatry because of its links with the messy problem of the validity of the concept of mental disorder. Reliability as a professional problem, in fact, gained its stature and legitimacy because it served as a limit on the more fundamental problem of validity. The researchers who were most concerned with these matters successfully shifted the focus toward reliability by outlining how these reliability problems might be resolved. Throughout these developments and central to the purpose of the field trials was the issue of reliability. Earlier, the validity of psychiatric classification had been solemnly wedded to its ability to show evidence that its use was reliable. This was no forced wedding. The significance of the ties between reliability and validity were regularly broadcast during the early struggles to create significant concern about unreliability. Following the publication of DSM-III, less and less was said about reliability, leaving the impression that somehow questions of validity had been settled as well. Most observers did not notice the trial separation or the eventual dissolution of the vows. Divorce came quickly and quietly. Understandably, the parents who had gone to such lengths to arrange the marriage were reluctant to spread the sad news.

Before examining the field trials data, let us continue to review the aftereffects of the introduction of DSM-III, not simply in the claims that were made, but in the actions that were taken or not taken. Even before DSM-III was officially released, discussions were underway about how to develop some ongoing mechanisms for continuing revisions that would undoubtedly be needed. To deflect criticism, DSM-III was described as only one "still frame" in a continuous film (APA, 1980:12,

1987:xvii; Talbott, 1980:32), constantly changing to reflect new knowledge. The image of DSM as a still frame has been used repeatedly to excuse shortcomings and deflect criticisms. But with any still frame, little can be understood about the meaning of the action or its direction. Still frames have the potential to obscure as much as to illuminate.

Shortly after the introduction of DSM-III, another task force was appointed to review it and suggest revisions that should be made prior to the publication of DSM-IV then expected in the early 1990s. The Task Force to Revise DSM-III, chaired again by Spitzer, began work in 1983 and produced another still frame in 1987: DSM-III-R (APA, 1987).

Although this revision began with a limited mandate to make minor changes, it became much more. DSM-III-R constituted a major, not a minor change. New diagnostic categories were added, diagnostic criteria were changed on the majority of categories, axes IV and V were modified, and so forth. Although field tests were conducted for DSM-III-R, and were referred to frequently in the preliminary discussions about the various drafts of the revised manual, less was known about them when the revision was published than about the original field trials for DSM-III. The field trials for DSM-III-R tended to focus on specific disorders, had low response rates, and only appeared in the journals years later (e.g., Spitzer, Williams, Kass, & Davies, 1989). More significantly for our purposes, the issue of reliability which was such a driving force in developing DSM-III, was hardly ever mentioned in the development of DSM-III-R.

Since no reliability studies of DSM-III were conducted by the APA or the DSM-III Task Force after it was published, one might have expected that the topic would be addressed when the manual underwent a major revision. However, no mention was made about the expectation or even the wisdom of conducting new studies of reliability on the final published version of DSM-III or on DSM-III-R. In fact, no new reliability studies were conducted by the DSM-III-R Task Force. (A reliability study of DSM-III-R was conducted as part of an attempt to revise a structured interview protocol, but the results were still unpublished as of December 1991. It will be reviewed in Chapter 9.) The reliability claims from the field trials of DSM-III appeared to have allayed anxieties about reliability, so that no one was pressing for new studies. When DSM-III-R was finally published in 1987, reference to reliability was made only in passing as something considered when making changes. No declarations about the reliability of DSM-III-R were made or any indications given that a reliability study was underway. More significantly, apparently no such studies were required or requested.

The problem of reliability, which merited a few pages in the Appendix of DSM-III, was completely dropped in DSM-III-R. By 1987, a connoisseur of reliability would have to find an outdated and out-of-print copy of the 1980 diagnostic manual to check claims about reliability. Few would see any need to do so. Issues of diagnostic reliability had become so much less prominent by the time DSM-III-R was published that it hardly merited serious attention, either negative or positive.

Shortly thereafter, the planning for DSM-IV began in earnest. Elaborate structures were again developed to solicit broad advice and channel discussion (for more, see Chapter 8). Emphasis was given to the need for synthesizing empirical evidence and requiring it for making changes in the manual. These beginnings prompted a brief, but revealing article by Spitzer and Williams (both members of the DSM-IV Task Force) about what would be the ideal research strategy for making DSM-IV as rigorously empirical as possible. Using the literary device of a "dream" to develop a governmental request for proposals (RFP), they outlined what they consider to be the ideal research strategy for developing knowledge for DSM-IV, if money and effort were no limitation (Spitzer & Williams, 1988). In the article, they emphasized the important role research played in DSM-III and its revision. They outlined the need for research on validity through the involvement of multiple collaborating research centers, multiple experts, using multiple diagnostic criteria sets and multiple external validity criteria. These are all important suggestions. It is an omission, however, that is telling: Not a word was said about the need for further studies of the diagnostic reliability of DSM-III-R or DSM-IV. After two decades and scores of journal articles emphasizing the crucial significance of reliability, there was an unmistakable impression that the problem was no longer of sufficient importance to merit attention in any comprehensive research agenda for DSM-IV.

The DSM-IV Task Force apparently shared that conclusion. At the beginning of its work, no plans were announced for a systematic and rigorous study of the reliability of the classification system that currently exists (DSM-III-R) or for comparing it with draft versions of alternative systems. Later, some preliminary plans were developed to address some reliability questions, but they were not a central concern for DSM-IV (see Chapter 8).

The reliability problem, as evident from the actions of the major committees of the APA, as described by leading spokespersons and as reflected in its journals, has a very different status a decade after the birth of DSM-III. Resolving the reliability problem marked a significant milestone in the evolution of American psychiatry. Reliability had served for at least two decades as a symbol of the weakness of psychiatry as a science and as a lightening rod for some of its political controversies. Now it was taken down and put away, to be polished up and displayed only on special occasions.

That closed chapter is viewed by many as the triumph of a scientific, empirically based psychiatry over a less rigorous nonempirical one. Although many would disagree with that characterization, few would disagree that there was a epic struggle involved in the development of DSM-III and that the goals of its developers were largely, if not completely, achieved. The APA's medical director (Sabshin, 1990) proudly described DSM-III and DSM-III-R as "one of the best symbols of late-century American psychiatry" (p. 1271) and as "amazing documents that did indeed change the shape of American psychiatry" (p. 1272). There is no question that they are amazing documents.

Reliability provided a crisis over which the old diagnostic system was dismantled and a new one raised. Was the evidence about this crucial problem of diagnostic reliability as clear and convincing as it was described by the proponents of DSM-III? Was the new diagnostic system with specific diagnostic criteria so much better at controlling error? Was the evidence so overwhelming that for all intents and purposes no further reliability studies needed to be done? Are mental health clinicians now much less likely to disagree about diagnoses than in the past? If the available evidence is examined more carefully, the answer to these critical questions is either No or We don't know. This gross inconsistency between the answers offered by the developers of DSM-III and the empirical facts regarding these questions will be addressed next.

Interpreting the Field Trials

So fundamental was the issue of reliability that it is interesting that among the vast literature about DSM-III that appeared within a few years after it was published, even among the literature that was critical (e.g., Brookes, 1982; Dumont, 1984; Eysenck, Wakefield, & Friedman, 1983; Taylor, 1983), there was no thorough review of the data on which the claims of far greater reliability rested. We undertake such a review here, which requires us to return to the world of kappa.

Not surprisingly, Spitzer and associates chose to report the extent of agreement using kappa. The actual computation of kappa in the DSM-III reliability studies is unclear. Weighted kappa is referred to, but it does not appear that it was used. The computation of "overall kappa" scores is never described in any of the articles reporting these data, although much is made of it. Although kappa requires that categories be independent, mutually exclusive, and exhaustive, DSM-III encourages multiple diagnoses both within and between axes, thus violating the mutually exclusive criterion (Cohen, 1960:38; APA, 1980:24). There are several ways this computation may have been handled in the analysis of the field trials data, but no clarification was described in any of the published reports. If the reliability studies accepted multiple diagnoses in computing agreement, the reliability estimates would have been inflated. Although significance tests have limited meaning in diagnostic studies (Grove, Andreasen, McDonald-Scott, Keller, & Shapiro, 1981), they are available for kappa; however, they were not reported in the field trials.

Interpreting Kappa

As we described in earlier chapters, there were no generally accepted standards for the interpretation of kappa beyond the anchor points of chance and perfect agreement. Similar kappas have been interpreted differently, depending on the spokesperson, the audience, and the objective. From the interpretations of the earlier reliability studies and those offered in the second wave of reliability reports, a few crude benchmarks can be inferred.

Instead of using these earlier standards, however, Spitzer and his associates proposed a new one in their first report of the field trials. In a brief remark about the field trials, and later reiterated in DSM-III, they make this important statement:

> Reliability is expressed using the kappa statistic, which indexes chance-corrected agreement. A *high* kappa (generally 0.7 and above) indicates *good* agreement as to whether or not the patient has a disorder within that diagnostic class. (Spitzer et al., 1979:816–817, emphasis added)

As will be discussed in some detail in the next chapter, the .7 standard is more lenient than that used in Spitzer and Fleiss's influential paper discrediting the earlier versions of DSM (Spitzer & Fleiss, 1974).

Quite apart from the evaluative standards used, the interpretation of kappa is also plagued by a series of statistical problems (also discussed in Chapter 2), which have been carefully described by others (Grove et al., 1981; Spitznagel & Helzer, 1985). The most serious problem is that the computed value of kappa is a function of sensitivity (the proportion of time a clinician will make a positive diagnosis when a disorder is present), specificity (the proportion of time a clinician will make a negative diagnosis when a disorder is absent), and the base rate (or prevalence) of the disorder in the population under study. Different values of kappa may be due entirely to differences in prevalence rates. Thus, simple comparisons of kappa need to take these and other factors into account, particularly when base rates are low. Grove et al.(1981:412), advise that kappas with very low base rates (below 5%) should not be reported because they can be misleading. Despite these problems in interpretation, we will accept the developers' post hoc standard of .70 as a guide to the interpretation of their data. What do the field trial data look like when viewed through the lens they suggest?

Reinterpreting the Field Trials

There are four original sources of information about the actual results of the field trials (Hyler et al., 1982; APA, 1980; Spitzer et al., 1979; Spitzer & Forman, 1979), as distinct from the many places where one can find an interpretation of the results. Table 6.1 presents the kappa statistics from three of the sources that were reported by the developers of DSM-III for adults on Axis I, Major Mental Disorders. The major diagnostic categories are listed with overall kappas for each one. If one accepts the .70 standard as the benchmark for good reliability that the researchers proposed after they analyzed their data, 31 of the kappas are above the mark and 49 are below their established level. The case summary results are striking: Not a single major diagnostic category achieved the .70 standard.

The results of the field trials on Axis I for children and adolescents, which are presented in Table 6.2, are lower. Only 8 of the 24 kappas achieved the .70 level of "goodness," and 4 of those that reported perfect agreement (1.0) are based on the assessment of *only one patient*. With only two exceptions, changes in reliability from Phase One to Phase Two show declines.

Axis II, Personality Disorders and Specific Developmental Disorders, is a particularly significant diagnostic dimension, because it attempts to identify individual traits that "are enduring patterns of perceiving, relating to, and thinking about the environment and oneself, and are exhibited in a wide range of important social and personal contexts" (APA, 1980:23, 305). Equally significant is that over half the adults and a quarter of the children and adolescents received a diagnosis on Axis II in the field trials. Table 6.3 presents these results. Only one of the seven individual kappas reached the .70 level. None of the overall kappas in Axes II did. Thus, the reliability for adults and children in Phase One and Phase Two must be considered less than good.

Although a prominent innovation of DSM-III was the multiaxial system, no information about reliability was provided for one of the five axes, Axis III, Physical Disorders. One of the developers (Williams, 1985) of the system claimed that no reliability studies were known to

Table 6.1. Kappa Coefficients of Agreement for Axis I, by Major Diagnostic Classes for Adults, in the Field Trials

Major Class of Disorder	Source of Data: 1 [a]			Source of Data: 2 [b]		Source of Data: 3 [c]
	Joint Interviews (n = 150)	Separate Interviews (n = 131)	Joint and Separate Interviews (n = 281) [d]	Phase One (n = 339) [d]	Phase Two (n = 331) [d]	Case Summaries (n = 46) [d]
Disorders Usually First Evident in Infancy, Childhood, or Adolescence	.66	.81	(16)	.65 (18)	.73 (12)	.44 (3)
Organic Mental Disorders	.74	.83	(36)	.79 (40)	.76 (33)	.30 (5)
Substance Use Disorders	.90	.74	(62)	.86 (72)	.80 (70)	.69 (14)
Schizophrenic Disorders	.82	.82	(36)	.81 (60)	.81 (77)	.54 (6)
Paranoid Disorders	1.0	1.0	(2)	.66 (4)	.75 (5)	.55 (2)
Psychotic Disorders Not Elsewhere Classified	.85	.43	(20)	.64 (38)	.69 (22)	.05 (3)
Schizoaffective Disorders	.56	.53	(13)	—	—	—
Affective Disorders	.77	.59	(125)	.69 (146)	.83 (128)	.59 (14)
Anxiety Disorders	.74	.43	(30)	.63 (31)	.72 (29)	.18 (2)

Somatoform Disorders	.53	.66	(12)	.54	(13)	.42	(11)	.53	(3)
Disassociative Disorders	1.0	−.004	(2)	.80	(3)	−.003	(2)	—	
Psychosexual Disorders	1.0	1.0	(6)	.92	(7)	.75	(5)		
Factitious Disorders	.49	1.0	(4)	.66	(4)	−.005	(3)	.34	(1)
Disorders of Impulse Control Not Elsewhere Classified	−.01	−.01	(5)	.28	(6)	.80	(6)	.00	(1)
Adjustment Disorder	.74	.60	(31)	.67	(41)	.68	(28)	.16	(2)
Psychological Factors Affecting Physical Conditions	—	—	—	.62	(11)	.44	(7)	−.05	(1)
V Codes for Conditions Not Attributable to a Mental Disorder	—	—	—	.56	(10)	.66	(10)	.00	(1)
Additional codes	—	—	—	.00	(2)	.28	(6)	.22	(1)
All others	—	—	—	—		—		.20	(5)

Notes:

[a] From R. Spitzer, J. Forman, and J. Nee, "DSM-III Field Trials: I. Initial Interrater Diagnostic Reliability," *American Journal of Psychiatry*, 136, pp. 815–817. Copyright © 1979.

[b] From *Diagnostic and Statistical Manual of Mental Disorders* (3rd ed.) (Washington, DC: American Psychiatric Association, 1980), p. 470.

[c] From S. Hyler, J. Williams, and R. Spitzer, "Reliability in the DSM-III Field Trials," *Archives of General Psychiatry*, 39 (November 1982), pp. 1275–1278.

[d] The numbers in parentheses in this column refer to the number of subjects given each diagnosis by at least one clinician.

Table 6.2. Kappa Coefficients of Agreement for Axis I, by Major Diagnostic Classes for Children and Adolescents, in the Field Trials[a]

Major Class of Disorder	Phase One (N = 71)[b]		Phase Two (N = 55)[b]	
Disorders Usually First Evident in Infancy, Childhood, or Adolescence	.69	(39)	.63	(37)
Organic Mental Disorders	—		.66	(2)
Substance Use Disorders	1.0	(4)	.54	(5)
Schizophrenic Disorders	1.0	(4)	.66	(2)
Psychotic Disorders Not Elsewhere Classified	.85	(4)	—	
Affective Disorders	.53	(12)	.30	(5)
Anxiety Disorders	1.0	(2)	1.0	(1)
Somatoform Disorders	1.0	(1)	−.009	(1)
Psychosexual Disorders	1.0	(1)	—	
Disorders of Impulse Control Not Elsewhere Classified	.66	(2)	—	
Adjustment Disorder	.66	(22)	.36	(18)
Psychological Factors Affecting Physical Conditions	−.01	(1)	−.02	(2)
V codes	−.02	(3)	.54	(5)
Additional codes	1.0	(1)	−.03	(3)

Notes:
[a] From *Diagnostic and Statistical Manual of Mental Disorders* (3rd ed.) (Washington, DC: American Psychiatric Association, 1980), p. 471. No data from the case summary study are reported for children and adolescents.
[b] The numbers in parentheses in this column refer to the number of subjects given each diagnosis by at least one clinician.

Table 6.3. Kappa Coefficients of Agreement for Axis II, Personality Disorders and Specific Developmental Disorders, in the Field Trials (number)[a]

	Adults		Children	
Category	Phase One[b]	Phase Two[b]	Phase One[b]	Phase Two[b]
Specific Developmental Disorders (includes 6 specific diagnoses)		.40 (4)	.77 (16)	.51 (16)
Personality Disorders (includes 12 specific diagnoses)	.56 (203)	.65 (165)	.56 (19)	.61 (10)
Overall kappa for Axis II	.56	.64	.66	.55

Notes:
[a] From *Diagnostic and Statistical Manual of Mental Disorders* (3rd ed.) (Washington, DC, American Psychiatric Association, 1980), pp. 470–471. No data from the case summary study or on the reliability of specific diagnoses have been published.
[b] The numbers in parentheses in this column refer to the number of subjects given each diagnosis by at least one clinician.

them, even though they reported earlier in DSM-III that reliability data had been collected on all five axes (APA, 1980:467). Apparently not all the data collected were analyzed or, if analyzed, reported.

Compared with the complexities of axes I, II, and III, axes IV and V were surprisingly simple: Each consisted of a single ordinal scale item. Axis IV asked the clinician to make a judgment of the severity of all psychosocial stressors on a single 7-point scale. The result was a single number that was supposed to represent the combined impact of all stresses from all sources. Axis V consisted of ratings of the patient's highest level of adaptive functioning in all aspects of life during the past year on a single seven-point ordinal scale. Tables 6.4 and 6.5 present the reliability of these axes in the field trials (using the intraclass correlations that were reported in DSM-III). For both axes, the picture was mixed, and the scores declined substantially for children between Phase One and Phase Two. Reliability for adults on Axis IV was below .70 and the scores on Axis V were the only ones that appeared to be good. Despite its higher scores, dissatisfaction with Axis V led to a complete revision in DSM-III-R.

Given that even the combined overall reliability for axes I and II did not reach the self-imposed .70 standard and that there were other reliability problems in various categories, one would expect serious concerns to have been raised about the reliability, and therefore the validity, of the classification system. But they were not. Instead, the data were interpreted liberally and inconsistently. The interpretation of the case summary study was particularly instructive. Instead of viewing the case summary study as a research method that permitted greater experimental control and therefore less chance for contamination between independent diagnosticians, the researchers (Hyler et al., 1982) went to great lengths to discredit the case summary methodology and an earlier re-

Table 6.4. Kappa Coefficients of Agreement for Axis IV, Severity of Psychosocial Stressors, in the Field Trials[a]

Adults and Children/Adolescents	Phase One[b]	Phase Two[b]
Adults	.60 (308)	.66 (293)
Children and adolescents	.75 (69)	.59 (53)

Notes:
[a] From *Diagnostic and Statistical Manual and Mental Disorders* (3rd ed.) (Washington, DC, American Psychiatric Association, 1980), p. 472. No data from the case summary study have been reported.
[b] The numbers in parentheses in this column refer to the number of patients in each category in each phase.

Table 6.5.   Kappa Coefficients of Agreement for Axis V,
Highest Level of Adaptive Functioning in the Past Year,
in the Field Trials[a]

Adults and Children/Adolescents	Phase One[b]	Phase Two[b]
Adults	.75 (321)	.80 (316)
Children and adolescents	.77 (67)	.52 (53)

Notes:
[a] From *Diagnostic and Statistical Manual and Mental Disorders* (3rd ed.)
(Washington, DC, American Psychiatric Association, 1980), p. 472. No
data from the case summary study have been reported.
[b] The numbers in parentheses in this column refer to the number of
patients in each category in each phase.

liability study by Cantwell et al. (1979) that had used it and found relatively low interrater agreement.

The Issue of Specific Diagnoses

The review of data from the field trials thus far has been in the terms
defined by the developers of DSM-III. Those terms obscure a fundamental issue regarding psychiatric diagnosis on axes I and II. In the field trial
reports, the reliability statistics were based on the "class" of the
disorder—not on the specific diagnosis. Although the developers of
DSM-III acknowledged this in their discussion of the results of the field
trials, its significance is usually blurred by subsequent interpretations
(APA, 1980:468).

When two field trial clinicians made different diagnoses, diagnostic
agreement was considered "perfect" if the diagnoses fell in the same
class. For example, if one clinician judged a series of patients to be
suffering from Agoraphobia with Panic Attacks and another clinician
thought all the same patients suffered from Obsessive Compulsive Disorder, their diagnoses would be considered in perfect agreement on the
diagnostic class of Anxiety Disorders and the kappa coefficient would be
1.0. Furthermore, the DSM-III multiaxial system encourages multiple
diagnoses both within and between axes I and II. Consequently, the
following could occur: One clinician could determine that a patient's
major disorder was an Axis I Dysthymic Disorder with a secondary Axis
II Borderline Personality Disorder, while a second clinician assessing the
same patient could make a diagnosis of Major Depression with a secondary diagnosis of Histrionic Personality Disorder. The foregoing diagnoses would be interpreted, using kappa statistics and class agreement,
as *perfect* diagnostic agreement even though there was *no agreement* on

specific diagnoses! There is every indication that the developers of DSM-III used these liberal definitions in computing diagnostic agreement and, by doing so, the practical meaning of reliability is confused. The most significant question about reliability is this: How frequently do clinicians using DSM-III agree in their diagnoses of specific disorders? The field trials data provide only a little information about this pivotal issue.

In Axis I, there were 17 different major *classes* of diagnoses for adults and children. For some of the major classes, there are *subclasses*, and for all the classes and subclasses, there are *specific discrete diagnoses*. For example, in the major class Disorders Usually First Evident in Infancy, Childhood or Adolescence, there were 9 subclasses and 39 discrete diagnoses. Table 6.6 presents each major class with the number of specific diagnoses available. Also in the table are the number of specific diag-

Table 6.6. Reliability of Specific Diagnoses for Axis I: Adults

Major Class of Disorder	Number of Specific Diagnoses Available	Number of Specific Diagnoses with Reported Kappa in Either Phase One or Phase Two
Disorders Usually First Evident in Infancy, Childhood, or Adolescence	39	7
Organic Mental Disorders	41	3
Substance Use Disorders	19	0
Schizophrenic Disorders	5	0
Paranoid Disorders	4	0
Psychotic Disorders Not Elsewhere Classified	4	0
Affective Disorders	9	3
Anxiety Disorders	10	0
Somatoform Disorders	5	0
Disassociative Disorders	5	0
Psychosexual Disorders	22	3
Factitious Disorders	3	0
Disorders of Impulse Control Not Elsewhere Classified	6	0
Adjustment Disorder	8	0
Psychological Factors Affecting Physical Conditions	1	0
V codes	13	0
Additional codes	3	0
Total	197	16

Note: From *Diagnostic and Statistical Manual of Mental Disorders* (3rd ed.) (Washington, DC: American Psychiatric Association, 1980), pp. 15–19, 470.

noses about which any reliability data were reported in DSM-III. In all, DSM-III allowed for nearly 200 specific diagnoses on Axis I. Kappas were reported for only 16 specific adult diagnoses. Only 9 of 26 kappas reported for these 16 specific adult diagnoses had reliability levels at or above .70. And for nearly 180 specific diagnoses, nothing was reported about the reliability of their use.

For Axis II, Personality Disorders and Specific Developmental Disorders, in which half the adult and a quarter of the child/adolescent diagnoses were made, no reliability data by specific diagnosis were provided in the DSM-III tables. But, even as a class, neither adult nor child/adolescent diagnoses reached the .70 level (see Table 6.3). There are 12 specific personality disorders for adults and 6 specific developmental disorders for children/adolescents, but no systematic reliability data were reported for them. Instead of giving the reader a full account, DSM-III provided the reader with selective information and an interpretation of the data as follows:

> Although Personality Disorder as a class is evaluated more reliably than previously, with the exception of Antisocial Personality Disorder (kappa 0.87 and 0.65 in Phase One and Phase Two, respectively), the kappas for the specific Personality Disorders are quite low and range from 0.26 to 0.75. (APA, 1980:468)

The decline in scores for antisocial personality should have stimulated some discussion, particularly since the other personality disorders, although not revealed, were quite low. Furthermore, since there have been serious controversies about the scientific basis for some of the specific personality disorders, one would have expected some extended probing. Instead, one gets the hint of bad news, presented in a way that avoids giving all the messy details. The reliability of this major class of disorders, therefore, for both the specific diagnoses and for the general class of personality disorders, cannot be described as good.

Small Numbers

Other questions about the analyses can be raised. *Many of the kappas reported are based on very small numbers.* For example, in the table on axes I and II, DSM-III Diagnostic Classes for Children and Adolescents, the reported kappa for the subclass diagnosis of Atypical Affective Disorders in Phase One was −.01 (less than chance agreement) on the basis of two cases. In Phase Two for the same diagnosis, a perfect kappa of 1.0 was reported on the basis of only one case (APA, 1980:471). Some may want to interpret such change between the two phases as improvement, but prudent researchers would simply report that the numbers were too small in both phases to draw any conclusions and the kappas would not even be given (Grove et al., 1981:412). In fact, 22 major categories (in Phase One and Phase Two and in the Case Summary study; see Table 6.1) have five or fewer cases; for children 19 out of 24 categories have five or fewer cases (Table 6.2). Obviously, if data for specific diagnoses had been presented, the few cases per cell might have highlighted the shakiness of drawing any general conclusions about reliability. Thus, the failure to report much data by specific diagnoses and the use of the aggregate major classes of disorders as the unit for computing reliability obscured two serious problems: that of small numbers and that of the unreliability or lack of data about specific diagnoses.

There are other serious problems with the data as presented. For example, the data about adults in Phase Two in the class Disorders Usually First Evident in Infancy, Childhood, or Adolescence reported a kappa of .73 based on 12 cases. Kappas were reported for only four of the seven subclasses and none were reported for any of the 39 specific diagnoses in this major class. Nevertheless, three of the four subclass kappas were at chance agreement ($-.003$, $-.003$, $.002$) and the fourth for mental retardation was .83 based on seven of the 12 cases. Consequently, the major class agreement was reported as good (.73) even though five of the 12 cases had only chance agreement. Moreover, the inclusion of mental retardation, which is determined primarily by test results, not clinical interviews, helped improve the kappa for the entire class, obscuring the complete unreliability of the other diagnoses in this class. This problem has also been noted by others (Rutter & Shaffer, 1980).

Thus, there were many grounds on which to question the sanguine interpretations of reliability given by the proponents of DSM-III. Certainly, the field trial data themselves offered no impressive endorsement that problems of reliability were things of the past. But, even if the field trial data were equivocal, were there other reliability studies of DSM-III that consistently showed that it had resolved the reliability problem?

Additional Reliability Studies

For a few years after the publication of DSM-III, other studies bearing on its diagnostic reliability appeared. Although few of these studies had the full scope of the field trials, they each provided some independent evidence of the reliability of DSM-III.

Adults

Mellsop and his colleagues (1982) studied the reliability of DSM-III Axis II diagnoses for adults using blind, independent ratings of three psychiatrists in everyday clinical settings. Agreement among them on the major class Personality Disorders, as measured by kappa, was .41, lower than in the field trials. Kappas for specific personality disorders ranged from chance to .49, poor agreement, and substantially less than the scores reported in the field trials. As Mellsop and Varghese concluded: "This study confirms the findings of the DSM-III field trials that there is relatively poor agreement on the diagnoses of specific personality disorder subtypes" (p. 268).

Lieberman and Baker (1985) studied 50 adult patients diagnosed in a psychiatric emergency service who were later admitted to an inpatient unit. Both clinical settings made DSM-III diagnoses on Axis I. Only the kappa for alcohol abuse achieved a level greater than .70 (.77). The other major classes had kappas ranging from .29 to .62; for example, for schizophrenia the kappa was .41; for organic brain syndrome, .37; and for other psychotic disorders, .32.

Hanada and Takahashi translated DSM-III into Japanese and conducted a reliability study of 345 adult patients in seven psychiatric facilities in Japan (Hanada & Takahashi, 1983). Participants were 103 experienced university-affiliated psychiatrists who participated in several seminars on using DSM-III for the evaluation of patients. Two clinicians interviewed the same patient and completed the diagnostic forms, noting Axes I and II diagnoses. Kappas for 10 of the 17 major diagnostic classes in Axis I were below .70. The kappa for Axis II (personality disorders) was .43.

In the second part of their study, Hanada and Takahashi selected 14 diagnostic categories and assigned 2 categories to each of the 7 psychiatric departments. Each department was asked to select patients who fit that assigned category, videotape interviews with them, and prepare two-page case vignettes for each of the two patients. These videotapes were edited to 30 minutes and, along with the case vignettes, were circulated to participants at the other six clinics who were instructed to evaluate them independently. In this part of the study, 140 clinicians participated, contributing 1,100 evaluations. Hanada and Takahashi did not provide information about how these clinicians were selected or how the independence of evaluations was assured. Also, they did not note the possibility (if not probability) that patients deliberately chosen because they clearly fit an assigned diagnostic category may be more easily diagnosed than are other patients. On Axis I, six major classes were above .70 and three were below. The other classes were lumped together and had only chance agreement. The Axis II kappa was a low .33.

Lipton and Simon used seven clinical experts to reevaluate the charts of 131 randomly selected patients following the introduction of DSM-III in New York State mental health facilities (Lipton & Simon, 1985). On reevaluation, only 16 out of 89 chart diagnoses of schizophrenia were confirmed; 50 rather than 15 diagnoses of affective disorder were made; and organic disorders were diagnosed in 26 patients, 19 more than had been so diagnosed in the charts. Lipton and Simon concluded that documentation of DSM-III criteria for the chart diagnosis was not present in 80% of the 131 charts reviewed. Although their study was not a controlled study of reliability as such, such evidence of misdiagnosis may be much more suggestive about the actual accuracy of the use of DSM-III in normal clinical settings.

As part of a case summary survey of sex bias in diagnosis, DeVault and Dambrot (1983) mailed a standard case from the DSM-III casebook to 369 clinicians. Among the 90 usable questionnaires returned, 77% correctly identified the diagnosis within the Affective Disorders class, but only 27% correctly made the specific diagnosis and only 4% agreed with the exact diagnosis listed in the DSM-III casebook.

Another study described the results of an intensive two-and-one-half-day training program designed to teach 251 experienced mental health professionals to use DSM-III (Webb et al., 1981). Training involved written material about DSM-III, a curriculum guide, slides, exercises, and discussions of written and videotaped case vignettes. Following this instruction, each participant viewed three of five videotaped case interviews. Four of the five tapes were simulations by actors, based on DSM-III criteria, for a given disorder. The "true" principal diagnosis for each of the five cases was determined by the faculty (expert opinion) of the training program. If any of the axis I or II diagnoses listed by the participants agreed with the principal diagnosis of the experts, agreement was obtained. Even with this intensive training, simulated interviews that illustrated obvious disorders, and liberal definition of agreement, less than 75% of these experienced participants could correctly make the diagnosis.

Skodal, working with other colleagues in the New York group, reported their experiences in teaching and supervising 10 psychiatric residents and 5 psychology interns to use DSM-III accurately (Skodal, Williams, & Spitzer, 1984). All trainees received didactic training in using DSM-III, and the residents had considerable additional exposure to DSM-III, including a three-month course in diagnostic interviewing. The trainees were supervised by the authors after about three diagnostic interviews with 200 new patients at an outpatient clinic during a one-year period. After the trainees completed each evaluation of a patient, they presented their multiaxial-axial diagnosis of the case to their supervisors (two of whom were Spitzer and Williams). After thorough discussion of the case, the supervisors recorded their DSM-III diagnosis of the case. Diagnostic disagreement occurred when the trainee's diagnosis differed from that of the supervisor. Although these judgments clearly were not "independent" in any way and the developers of DSM-III were themselves participants in the study, Skodal et al. reported that 36% of Axis I diagnoses were in error; 11% of Axis II; 3.5% of Axis III; 22% of Axis IV; and 13% of Axis V. The authors admitted that these trainees had more exposure to DSM-III than had most clinicians, that they undoubtedly paid more attention to diagnostic issues because they knew they had to substantiate carefully their diagnoses for their supervisor, and that, consequently, in a normal outpatient clinic without such training or supervision, "the frequency of errors is probably much higher" (p. 254).

There are two studies that have indirectly examined the reliability of DSM's Axis III, Physical Illnesses Relevant to Mental Disorders. Both studies appeared years after DSM-III was published. In one, Maricle, Leung, & Bloom (1987) retrospectively studied the charts of 50 randomly selected discharged psychiatric inpatients. They found that medical findings were poorly reflected by the diagnoses listed on Axis III. Only 12% of the total sample received Axis III diagnoses that accurately reflected abnormal results of physical exams and laboratory tests. Similarly, a prospective study by D'Ercole, Skodal, Struening, Curtis, & Millman (1991) studied the use of Axis III by psychiatrists who diagnosed a random sample of 357 primarily black and unemployed persons shortly after they were admitted to an inpatient facility in Harlem. The patients' health status was independently assessed by a physician's assistant using a standardized health status form. They compared the psychiatrists' Axis III diagnoses with those obtained by the physician's assistant and found that psychiatrists had significantly underreported physical illnesses on Axis III. Only 24% of the physical illnesses that were apparently present were identified on Axis III, calling into question not only the reliability, but the validity of this axis.

A study at the University of British Columbia followed a cohort of 154 patients who experienced their first episodes of psychosis during 1982 to 1984 (Bassett & Beiser, 1991). An initial assessment was made by a research clinician using a semistructured clinical interview. Additional information was gathered by research assistants from each subject, from significant others, and from referral sources. These data were then evaluated by at least two clinicians to record the presence or absence of all the criteria relevant to each DSM-III diagnosis. Using a strict application of the DSM-III rules, diagnoses were made for each patient. These research diagnoses were then compared with the community-based clinicians' diagnoses for these same patients. The kappa scores were all considerably lower than in the DSM-III field trials. For Axis I, the kappa were .26 for Schizophrenic Disorders, .53 for affective disorders, .08 for Psychotic Disorders Not Elsewhere Classified, .05 for Paranoid Disorders; the overall kappa was .21. For Axis II, the kappa was .24 and for Axis III it was .41.

One of the most important psychiatric research efforts undertaken in the early 1980s was the NIMH-sponsored Epidemiological Catchment Area study, a gigantic community survey in five cities to document the distribution of mental disorders in the population. The entire study was grounded on DSM-III diagnostic criteria and used a carefully constructed structured interview schedule. The Baltimore site included a check for the reliability of the diagnoses made on 810 community residents (Anthony et al., 1985). Residents were first interviewed by highly trained lay interviewers using the structured Diagnostic Interview Schedule, based on DSM-III criteria, and later were interviewed by one of four research psychiatrists, also well trained in using DSM-III criteria. Agreement between the lay and psychiatric interviewers was reported by kappa. Among the eight major diagnostic categories, no category obtained a kappa above .35 and seven of the eight kappas were below .26.

Children/Adolescents

Cantwell et al. (1979) asked 20 child psychiatrists at the Department of Child Psychiatry, University of California at Los Angeles, independently to complete diagnostic questionnaires for 24 actual case histories. All the clinicians were using an early draft of DSM-III for the first time. The overall level of agreement among the raters with the expected diagnosis was 49%, and there was a striking inconsistency within the diagnostic groups. The authors also computed interrater agreement using both DSM-III and DSM-II. (Unfortunately, as with some of the other studies, kappas were not computed, which makes comparisons difficult. However, this was one of the few studies that actually compared the reliability of DSM-II and DSM-III.) Interrater agreement for DSM-II was 57% (range 20–95%) and for Axis I of DSM-III it was slightly *lower*—54% (range 20–100%). The authors concluded that DSM-III Axis I was only slightly less reliable than DSM-II, but looked promising. Interrater agreement on the other axes ranged from 63 to 90%.

Strober, Green, and Carlson (1981) jointly interviewed 95 adolescent consecutive first admissions at a university inpatient unit using a structured interview. Prior to the interview, they reviewed all available collateral information, including school records, referral notes from prior psychiatric contacts, detailed nursing notes on the patient's initial days of hospitalization, and so forth. Each of the two raters then made a DSM-III diagnosis. Only the primary diagnoses were reported in the study. Kappas were reported by major diagnostic class after the data were collapsed into a series of 2 × 2 contingency tables (such as schizophrenic versus nonschizophrenic). The kappa coefficients for major classes ranged from .47 to 1.0 and had an overall kappa of .74. When there were sufficient data available on more specific diagnoses, the kappa ranged from .46 to 1.0. Only 4 of 10 specific diagnoses were greater than .70.

Werry et al. (1983) diagnosed 195 admissions to a child psychiatric inpatient unit in New Zealand. The DSM-III diagnoses were made by two to four clinicians on the basis of case presentations at ward rounds, part of the normal clinical procedures. Reliability was calculated using kappa. Using 17 major diagnostic categories, the researchers found that 7 had kappas greater than .70. They also reported kappas for 41 specific diagnoses, only 7 of which were greater than .70. They concluded that there are serious problems with the reliability of the specific diagnoses in DSM-III.

One study (Rey, Plapp, Stewart, Richard, & Bashir, 1987) examined the reliability of the use of DSM-III axes IV and V on an adolescent unit at a hospital in Australia. Two clinicians who had three years of experience using DSM-III rated 140 adolescents on axes IV and V. Using two related intraclass correlations, they got reliability coefficients of .44 and .46 for Axis IV and .58 and .58 for Axis V. This level of reliability was lower than they obtained using an alternative system, the Psychosocial Adversity Index. They concluded that their data "are best interpreted as independent evidence of the relatively poor reliability of axes IV and V in adolescent patients" (p. 232).

Claiming Success

As we have seen, following the publication of DSM-III, a broad scattering of studies with both adults and children reported data that were not better and usually somewhat worse than the reliability levels reported in the field trials. More significantly, neither the data from the field trials nor the other studies strongly supported the remarkable claims that were made about the reliability of DSM-III.

The developers of DSM-III repeatedly asserted that careful, systematic field trials established the improved scientific reliability of DSM-III. However, important information about the methods and findings of the field trials was never reported. Some of the reports were inconsistent and unclear. The field trials themselves could more accurately be described as uncontrolled, nonrandom surveys in which several hundred self-selected and unsupervised pairs of clinicians throughout the country attempted to diagnose nonrandomly selected patients and, after some sharing of information, made "independent" assessments of these patients. The possibility for contamination between clinicians obviously was great, although this was dismissed as a minor problem based on the self-reports of the participants to the developers (Hyler et al., 1982). Other than the researchers' through-the-mail admonitions that participants should avoid conferring about their diagnoses, the researchers had no way to control either deliberate or unintentional contamination that would bias the data in the direction of higher reliability scores (Grove et al., 1981). Furthermore, nowhere is it reported how many clinicians initially agreed to participate in the reliability studies versus how many eventually submitted usable data. Were the participants more likely to be close colleagues, who had similar training and experience and similar orientations? Were those who had more difficulty with the diagnostic system or those pairs who found that their diagnostic judgments were in disagreement less likely to submit their results than were others? It would appear to be a plausible hypothesis. If this happened, then even the levels of reliability that were reported may have been overestimates.

Rutter and Shaffer, who were among the researchers to comment on the methodological quality of the field trials, concluded:

> as pieces of research they leave much to be desired. [The reliability was based on] agreements only between close colleagues . . . an unknown data base which differed from pair to pair . . . no uniformity in the information provided . . . no control over adherence to the rules and no means of preventing consultation between two clinicians making supposedly independent diagnostic codings. [Thus, the field trial findings] do little to provide a scientific basis for DSM-III. (1980:386)

Despite the fact that aspects of the methodology of the field trials may have inflated diagnostic agreement, the reliability for major classes of disorders was questionable even if the developers' own standards were applied. On no axis were the reliability data (as expressed in kappa) consistently good. And in some important areas, such as personality disorders and diagnoses for children and adolescents, the reliability data often were poor. Moreover, by using major classes of disorders as the categories on which to calculate diagnostic agreement, even when there was little or no agreement on specific diagnoses, the entire presentation of reliability appeared higher than it really was for specific diagnoses.

The standards to be used in judging levels of reliability should depend on how the measure will be used. Standards of reliability should depend on the purposes of the assessment and their consequences. Take an example from another field. In our criminal justice system, the standards of evidence to make an arrest are much more liberal than the standards for convicting someone of murder and subjecting them to capital punishment. In psychiatry, the consequences of diagnostic decisions vary tremendously. At times, a psychiatric diagnosis can be harmless and at other times can deprive a person of personal liberties, as in the duPont case. Standards of certainty should vary accordingly. One prominent psychometrician argued that standards of reliability for various tests and measures could be relatively low for exploratory research purposes, but should be considerably higher when used in applied settings to study differences between groups or when the diagnostic decisions about individuals will have important consequences (Nunnally, 1978:245–246). For example, in using IQ or other aptitude tests to select students for special classes or where important decisions are made, he argues that a reliability coefficient should be very high and that low ones should not be tolerated.

In this chapter, we have accepted the developers' interpretation of what constitutes good reliability (i.e., .70), but the .70 standard is not sacred. We initially considered the field trial results in relation to it because this was the only standard of good reliability suggested by the developers of DSM-III. It may be too high or too low to use for psychiatric diagnoses, whether major classes or specific diagnoses are used. Or, as Spitznagel and Helzer (1985) suggested, it may even be meaningless without reference to the prevalence of the disorder in the study population. We have found only one paper that proposes explicit interpretive standards for kappa. It was published by researchers in New York a decade later (Mannuzza et al., 1989), but its authors are quick to emphasize that a specific kappa value may suggest good reliability in one type of study and only fair reliability in another (p. 1095) and that "it can be misleading to compare kappa values across studies (even studies reporting on the same diagnoses)" (p. 1100).

In fact, "meaninglessness" may be close to what can be claimed about the reliability field trials. Without consideration of the statistical complexities of sensitivity, specificity, and base rates in the DSM-III studies, any generalization is hazardous. The lack of data on most specific diagnoses, combined with the small numbers for some classes, suggests that the claims of good reliability were, at best, premature.

Even more problematic was the confluence of statistical and methodological problems in the field trials. Statisticians know, for example, that the standard error of proportions increases as the proportion in the population of a binomial (e.g., disorder vs. no disorder) declines or is skewed (as in low base rates) and as the number of cases declines (Kachigan, 1986). Or in layman language, studies of diagnosis using small and skewed samples contain more errors. Therefore, some statistics, like kappa, that are based on proportions are particularly affected by low base rates and small numbers of subjects. The field trials encountered both of these problems, although they were never explicitly acknowledged.

Furthermore, kappas derived from different studies or from different settings that may have had different base rates and different sample sizes cannot be easily or meaningfully compared. Indiscriminate interpretation of kappa across disparate studies can lead to false conclusions (Mannuzza et al., 1989). Since the field trial data were gathered at multiple sites, each with different or unknown base rates and with unknown rates of diagnostic practices (tendencies toward making more of particular types of diagnoses), the pooling of results creates problems. For example, if the diagnoses of two clinicians working at an anxiety clinic where 90% of their patients present with some "anxiety disorder" are lumped with the diagnoses of two clinicians working in a general mental health center where only 20% of their patients are expected to have some "anxiety disorder," the results can be misleading. Similarly, analyzing the data from the two clinics separately, while controlling for the base rate problem, will not lead to kappas that can be meaningfully compared with each other (Carey & Gottesman, 1978). The presentation of the field trial data ignored these issues, lumped all data from all sites together, calculated kappa without specifying exactly how the data were handled, and reported partial results with sanguine interpretations.

Despite all these problems, the claims of greatly improved reliability were not the focus of debate or scrutiny but, rather, as we have discussed at the beginning of this chapter, the object of adoration. Gerald Klerman, who was the administrator of the Alcohol, Drug and Mental Health Administration during the time the agency funded the field studies, and who often served as a promoter and defender of DSM-III, praised the results of the field trials. He went so far as to declare that the problem of reliability was "solved," that DSM-III marked a "great scientific achievement," that debate about it was an "anachronism," and that DSM-III had already been "declared a victory" by psychiatrists, psychologists, and other mental health professionals (Klerman, 1984:541–542, 1987; Kutchins & Kirk, 1987a). What is noteworthy is Klerman's bold use of the rhetoric of politics, not the observations of scientific method, to claim victory when the actual data suggested, at the very best, a slight and difficult advance.

It was the claims of success, however, that were successful. Few questioned the methodology or the data presented, few suggested that major new independent reliability studies should be undertaken, and most observers persisted in believing that diagnostic reliability took a giant step forward with DSM-III. So successful have the claims been that no one seems to have noticed that many diagnostic categories were retained in DSM-III regardless of their reliability. High, only satisfactory, or poor reliability appears to have had little effect on the decisions about what was included in the diagnostic system.

DSM and psychiatry are by no means alone in reporting and then embracing dubious research findings. Flawed research is widespread throughout the medical literature (Lipton & Hershaft, 1985). A survey of 760 articles on medicine found that 58% reported no statistics or only descriptive statistics. Another study of articles in medical journals found that 52% of the studies did not present clear statistics and in only 19% was there any recognition that uncontrolled factors may have contaminated the results (Lipton & Hershaft, 1985). Similar weaknesses have been raised about articles in social work journals as well (Huxley, 1986, 1988). Blame for these limitations can be shared by authors, journal editors, and manuscript reviewers. Methodological weaknesses are not easily detected by unsophisticated readers or even by overworked journal referees. Nevertheless, the complete success of DSM-III cannot be attributed only to busy schedules and hasty reviews. The developers must be given some of the credit.

In the next chapter, we attempt to explain the developers' remarkable achievement by examining how these potentially troublesome reliability findings were presented so effectively in claiming success and persuading others that reliability was no longer considered to be a serious threat to psychiatry. To do this, we look carefully at the rhetoric of science used to present these findings and how the process was managed.

7

THE ART OF CLAIM-MAKING

Perhaps the most important part of the study was the evaluation of diagnostic reliability. . . . The results . . . generally indicate far greater reliability than had previously been obtained with DSM-II.

Robert L. Spitzer, *Introduction to DSM-III*

By itself a given sentence is neither fact nor a fiction; it is made so by others, later on.

Bruno Latour, *Science in Action*

[T]he DSM-III committees and task forces of APA produced amazing documents that did indeed change the shape of American Psychiatry. While it was a brilliant tour de force, its acceptance was deeply influenced by the dire need for objectification in American psychiatry. We needed to prove to many people that psychiatric disorders could be diagnosed and that a rational basis for determining how to deal with psychiatric patients could be developed.

Melvin Sabshin, *American Journal of Psychiatry*

In an ingenious study, a researcher examined the content of the speeches of ten recent United States presidents (Tetlock, 1981), both before they were elected and at several time periods after they were elected to office. The focus was on presidential rhetoric, particularly the extent to which the candidates (and then later as officeholders) discussed public policy issues in simplistic or complex ways. The study found support for an "impression management" hypothesis, which predicted that candidates talk about issues in deliberately simplistic ways during election campaigns but in more complex ways upon assuming office when they face the necessity of justifying sometimes unpopular decisions to skeptical constituencies. Transitions from simplicity to garner support to complexity to ward off skeptics is not confined to presidential politics.

Complaints about diagnostic reliability had initially provided a simple rhetoric to talk about problems in American psychiatry. As the problem was pushed to the forefront by a small group of researchers who gained prominence and power within the APA, the problem was converted into a more complex technical problem for which solutions could be constructed—at least in controlled research settings. As we have illustrated in the previous chapter, they then claimed successfully that the reliability problem had been solved, even though the actual data presented and the other available research were equivocal.

In this chapter, we extend the analysis in three ways: First, we look at the use of language in key articles that presented the field trial findings, language that encouraged a favorable interpretation of the data. Second, we examine the way in which the standards of what constituted good reliability were shifted dramatically in order to sell DSM-III. We show, for example, that the DSM-III results were little better than the early reliability studies and not nearly as good as what had been achieved in the RDC research. Finally, we review several aspects of the management of science that helped to facilitate the remarkable achievements of the DSM-III Task Force.

Claim-Making and the Scientific Article

Major scientific achievements are rarely the result of a discrete, single, isolated occurrence. Few breakthroughs come from a single laboratory finding so robust and unambiguous that the investigators know immediately what has happened. Discovery is a reiterative process of observation, inference, interpretation, and communication. Interpretation and communication occur among members of a team working on a scientific problem and between that team and interested outside audiences. Within the investigating group, decisions must be made about what observations to make, when to make them, how the preliminary results should be interpreted, and with what degree of confidence or skepticism. Making sense of their observations is a complex social interaction, not just a technical process. Hundreds of microdecisions confront researchers. Decisions must be made about how to describe the observations they have chosen to make, and how and when to communicate with other interested researchers. Although established scientific procedures guide the general process of research (e.g., how to gather information, how to organize it for statistical analysis, and how to decide how much information should be included in a journal article), numerous small decisions are made throughout every research project that are never revealed in the final report, either because they are so routine that the investigators are not conscious of them as research decisions or because there are too many of them to describe in journals demanding brevity (Kuhn, 1970; Latour & Woolgar, 1986; Latour, 1987, 1988).

Claims about scientific findings are not captured by any one specific development occurring in one place or at one time, but rather involve a process that unfolds over many years and includes many people and occasions (Watson, 1968; Kuhn, 1970; Latour & Woolgar, 1986; Latour, 1987, 1988). Most of those developments are private and leave no readily accessible archival record. They occur in the scientific lab, in the library, at the computer center, and in small group discussions among the primary investigators. The process of constructing scientific findings happens in private discussions among close colleagues, personal memos, telephone calls, staff meetings, chance encounters, and other normal social interaction. Those interested in studying the process of scientific discovery either must be participant observers of these processes at the time (cf. Latour & Woolgar, 1986) or rely on the ex post facto reports of the participants themselves to reconstruct the unfolding of discovery and claim-making (cf. Hazen, 1988).

Reconstructing the claims made about the reliability of DSM-III faces these same limitations. No outside, disinterested observer participated in the process and recorded the development of the reliability claims. The members of the DSM-III Task Force have written few insider accounts and those accounts have not focused at all on the reliability field trials but on more controversial topics such as the diagnosis of homosexuality, neurosis, or self-defeating personality disorder (Millon, 1986; Bayer & Spitzer, 1982, 1985; Bayer, 1981; Walker, 1986).

Thus, we are left to examine claims about reliability that were made publicly. Whatever the early microprocess of developing scientific claims, the phase of "going public" is the critical one. If the claims are rejected, ignored, or seriously questioned, the time-consuming efforts behind them may have been in vain. If the claims are rejected because of methodological or statistical errors or oversights, the reputations of the researchers may be tarnished. Consequently, investigators usually take great care in determining what claims they are going to make, how they are going to make them, and what information about their methodology or procedures they are going to reveal. They also carefully consider how to persuade outside audiences of the wisdom of their interpretations of the findings. In short, an enormously important part of any scientific achievement is how and what the principal investigators say about their work as they offer it to the scientific and professional community (Gusfield, 1981).

The standard, widely accepted mechanism for making scientific claims is to publish an article in a scientific or professional journal. This follows the recognized norms of science, which emphasize (1) universalism (that claims are subjected to preestablished impersonal criteria), (2) communalism (that scientific findings become public intellectual property), (3) disinterestedness (enforced through the "exacting scrutiny of fellow experts"), and (4) organized skepticism (in which the scientist can question beliefs often ritualized by others) (Merton, 1973). Publication officially places the intellectual property in public space and allows other experts to judge the extent to which claims are well founded in impersonal criteria and are disinterested. Publications are bids for scientific legitimacy.

Scientific journal articles are more than dry, disembodied reports, full of facts without soul. To the contrary, the scientific article is itself an intricate method of persuasion, a form of rhetoric (Latour, 1987). Every author must make a series of choices about what types of information to convey about the subject under study, what symbols to use, and how tight to make the fit between language and object. Through explicit citations and implicit assumptions, authors connects their work to the previous literature on the subject, placing their articles where they think they belong in the realm of knowledge. Each article is an argument addressed to certain readers, and assumptions have to be made about the audience's level of knowledge and attitudes about the subject. The author conveys some charge to the readers, something they should believe or do after being convinced by the argument. Finally, by making statements about personal thoughts, purposes and feelings, an author conveys a unique persona, a public face, and becomes a distinctive person with a point of view:

> A text is, in a sense, a solution to the problem of how to make a statement that attends through the symbols of language to all essential contexts appropriately. More explicitly, an article is an answer to the question, "Against the background of accumulated knowledge of the discipline, how can I present an original claim about a phenomenon to the appropriate audience convincingly so that thinking and behaviour will be modified accordingly?" A successful answer is rewarded by its becoming an accepted formulation. (Bazerman, 1981:363–364)

In the previous chapter we examined reliability claims in relation to the standards offered by the primary investigators. Here we will go beyond the standards for judging reliability that were offered, and discuss several prominent aspects of the rhetoric used in making claims. Examining key journal articles capitalizes on the fact that these articles represented finely tuned, public announcements of scientific achievements. Since they appeared in leading professional journals, they were readily accessible. Moreover, as archival information, they reflect the spirit of their time, undistorted by selective reminisces or the modesty that comes with future wisdom.

The First Word

The claims about the reliability of DSM-III became an accepted formulation. There are six primary sources that contain claims about the reliability of DSM-III: two early reports about the field trials (Spitzer et al., 1979; Spitzer & Forman, 1979); a later report about the field trials (Hyler et al., 1982); a published interview with Spitzer as DSM-III was published (Talbot, 1980); a lengthy article about DSM-III by the developers published in the *American Journal of Psychiatry* as DSM was released (Spitzer et al., 1980); and DSM-III itself (APA, 1980). Four of these texts report at least some new data; two only refer to and interpret that data. Spitzer and his close associates were the primary authors of all of them. All but one article (Hyler et al., 1982) were published on the eve of the release of DSM-III. Although each contains some discussion and information that the others do not, with regard to reliability, there is considerable redundancy in both content and style of presentation. Since, as we have argued, these articles played an important role in persuading others that a critical and controversial problem had been greatly resolved, how was that accomplished?

The very first article published about the field trials might well have served as the final word, since it contained most of the major claims that would be echoed for years in other publications. More significantly, the manner in which those claims were made set the pattern for the future rhetoric of reliability. The article, "DSM-III Field Trials: I. Initial Interrater Diagnostic Reliability" (Spitzer et al, 1979), is noteworthy on many counts. It was the first public report of the results of the field trials. It was published in the most visible journal in the field, the *American Journal of Psychiatry* (AJP), the major official periodical of the APA, under whose auspices DSM was being revised. The article contained the first public claims about the reliability of DSM-III. Finally, the title of the article itself reveals the centrality of the reliability issue to DSM-III, showing deference to the problem that had for three decades set the stage for DSM-III.

The publication schedule for the article would be the envy of every journal author. As is the custom at AJP, the dates of submission and acceptance are provided on the first page of the article. AJP received the original manuscript on December 11, 1978. Despite the holidays, which normally delay the review and processing of journal articles, it must have received quick attention, because it had been initially reviewed, returned to the authors, revised, and resubmitted in less than three months, by March 8, 1979. Apparently the resubmission received an instant second review, because it was accepted for publication four days after resubmission and sent immediately to press to appear in the June 1979 issue. This brief four-day elapsed time between resubmission and the decision to accept was highly unusual. For example, every other resubmitted article that appeared in either the May or June issue of AJP took considerably longer before it was accepted. Major articles averaged over ten times longer (about 50 days), topical papers averaged about eight times longer (about 35 days), and brief communications took nine times longer (over 36 days). In fact, no article published in the May or June issue came anywhere close to enjoying an acceptance decision in only four days.

Interestingly, the article was extremely brief, not at all in keeping with the complexity of the issues that it addressed or the very lengthy discussions that had preceded it. The entire article was less than three pages in length and contained less than two pages of text. It was published in a section of the journal called *Brief Communications*, a peculiar location for the first report about what had been a central and long-standing problem. The article was the first of a two-part piece, but both parts were published back-to-back in the same issue. The second part dealt primarily with information about the multiaxial character of DSM-III and will not concern us here.

The article contained only three references, all to papers in which Spitzer was the senior author: the 1967 article that had introduced kappa (Spitzer et al., 1967); the 1974 article that had used kappa to reinterpret the early reliability studies (Spitzer & Fleiss, 1974); and, finally, the companion article to the present one, which appeared immediately following it in the journal (Spitzer & Forman, 1979). Symbolically, few other citations were needed. Two enormously important events were footnoted: the introduction of kappa as the quantitative language to be spoken when discussing reliability and the very influential reanalysis of the early reliability studies in which the profession's credibility was said to be at stake. The fact that the footnotes all consisted of self-citations was not unnecessary. Spitzer had, in fact, contributed important papers at the key turning points in the history of the reliability problem and his use of self-citations was justified.

Almost every aspect of the article conveyed something significant about the drama that was unfolding, however routine or modest the presentation. The abstract of the article, frequently the only part actually scanned by busy readers, contained a series of important rhetorical points.

The interrater agreement for major diagnostic categories in studies using DSM-I and DSM-II was usually only fair or poor. In phase one of the DSM-III field trials the overall kappa coefficient of agreement for axis I diagnoses of 281 adult patients was .78 for joint interviews and .66 for diagnoses made after separate interviews; for axis II—personality disorders and specific developmental disorders—the coefficients of agreement were .61 and .54. The interrater reliability of DSM-III is, in general, higher than that previously achieved and may be due to changes in the classification itself, the separation of axis I from axis II conditions, the systematic description of the various disorders, and the inclusion of diagnostic criteria. (Spitzer et al., 1979:815)

The brief article expanded on these points. It described the field trials, emphasizing that everyone in the country was invited to participate and all who volunteered were accepted. They came from everywhere, "from Maine to Hawaii." It briefly described the instructions to those who participated in the reliability study.

The findings were then presented in two paragraphs and one large table. The first paragraph told how many participated and who they were in terms of race/ethnicity, clinical setting, and type of facility. The second paragraph referred to the table, which listed major diagnostic classes and the results of patients interviewed jointly and those done sequentially (test-retest), introduced for the first time the .70 kappa standard as an indicator of good agreement, and introduced the concept of the overall kappa for major classes as "the extent to which there is agreement across all diagnostic classes for all patients given an axis I diagnosis by at least one of the clinicians and is thus an overall index of diagnostic agreement" (pp. 816–817). In the concluding discussion, the authors say:

> For most of the classes, the reliability for both interview situations is quite good and, in general, is higher than that previously achieved using DSM-I and DSM-II. These results were so much better than we had expected that we wondered if our instructions for avoiding bias might have gone unheeded in many cases. (p. 817)

They then reassure the reader that they checked this out by mailing a questionnaire to participants asking them if they had in fact followed the instructions. The reader is told not to worry—participants had reassured the developers that they had not fudged their responses. They conclude by promising:

> In future reports we will present the reliability of the individual diagnostic categories and the results of phase two of the field trial, which involves

reliability interviews to assess the effects of changes made in the DSM-III
classification and in the diagnostic criteria. (p. 817)

The article is very efficient. With modesty and brevity, the authors
presented an upbeat report of a major study that purported to have gone
a long way in remedying the problem of unreliability. Their claims con-
formed nicely with their earlier promises about what a revamped diagnostic system would do and with their advocacy on behalf of the soon-
to-be unveiled DSM-III.

The Uses of Broad Participation

The articles about reliability persuaded not merely by offering statistics, but by the use of language in which the numbers were embedded.
Numbers cannot speak for themselves; the architects of DSM were quick
to provide them a voice that would be heard and a message that would
convince.

In this first article and in subsequent presentations, the developers
frequently referred to the field trials as the largest reliability study ever
undertaken, and they made a point to thank "the field trial clinicians for
their efforts in this work." Although they used different and inconsistent numbers as they made these claims, the rhetorical intent remained
the same: to claim methodological and political legitimacy on the basis of
numerical and geographical vastness. By referring to the diversity of
participants, the authors attempted to buttress their claims about the
methodological quality of the research, particularly about its generalizability. In fact, broad participation in a field trial, if it involved randomly selected clinicians and patients (which the field trials did not),
would allow for generalization from the study sample to the wider uni-
verse of clinicians, clients, and settings. National opinion polls are examples of the systematic use of small samples that are representative of
broader populations.

Large numbers by themselves, however, are of no particular scientific
use, even when they are gathered from participants far and wide. Jimmy
and Tammy Bakker had millions of willing participants from "Maine to
Hawaii," who would dutifully follow instructions by sending money to
the evangelists. We would be hesitant, however, to confer on these
donors the status of being representative of all people or of all Christians
in the United States. Similarly, volunteer, self-selected clinicians from
across the country who heard the call of the developers of DSM-III and
who diagnosed their clients using the new system and then mailed in
their contributions may be appreciated for their cooperation, but their

participation should not be confused with representativeness. Having supporters and contributors from "California to the New York islands" is not necessarily relevant to the methodological quality of a study of diagnostic reliability.

Stressing broad participation, however, has important rhetorical effects that transcend scientific aims. It suggests openness and diversity—a democratization of effort—that helps to establish legitimacy. The field trials were presented as a national effort of many dedicated people, rather than the laboratory work of a few. Although as we have said in Chapter 4, the architecture of DSM-III was primarily the design of a few, it was politically wiser to emphasize its ties to a broader constituency.

The notion of broad participation made frequent appearances in the development and selling of DSM-III. The various DSM-III Task Force advisory groups allowed many to feel that they had a hand in the making of DSM-III. Drafts of the manual were shared widely among others in addition to the participants in the field trials. Lists of names of people who were involved in the making of DSM-III and the credentials (authority) of the participants were dutifully listed in the final manual. The effect was to gain legitimacy by the numbers. The more people involved, the more credible the product.

So Much Better Than We Had Expected

Throughout the discussion about reliability in the field trials, we find the proclamation regularly repeated that the results were "so much better than we had expected" (Spitzer et al., 1979:817). By claiming that the reliability results were so much better than they had expected, they conveyed pleasant surprise. Why should they be surprised? What is gained by claiming surprise? There are two possible ways in which they may have been genuinely surprised at their results.

First, they may have been genuinely surprised because, despite their earlier bold claims about knowing how to improve reliability, they actually did not believe their own rhetoric. Their surprise was the astonishment of former, secret disbelievers.

A second possibility is that they believed that some kind of new diagnostic system might improve reliability, but they never really expected that DSM-III would do the trick or that the field trials would show it. In this case, their surprise was not that reliability was improved, but that this complex manual called DSM-III was responsible for it. In this case, their surprise would stem from their initial lack of faith in the product that they had so painstakingly developed for five years; it would be the surprise born of low expectations.

There is a third possibility: They were not really surprised at all. From the beginning, promises were made about the handsome return that would be reaped by a major investment in diagnostic criteria and structured decision-making. The developers knew well the difficulty of actually achieving that goal; they knew as well the consequences of failing after so much effort. The reliability problem had not at all been solved and yet the promissory note was now due. Under the circumstances, they made the best of field trial outcomes by emphasizing gains where they could be found and trying not to highlight losses. "So much better than we had expected" was part of the rhetoric of success that enveloped DSM-III.

Surprise does have a legitimate role in scientific discovery. Occasionally there are serendipitous findings that surprise the investigator and lead to significant discoveries or the results of a study are found to be the opposite of what was hypothesized. But claiming to improve reliability with DSM-III can hardly be presented as either the result of serendipity (since it was deliberately sought) or a reversal of expectations (since they never predicted that reliability would get worse). Thus, conveying surprise by noting that the results were "so much better than we had expected" is best viewed as a rhetorical device rather than as a scientifically meaningful assertion.

Since the developers had never publicly established, either before or after the field trials, what exactly it was that they expected to find, claiming that what they now found was better than what they may have privately conjured provides no useful information about reliability, but it does provide them with a useful rhetorical platform. Why should the reader care what they privately expected? The reader is made to care by learning that what they are reporting to us is "so much better." It is the "so much better" that constitutes the active ingredient of the phrase. Better than what? the reader might ask. Claiming that something is better always implies a comparison. Consequently, in order to describe the results as "so much better" requires the use of some comparative standard. Since they had not explicitly promulgated any prior standard for reliability, their own expectations thus became a rhetorical vehicle of convenience. It permitted statements about DSM-III to include words like better without immediately exposing them to any verifiable standard.

Throughout the presentation of the field trials articles, the authors use the language of pleasant news. For example, in the first article they state: "It is *particularly encouraging* that the reliability for such categories as schizophrenia and major affective disorders is *so high* (Spitzer et al., 1979:817, emphasis added). This conveys relief and surprise. The reader is made conscious that the authors are proud parents of these findings.

This is an announcement of good, not troubling news. The brevity of the article itself as well as these interpretive statements communicate that the news required little elaboration; readers should surely hear the cheerful message.

The Slippery Standard of "Good"

Another reason why the "so much better than expected" phrase was effective was because no consistent interpretive standard of reliability had ever been established. The reader of the reliability literature looks in vain for standards of what should constitute good reliability.

During the 1950s and 1960s there were clearly no explicit standards. Commentators on reliability wavered in their evaluation of the seriousness of the reliability problem. By the 1970s and the publication of the second wave of reliability studies that used diagnostic criteria and structured interviews, however, a growing consensus developed that reliability had been low previously and that the new diagnostic technologies promised much higher levels. But by the time the field trial results were prepared for public consumption a few years later, the standard for good reliability became particularly slippery. Slipperiness is not, of course, confined to psychiatry; it can be found even among disciplines that pride themselves on their objectivity, such as economics (cf. McCloskey, 1983:496). The focus here is on the instrumental uses to which slipperiness was put in making claims about the reliability of DSM-III.

Let us look at another statement from this first article about the field trials: "For most of the classes, the reliability . . . is *quite good* and, in general, is higher than that previously achieved" (Spitzer et al., 1979:817, emphasis added).

When the authors state that reliability, in general, is higher than that previously achieved, they are making a comparison that appears to be more concrete and verifiable than one involving their private hunches. On the other hand, "previously achieved" covers a lot of territory. Achieved by whom, when, how? No specific reference is offered for this bold comparative conclusion. It is assumed that the reader knows what was previously achieved and will readily accept these new findings as better. The style of presentation invites the reader to be admitted into the inner circle of knowledgeable exerts by accepting these claims of great improvement.

But exactly what had been previously achieved? And how do the current data lead to the conclusion of higher and better reliability? We have already examined in the previous chapter how the data presented compared to the standard of good reliability that they invented after the field trials data were in. We now turn to an examination of how the field trials compare with the findings from earlier studies. It is these previous studies against which DSM-III is claimed to be higher or better.

The critical "previously achieved" studies are: (1) the early reliability studies of the 1950s and 1960s, especially as they were reanalyzed and interpreted by Spitzer and Fleiss (1974); (2) the "classic" study by Helzer et al. (1977a, 1977b) using the Feighner criteria; and (3) the three studies reported by Spitzer et al. (1978) using the RDC. These will be compared with the DSM-III reliability data.

There are no standard methods of making these comparisons, other than by examining kappas and seeing which ones are higher or lower. And since the number of diagnostic categories available varies across studies as does the definition of the different diagnoses, even this seemingly simple comparison is fraught with ambiguity. Although we have described and compared these studies earlier, we now want to compare them with the DSM-III field trials data in order to show how the slippery standard of good reliability has evolved. We refer back to Figure 3.5 (Chapter 3), which shows a summary of the ranges of kappa from each article (when those data were presented) and calculates the average (mean) kappas from those ranges. In addition, each kappa range is described using *exact quotations* that were given in the articles. It is both the interpretive language as well as the kappa scores that will receive our attention.

The 1974 reanalysis (Spitzer & Fleiss, 1974), which reviewed studies from the 1950s and 1960s, used negatively loaded language to describe these early studies. Despite the variation in terminology, there appears to be some structural consistency in the interpretations (see Chapter 3). Despite the ambiguity about the meaning of "poor," "no better than fair" and "only satisfactory," the empirical data give those three vague labels an internal *structural interpretation* whereby each term can be matched to kappa scores that are higher in several simple statistical ways. Despite substantial overlap, the kappa scores that are referred to by those terms are different in terms of low and high end of the ranges and the mean scores. Thus, without deliberately seeking to provide a consistent set of standards for interpretation, the article implicitly does so. And, since the early studies as interpreted by Spitzer and Fleiss are used continuously as ammunition to bombard the weak state of reliability before the advent of diagnostic criteria and structured interviews, it is quite proper to use this framework to interpret subsequent studies. Moreover, since no other consistent set of interpretive guidelines was ever offered, we are left little choice.

The Helzer et al. (1977b) article, which served as a call to action for the use of diagnostic criteria, did not intend explicitly to establish any standards for the interpretation of kappa. Like the Spitzer and Fleiss piece, it almost completely avoided offering a specific interpretation that would allow one to anchor adjectives to kappa scores, and instead roamed in a rhetorical free zone by talking generally about results being "better" or "higher" than before. For example, it was far safer to claim that a kappa score for schizophrenia of .58 was higher than an earlier score of .57 (a claim they make on pp. 138–139) than to tell us that a kappa of .58 is low, poor, barely acceptable, good, or whatever.

All of the reliability reports have a fondness for this free zone and wander in it frequently. But Helzer et al., like the others, described their results in some evaluative language in order to promote their solution to the reliability problem. Thus, inevitably, they offered some adjectives in referring to their own data. Their use of these terms allows us to anchor their language in their own data.

The interpretations in the Helzer et al. article are difficult to reconcile with each other or with the earlier interpretations of kappa of Spitzer and Fleiss. Their use of "low" to describe several kappas in the .2–.3 range is by itself reasonable; they are scores that cluster at the lower end of a broad range (.1–.6). Recall that Spitzer and Fleiss refer to scores in this range as "poor." But the terms *low* and *poor* are at least not inconsistent; one refers to a place toward an end of a continuum, while the other makes an evaluative interpretation of that end of the continuum. Helzer et al. apparently consider a kappa of .4 "unacceptable," while Spitzer and Fleiss blanket that score in both their "poor" and "no better than fair" characterizations. On the surface, one could reconcile the terms *unacceptable, poor*, and *no better than fair* for similar scores, although it appears that Helzer et al. may be using higher standards, since *unacceptable* is a less forgiving term than *no better than fair*. But even if the reader can hold together some consistent interpretive framework up to this point, hereafter confusion triumphs.

Two kappas of .5 are described as "low end," but without specifying "of what." Low end of a high-low continuum? Low end of acceptability? Low end of good? We know from their data that .5 is not the low end of all the kappas. Therefore, we must assume that they are referring to the low end of some other unspecified scale, the middle or high end of which is left to the reader's imagination. But the confusion intensifies when they begin to present the data about which they are obviously most pleased.

The kappas they present range from .2 to .8 with an average of .66. The low end of that range matches Spitzer and Fleiss's "poor" and stretches to the top of their "only satisfactory." The average falls square between what Spitzer and Fleiss described as "no better than fair" and "only satisfactory." But Helzer et al. do not have the motivation that Spitzer and Fleiss did to disparage the results or to make them grudgingly acceptable. Spitzer and Fleiss were reviewing old studies and decrying the poor state of reliability, as a backdrop for a different approach that they would later propose. Helzer et al., in contrast, were reporting data about an approach that they obviously want to promote. Indeed, they were quick to claim not only that their kappa scores were higher than previous studies, but that they were unequivocally "good" and that they were "high.'

Thus, data that would be considered by the Spitzer and Fleiss standards as no better than fair or only satisfactory, were, *three years later*, described as both good and high. More perplexing, Helzer et al. proudly documented their success using average kappas that were only slightly better than ones they described in the same article as low end. Apparently, their implicit, unspecified continuum had a low end at .5 and a high end a notch higher at .6.

Perhaps it is unfair to hold researchers to the standards of interpretation that were used by other researchers. Authors need not be constrained by the implicit interpretive standards of others. Inevitably, any researchers working in an arena where there are no set standards are free to develop, articulate, and defend their own. The purpose of placing the Helzer et al. findings within the interpretive standards of Spitzer and Fleiss is to demonstrate how elusive those standards were and how easily they were arranged to denigrate or promote the data at hand.

The general elusiveness of interpretive standards clearly helps authors achieve their instrumental purposes. The Helzer et al. report was not an attempt to clarify the meaning or use of kappa. The purpose was to promote the benefits of two innovations: operational criteria and structured interviews. Their data, represented by kappas, benefited from inconsistency and ambiguity. They had no more need to be consistent than the promoter of any new product that is fighting for a market niche. Inconsistency and vagueness have their uses.

The third important article published prior to the release of DSM-III that claimed success in solving the reliability problem was the RDC article (Spitzer et al., 1978), which appeared just one year before the first reports of the field trials. Chapter 3 described this influential article, which argued the case for the RDC and structured interviews as technical instruments that were moving the profession a long way toward solving the reliability problem. Recall that the paper reported reliability results from three studies. Here, as with the two articles reviewed above, we are primarily interested in the standard of good reliability that was implicitly offered in the interpretation of the data. How was the authors' interpretive language connected to the kappa scores they presented? Figure 3.5 reports that language and ties it to kappa scores.

As we said in Chapter 3, one of the major purposes of the RDC paper was to signal that the way had been found to solve the reliability problem. Describing kappas as very or amazingly high is a way of proclaiming success and setting the tone for what should be expected. Thus, the 1974 review of the early studies and the RDC report of success established the approach for solving the reliability problem with DSM-III.

Using Slippery Standards

DSM-III and its field trials delivered on these promises. After publishing only partial reliability data in the 1979 articles (Spitzer et al., 1979; Spitzer & Forman, 1979)—avoiding, for example, reporting unsatisfactory findings on specific personality disorders or children—the developers pledged that other reports would be made. However, no other public reports were made prior to the approval and publication of DSM-III. More complete reliability data were reported in an appendix of the manual itself (APA, 1980) along with some interpretive language. Two years later, in a separate paper, the case summary data were published (Hyler et al., 1982).

How were the field trials data interpreted in DSM-III? The introduction to the manual itself claimed that there is *"far greater reliability* than had previously been obtained with DSM-II" (APA, 1980:5, emphasis added). In the reliability appendix there were claims that "reliability for most classes in both phases is quite good" (p. 468). Two years later, the developers spoke in the past tense and confidently inflated their interpretation: "the reliability of the major diagnostic classes of DSM-III was *extremely good"* (Hyler et al., 1982:1276, emphasis added). Only in reporting the children's diagnoses did they use a more cautious, if upbeat interpretation: "Although the reliability . . . is only fair, it is still far higher than [other systems]" (APA, 1980:469).

In short, DSM-III is introduced to the world through *the language of success*. It has a very familiar ring to it because it is the same language that was used by the St. Louis and New York groups throughout the 1970s to herald the invention and testing of diagnostic criteria and structured interviews. More importantly, the language promoted the product that had been promised by the DSM-III Task Force: a diagnostic system that would solve the reliability problem and remove it as a fundamental threat to psychiatry. DSM-III was described as largely fulfilling those promises.

The interpretation of the reliability of DSM-III used both favorable comparisons with the past ("far greater" and "far higher") as well as straight assessments ("quite good" and "extremely good") to make its case for the success of the new manual. Since the standard of good had never been made explicit and the interpretive language was ambiguous, there were no readily available grounds on which to dispute those claims. Prior success in mystifying reliability and its interpretation permitted claims about its improvement to be made with impunity.

There are several ways to examine the claims about DSM-III's reliability. In the preceding chapter, we used the developers' self-imposed standard of .70 as an indicator of good reliability to evaluate kappa scores. An alternative method is to compare the field trials data to the interpretive standards used with the early reliability studies. This is what we will do now. Figure 7.1 presents the ranges and averages (means) of kappa for the reliability data offered in support of DSM-III. It is presented by Axes I and II, by field trial phases, and for adults and children. Also included are field trials data published later in a separate article (Hyler et al., 1982).

As can be seen in Figure 7.1, the ranges of reliability for major diagnostic categories (as measured by kappa) are very broad and in some cases range from 0 to 1—the entire spectrum from chance to perfect agreement. In three of the four comparisons that can be made in Figure 7.1, there appears to be a pattern of lower average reliabilities in the later, second phase than in the more preliminary first phase of the field trials. The data in Figure 7.1 were the raw information on which the claim rested that DSM-III was so much better than previous studies of earlier diagnostic systems. This is the core claim on which the scientific success of DSM-III hung. How does the reliability of DSM-III compare with the results of the early reliability studies, as presented in the reanalysis paper of 1974? Comparing the DSM-III data with this 1974 report, both authored by the chair of the DSM-III Task Force, is enormously telling.

Figure 7.1 presents a graphic comparison of the field trials data and the reanalysis of the early studies. The claims usually made about DSM-III appear to be inconsistent with the actual data. The standards implicit in the 1974 article, if applied to the results of DSM-III, would lead to an interpretation that DSM-III's reliability was *no better than fair and highly variable*. Or, depending on how one wanted to select, summarize and array the kappa scores, one could argue that the field trials data suggested a slight improvement in reliability, perhaps bumping overall mean kappas from the .5 to the .6 range, both still within the earlier "no better than fair" range. The field trials data could have been interpreted in a variety of other ways, for example, as "about what we expected," "similar to earlier studies," "no worse than the 1950s and maybe better," or as "uneven, but promising."

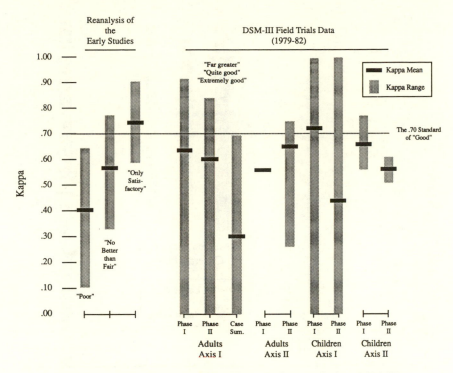

Figure 7.1. Interpreting kappa scores before and after DSM-III.

If the field trials data are compared with the Feighner (Helzer et al., 1977a, 1977b) or the RDC (Spitzer et al., 1978) reports, which touted diagnostic criteria and improved reliability, the DSM-III results are clearly less, not more, reliable (see Figure 7.2). Rather than being better or higher than previous findings, *the DSM-III results could more accurately be described as no better than the early studies and not as good as what had been achieved in the RDC studies.*

The *language of failure* might have been more accurate than the language of success. Or, at best, the language of partial and severely limited improvement might have been employed. Compromise, however, does not provide a very powerful language; it is full of qualifiers, caveats, and technical imponderables. It would hardly justify the Draconian and hard-won revisions that had been made in the official manual, or would it silence the critics nor deliver on the core promise to place psychiatric diagnosis on a firm, reliable foundation. No one wanted to hear equivocal language about equivocal data. The launching of DSM-III after five years of bitter struggle was not a time for raising more doubts about it. It was certainly not the time for suggesting that the old bogeyman of unreliability was still around, big as life.

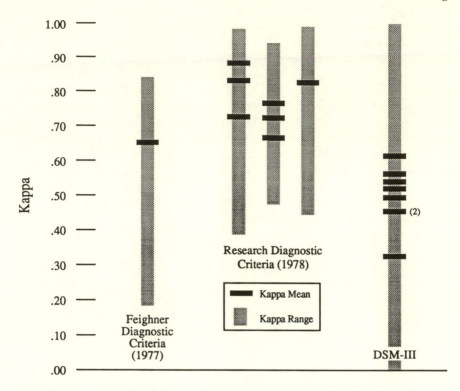

Figure 7.2. Comparing studies of the Feighner diagnostic criteria, the RDC, and DSM-III.

Accuracy in interpretation may not have served the purposes of the DSM-III Task Force as it prepared to defend and disseminate a controversial new manual. Why admit that the critical problem was far from resolved? Why hand opponents a lethal weapon? A controversial product had to be sold to the world of practitioners and agencies. Too much investment had been made in developing this manual, in justifying diagnostic criteria, and in promoting the latest technologies to allow the field trials to raise serious old questions.

The Art of Managing Science

The process of mystifying reliability and its measurement reached full flower by the late 1970s.It produced its first fruit with DSM-III. While clever wording, skillful rhetoric, and shifting interpretive standards were important in selling DSM-III, other contextual factors assisted with the harvest.

Data do not speak for themselves, nor do they speak consistently. Researchers give them a voice and purpose. They describe for the audience what the data mean and how they should be understood. But just as data do not talk by themselves, audiences do not necessarily listen. These are common problems for scientists who want to speak to those outside their small research communities. Speaking to wider audiences has special risks, as when unsophisticated listeners unintentionally misinterpret the findings or generalize them inappropriately to other circumstances.

Speaking to relatively naive audiences, however, also has its advantages. Listeners are not in a good position critically to assess scientific data, the methods used to gather them, or the faithfulness of their interpretation. This provides scientists with some license. [For case studies of some of these problems see Brodeur's (1989) *Currents of Death*, involving the controversy about the dangers of electromagnetic fields; or see David Owen (1985), *None of the Above: Behind the Myth of Scholastic Aptitude*, about the validity of the SAT.] These advantages can be magnified if scientists can maintain some control over how, when, and where the findings are presented. All these advantages were enjoyed by the developers of DSM-III.

Managing Data

One of the legacies of the DSM-III field trials, described as the largest field trials in psychiatric history, is how little is actually known about such an ostensibly important study. No book was written, no complete technical report was made available to other researchers, no final summary report was produced, and the data set was not made available for reanalysis by other investigators. More significantly, virtually nothing was available before final decisions were being made about DSM-III, when such information could have been appropriately used. But even if such a report had been produced after DSM-III was published, it would have been as inconsequential as a football game film that shows an unrecognized crucial clipping offense that could have altered the course of the game had it been called.

As described in Chapter 6, the reports of the field trials are inconsistent and incomplete. This is by no means a disadvantage for advocates, but it is for would-be critics who must contend with unrelenting ambiguity. Increasing the difficulty for an attentive audience, if there was one, was the fact that the field trials data were published in pieces. The first public appearance of any "findings" from the field trials was in two brief articles (Spitzer et al., 1979; Spitzer & Forman, 1979). In them, data from Phase One about Axis I and Axis II for adults by major diagnostic category were presented; and in the second article, four intraclass correlation coefficients were presented for the reliability of axes IV and V and some survey data reporting clinician's initial reactions to the draft manual. All this was presented in a favorable and positive light. These brief preliminary reports constituted *all* of the field trials data that were publicly available before DSM-III was officially adopted by the APA and presented to the mental health professions.

What data were not released before adoption and dissemination of DSM-III? The following information was gathered in the field trials, but was not published during the debates about the manual or before the manual was published:

- data about the reliability of specific Axis I diagnoses for adults in Phase One
- data about the reliability of specific Axis II diagnoses for adults in Phase One
- data about the reliability of Axis I diagnoses (major class or specific) for children and adolescents in Phase One
- data about the reliability of Axis II diagnoses (major class or specific) for children and adolescents in Phase One
- data about the reliability of Axis III
- data about the reliability of Axis I diagnoses (major class or specific) for adults in Phase Two
- data about the reliability of Axis II diagnoses (major class or specific) for adults in Phase Two
- data about the reliability of Axis I diagnoses (major class or specific) for children and adolescents in Phase Two
- data about the reliability of Axis II diagnoses (major class or specific) for children and adolescents in Phase Two.

Thus, by the time DSM-III was approved, relatively little data had been presented or available to those who may have been interested. Only a small slice of Phase One data was published, data that looked somewhat better than some of the rest. The point is not that data may have been deliberately withheld, but the more significant observation that no one apparently felt the need for more information. The language of success not only soothed anxieties, it dulled curiosity.

Additional data were eventually published, as needles in a mammoth haystack. DSM-III (published in 1980) is the five-hundred-page haystack and the last six-page appendix contains the needles. Those six pages contain three pages of text drawn primarily from the initial 1979 field trial report and three pages of kappa scores from phases One and Two. Here for the first time are the summary data about Phase Two and about the reliability of diagnoses for children and adolescents. These few pages contain what is to this day the only final report on the field trials. And even here, no reliabilities are presented for many specific diagnoses in Axis I and none for Axis II, even though they were known and available to the developers. The specific diagnoses by their very nature, of course, would have revealed kappas that were lower than the ones presented for major classes of disorders.

The omission of the more complete data was not for lack of space. For example, in what is almost unprecedented in research reports, the six-page reliability report was followed by nine pages listing the names, academic degrees, and organizational affiliations of all the participating clinicians in the field trials. This is a nice gesture on the part of the developers to acknowledge all the clinicians who had voluntarily agreed to participate in the surveys. Surely it must have made all the participants feel proud to have their names printed in such an important sourcebook. But since participants in scientific studies are almost never identified in publications (and, in fact, human subjects review committees usually require that the identities of respondents be carefully masked), this unusual display of names clearly has functions beyond expressing gratitude.

Acknowledgments build legitimacy. The development and dissemination of DSM-III needed all the legitimacy it could muster, since it departed in so many significant ways from its predecessor and the road to its success had been troubled. The opening four pages of DSM-III, pages preceding the table of contents, are lists of the names of those psychiatrists who served on the various subcommittees that had a hand in developing DSM-III. The final nine pages contain the names of field trial participants. The text of the manual is sandwiched between these superfluous acknowledgments, conveying legitimacy through broad association . . . from Maine to Hawaii.

Listing all the field trial participants in the reliability appendix promotes legitimacy in another way. Not all of the field trial participants were involved in the reliability studies. The published reports of the exact number of field trial participants and the exact number of participants in the reliability studies are either inconsistent, approximations or unstated (see APA, 1980:5; Spitzer et al., 1979:816). By inference from the published articles, it appears that approximately 300 clinicians actually participated in the reliability studies. The reliability appendix, however, lists the names of 679 participants. The effect is to make the reliability studies appear to have involved twice as many clinicians as actually participated, thus broadening through acknowledgments the appearance of legitimacy.

Having the reliability report within the manual, even in the final appendix, serves important symbolic functions. The appendix gives the manual a scientific patina since it is one of the few places that present "data." It suggests, by implication, that the other five hundred pages of the manual rest on some similar empirical basis. Since few clinicians understand the language of kappa or the complexities of the problems embedded in reliability studies, Appendix F offers for those who browse through the manual a peek at the quantitative mysteries of reliability. Two full, numbing pages of numbers, they are told, attest to the good reliability of the new diagnostic system. Who would not be impressed? Certainly very few could fully or critically understand. Moreover, with the publication of DSM-III and its small final appendix, future references to the good reliability of the new system needed only to cite the manual. The final pages that close DSM-III were meant to close the book on the problem of reliability.

Managing Timing

Timing is everything. The DSM-III Task Force, working under tight time schedules, had moved back the publication date of DSM-III several times. Controversies continued to swirl around such issues as the elimination of neuroses, and tobacco. The field trials through which empirical legitimacy was sought became an important element in the unfolding drama. The results of the field trials would only become available after almost all of the major decisions about DSM-III had been made. By 1979 when the field trials concluded, the multiaxial system had been adopted, almost all of the diagnostic categories were decided upon, the great bulk of the diagnostic criteria were in place, and many of the controversies had been resolved. Equally important, the schedule of decision-making leading to the adoption of DSM-III by the APA board had been set. The field trials needed to confirm these prior decisions, not to raise more questions about them. They were less a form of testing than of sanctification. Blessings are needed at some times more than at others.

The two-part article describing the initial results of the field trials that was rushed into print in June 1979 hit at a strategic time. The review process of the DSM-III Task Force was in a critical phase. Empirical evidence was needed that the manual "worked." Moreover, empirical data that suggested that it worked better than its predecessor were crucial. Furthermore, the APA membership, having been aware of the lengthy process of development of DSM-III, was awaiting news of the final product, due within a year. In this context, a brief report of success just prior to final adoption of DSM-III was undoubtedly reassuring to the DSM-III Task Force participants and to the membership waiting for the new manual. The brief report would have been considerably less important if it had been published in 1982, two years after DSM-III's arrival. If it had been published later, it would have served merely as an historical footnote. In 1979, it was campaign literature.

Campaign literature promotes. It challenges disbelievers, sways the undecided, and reassures the committed. It never suggests that the campaign may be misdirected or that the candidate may not be the best one. The selection has been made; it is irreversible. Just before the election, unwanted news about the candidate's financial or sexual indiscretions are suppressed, vehemently denied, or finessed as "blown out of proportion." Good news, if not available, is manufactured and savored, whatever its origins. The issues are made simple, the direction clear-cut.

The 1979 brief report about the field trials could only have contained good news. It would have been unthinkable for those who raised the reliability problem to a new art form, who developed the technology to solve it, who promised that they would solve it if given a chance to revamp DSM, who fought for five years to produce a product they believed in, to announce, shortly before the final publication, that the new manual did not work too well or that reliability problems were far from resolved. It was unthinkable. The eve of the publication of DSM-III was no time for misgivings, or for complete disclosure. The brief report of success was all anyone would see or wanted to see until after the election when the candidate was safely in office, and the issues appeared not so simple anymore.

Managing Publications

Journal articles are the currency of intellectual exchange in science. Journals provide a controlled, neutral forum for the competition involved in scientific discovery, for reasoned debate, for the display of intellectual wares, and for determining or reaffirming status. The most important journal in American psychiatry is the *American Journal of Psychiatry,* the official and primary publication of the APA. Every member of the association receives a copy by virtue of membership, making it one of the most widely disseminated journals in psychiatry. It is considered by many people to be the most prestigious psychiatric journal.

The owners of professional journals are supposed to be disinterested parties to the fate of the research articles that they publish. Understandably, journal editors want to publish the latest and most important research. In that indirect way editors are dependent on the quality of the research articles they select for publication. Rarely does the owner of a journal have a direct pecuniary stake in the persuasive appeal of its

articles. With the impending publication of DSM-III as an official product of the APA, however, the AJP was cast in a different role: that of
house organ. Having the initial data about the field trials reported in AJP
served the interests not only of the developers of DSM-III, but also of the
APA, whose credibility was also closely tied to what was to become by
far its most visible and lucrative consumer product. The APA and its
primary journal were not disinterested parties to the initial articles about
DSM-III; they were prime sponsors.

The relationship of the DSM articles to AJP more closely approximates
that between an advertisement for a product and a magazine that not
only publishes the ad, but also has a financial stake in the product's
success. And with DSM-III, one advertisement was not enough. In 1980,
on the eve of the publication of DSM-III, the APA issued two more
promotions. One was published by the developers of DSM-III in the AJP
and was immodestly titled, "DSM-III: The Major Achievements and an
Overview" (Spitzer et al., 1980). This article, described in Chapter 6, was
a 15-page advertisement for DSM-III, using all of the rhetorical power
that could be mustered for the unveiling of the latest model of the
diagnostic manual.

The "major achievements" article sported a telling footnote on the first
page, which revealed the ownership of and pecuniary interests in the
product. Customarily, reprints of scientific articles can be obtained by
simply writing the authors, who will gladly send copies free of charge to
all who request them. The "major achievements" article, by contrast,
was published with a footnote explaining that copies could be obtained
from the Publication Sales Department of the APA, listing the prices for
multiple copies and indicating that prepayment was required. This is
highly unusual for articles in mental health journals. The APA and the
authors were apparently comfortable with the joint ownership of the
article and their expectation that there was a market waiting and money
to be made.

The other promotion was published in another APA journal, *Hospital
& Community Psychiatry*, in the form of an interview, "An In-Depth Look
at DSM-III: An Interview With Robert Spitzer" (Talbott, 1980). This was
also described in Chapter 6. The "interview" was conducted by John
Talbott, a member of the editorial board of the journal and a trustee of
the APA. This was not the kind of interview that political candidates get
from a hostile press, but rather the kind that victors receive from those
who admire their achievements. The interview also comes with a front-
page footnote: this time with a complete price list for copies of DSM-III,
offering a 20% discount for orders of more than one hundred copies and
directing that the money be sent to the APA's Publication Sales Office in
Washington D.C. Under the circumstances, a probing interview would
have been most awkward.

The "in-depth interview" and the "major achievements" article are exquisitely timed and placed. They appeared in the months preceding the long-awaited manual; they are placed in the leading journals of the APA; and they are accompanied by no critical or questioning commentaries. Readers are encouraged to buy the product, advice more frequently found in mailings from stockbrokers than in articles in a leading research journal. And as expected, both promotional articles reassure the readers that the reliability of DSM-III is "so much better than expected."

Managing and interpreting the reliability data, strategically timing and placing the promotional articles required a singleness of purpose. Similar to the management of the DSM-III Task Force, the management of its main product required oversight, coordination, unity of purpose, and control of information. The field trials that served such an important symbolic purpose in the development of DSM-III could not be delegated to others. Too much depended on the results for them to be farmed out to others who might create problems. The field trials were not trials in the sense that something was tested that might fail, but rather they were activities that would reinforce the solutions that already had been framed. Their management was another important element in the development of DSM-III.

Managing Testing

For consumer protection, the introduction of new products or new pharmaceutical drugs is preceded by independent testing of the products for safety and efficacy. Independent laboratories test electrical devices for safety. Automobiles are tested for crashworthiness. Unanticipated harm to those using a product can open the producer to expensive liability claims. So stringent and time consuming are some of these protections that, for example, the elaborate testing procedures of the Federal Drug Administration have been criticized as unnecessarily delaying the availability of drugs to treat AIDS victims.

These developments are designed to protect the public from charlatans, tricksters, and crooks. Psychiatric treatments are subject to few such requirements. Malpractice is extraordinarily difficult to prove, although recent cases have alerted psychiatrists to these issues (Klerman, 1990; Stone, 1990). There was no testing for efficacy of the more than four hundred psychotherapeutic techniques before they were used. Similarly, there are no restrictions, beyond public tolerance, on what the APA may claim as mental disorders. The validity or reliability of its claims is of little importance, as long as most psychiatrists consent to their use and no other interested parties create embarrassing public disputes. The constantly changing mix of diagnostic categories attests to this fluidity, in which many new categories were added to DSM-III and some categories of DSM-II simultaneously ceased to exist. The same thing happened with DSM-III-R and appears to be happening with DSM-IV. There are no limits to these changes beyond the internal negotiations within the APA and the desire of the profession to avoid public ridicule.

In this free market for diagnoses, there are few calls for testing or for outside, independent study. Conducting the DSM-III field trials, then, went beyond what was customary or required. It went beyond what was technically needed as well, since no previous version of the manual had undergone such extensive field testing. Thus, the developers did indeed go beyond customary practice in testing DSM-III, and that effort itself, quite apart from its results, redounded to the credibility and benefit of the new manual. While the developers of DSM-III were appropriately self-congratulatory about the field trials, this form of testing does not constitute independent scrutiny.

Spitzer was both the prime mover in the development of DSM-III and the principal investigator in the National Institute of Mental Health–funded field trials. He was testing a system he had the major hand in developing and about which he had promised much. This arrangement is not at all uncommon in psychiatric, behavioral, or social research, where the originator of a measurement scale or structured interview schedule or treatment gathers and offers the initial evidence of its utility. It is, in fact, the manner in which most scientific findings are disseminated to others for their review and replication. The flurry of scientific activity in 1989 that surrounded the claims of University of Utah scientists about cold fusion illustrates the normal manner in which claims are tested by others before they are accepted or rejected and before industrial or federal policies are revised.

The merger of the roles of developer and tester are typical in early reports of scientific findings. If public decisions are to be made that will be binding on many others in the scientific or professional community, the developers' claims about data are seldom the only evidence that is available. In the case of the DSM-III field trials, however, not only were the field trials data made available late in the decision process, but only selected parts of the data gathered under the developer's watchful eye were available. A mildly challenging study by Cantwell et al. (1979), participants in the field trials, appeared the same year as the field trials data, but it was ignored and later discounted (Hyler et al., 1982). Few if any independent studies of the reliability of DSM-III were available when the crucial decisions about the new manual were made by the DSM-III Task Force or by the APA.

Testing of DSM-III was an in-house operation conducted by those most invested personally and professionally in its success. But this arrangement was not nearly as important as the fact that the testing was done when there was so little time to use its results to do anything more than spruce up the diagnostic criteria and instructions. By 1979, the field trials were not an attempt to find the proper gown for the profession to wear—those decisions had already been made—but to conduct a final fitting of the garment in which a tuck here and a seam there needed last minute attention before being sent to the cotillion ball. The debutante was marred by a few blemishes, but these were skillfully excused, touched up, underplayed, or shielded from view.

Managing Counterevidence

All scientific endeavors confront occasional anomalies, findings that are not consistent with the guiding theoretical approach. These can be ignored, attributed to procedural and measurement error, or reinterpreted as actually supporting a position that at first they appear to contradict. As DSM-III was published, potentially discouraging findings were often embedded in very positive pronouncements. In the 1979 initial report on reliability, for example, the developers acknowledge that "several important classes still have only fair reliability—schizoaffective disorder, chronic minor affective disorder, and personality disorder" (Spitzer et al., 1979:817). But this statement is followed immediately by one that indicates that these latter categories are still being reworked and that they "hope this will result in improved reliability" (p. 817). For personality disorders, they confess that they do not know how to improve reliability, but reassuringly claim that as a category of disorder, it "is more reliably judged than previously" (p. 817). They offer no citation for this claim. And, in general, they do not dwell on categories with low reliabilities or ever suggest that anything more than fine-tuning should be necessary to improve them. Problems with reliability, where and when they must be acknowledged, are never fundamental problems of approach or validity. They are always presented as technical problems requiring slight revisions of diagnostic criteria to control errant clinicians. The authors' explanations for counterevidence sooth; they promise to try harder and do better the next time.

These promises are effective because there is always a next time. When Phase One of the field trials data were reported, they were already revising criteria and categories for Phase Two. When DSM-III was published, they were about ready to start the revisions that would result in DSM-III-R. By the time DSM-III-R was published they were planning for DSM-IV. The rapid revision process itself allows the developers to deflect criticism and downplay negative evidence of the old version by claiming that changes are being made and that hopefully the next version will be better.

The most serious counterevidence that emerged from the field trials was published in 1982 by the developers themselves (Hyler et al., 1982), although it had been submitted for publication more than a year before and the data were obviously available to the investigators some months before that. This article reported data from the most methodologically rigorous test of the reliability of DSM-III. But the article is not presented as a test of DSM-III as much as a comparison of two methods of studying reliability: through live interviews versus written case summaries.

The study was done as part of the field trials and simultaneously with them. As described in Chapter 5, clinicians participating in the field trials were asked to prepare written case summaries. The researchers selected 46 of these case summaries and 5 of these were sent to each of the clinicians who had contributed one of the 46 cases. These clinicians were asked to make diagnoses based on these summaries. Only Axis I diagnoses were reported in the article and these were compared with the Axis I diagnoses through live interviews.

Remember that one major common source of diagnostic error is information variance, the exposure of different diagnosticians to different information about a patient. Using written summaries usually is viewed as one research method that controls for this source of error and thereby is usually considered to yield higher levels of reliability than studies using separate live interviews.

What they report is unexpected. The kappas for major categories of disorder on Axis I range from −.05 to .69 and average .47 for the case summaries. The live interviews had an even broader range, but averaged .67. For all but one of the categories, the case summary kappas are lower than the live interviews. Both sets of scores are not particularly good, but the case summaries are unexpectedly worse than the interviews.

The authors go to great lengths to explain this difference between the case summaries and the live interviews. They explore and reject several possible hypotheses. But the thrust of their exploration is to account for the *higher* reliability in the live interviews, that is, to buttress the validity of the method that produced higher kappas. This is instructive. Instead of viewing the case summary study as a method of permitting greater experimental control and therefore less chance for contamination between independent diagnosticians, they went to great lengths to discredit the case summary methodology and an earlier reliability study by Cantwell et al. (1979) that had used case summaries to test an earlier version of DSM-III and also found relatively low interrater agreement. They did so despite the fact that some researchers believe that case vignette methods usually produce relatively higher reliability estimates than do *in vivo* studies (Grove et al., 1981). Ironically, although they had suggested for years that control of information variance was one of the golden bricks in the road to greater reliability, they were now arguing that control of information variance in the case summaries was a pothole and the reason for low reliability!

In the end, they offered the explanation that a mental disorder is like a rose (their metaphor). The clinical interview, they explained, is like seeing a rose. The case summaries are like reading a description of a rose. Observers are better able to identify a rose than are those who only read about one. Their "flower defense" was a clever way of dealing with evidence that they had gone to great lengths to cultivate, but now having plucked it, they discovered that it had an unexpected odor. Through a combination of downplaying negative findings, revealing only partial data, at different times and places, and by withholding information, counterevidence was effectively managed and DSM-III came out smelling like a rose.

Managing Outside Critics

Managing critics is a more complex task, an activity in which control is much less secure. The developers were ruffling the feathers of many birds both within and outside psychiatry. When, where, and how they would squawk was not entirely predictable. Controversy and debate was clearly expected within the DSM-III Task Force. As we discussed in Chapter 4, the design of the DSM-III Task Force and its many advisory committees, and the selection of members was a method of containing and channeling disagreement so that a consensus document would emerge. Critics within the DSM-III flock were coopted and, if not completely mollified, their squeaks were at least not heard outside.

Managing outside critics was more difficult. Those who were not participants in the development of DSM-III had no loyalty to the product. Moreover, they were not constrained by the task force process or even the way in which the central issues were defined. Furthermore, they were under no obligations to accept the assumptions that underlay the development of DSM-III. Outside critics could be lurking anywhere and could fire from any angle at any time. They would have to be taken on individually. Such firefights occurred frequently during and after the development of DSM-III.

There were, however, no such direct assaults on the quality of the field trials or on the reliability of diagnosis. Prior to the publication of DSM-III, of course, little information was published that could be reviewed and questioned. After the publication of field trials data, so complete was the mystification, so incomplete was the reporting of research details, and so frequent was the reiteration that reliability was so much better than before that few outside critics bothered to contest the claim. Critics as well as proponents of DSM-III were likely to accept the claims of high reliability, but to complain that the emphasis on improved reliability had occurred at the expense of diagnostic validity (Michels, 1984a, 1984b; Vaillant, 1984). For six years after DSM-III was published, there were only a few outside critics who raised questions about its reliability (Scheff, 1986; Kutchins & Kirk, 1986). Most observers simply accepted the claims of success.

That reliability claims were accepted did not mean that there were not other issues about which critics had serious misgivings. Eysenck (1986) was hostile to the entire DSM-III approach to classification. Strauss (1986) believed that DSM-III neglected longitudinal processes. Other critics found a variety of weaknesses in the new diagnostic system (cf. Garfield, 1986; Salzinger, 1986; Bemporad & Schwab, 1986; Rothblum et al., 1986). Many critics were not answered, particularly those who raised questions many years after the victory of securing acceptance of DSM-III. But while the campaign to sell DSM-III was in full gear, many critics could expect to be challenged. Several such exchanges with critics while the manual was being developed were mentioned in Chapter 4. After it was published, other critics emerged and had to be managed.

The way that DSM-III's proponents handled psychologists is an excellent illustration of how postpublication controversy was managed. There had been a steady drumbeat of criticism before the manual was published. Psychologists produced a number of challenges with provocative titles such as "Whatever Happened to Interpersonal Diagnosis? A Psychosocial Alternative to DSM-III" (McLemore & Benjamin, 1979), "But Is It Good for Psychologists? Appraisal and Status of DSM-III" (Schacht & Nathan, 1977), "Never Mind the Psychologists; Is It Good for Children?" (Garmenzy, 1978), "But Is It Good for Science?" (Zubin, 1978), and "But Is It Good for the Patient?" (Salzinger, 1977).

After DSM-III was published, Spitzer (1981b) executed a preemptive strike and published "Nonmedical Myths and the DSM-III" in the *American Psychological Association Monitor*, the newsletter distributed to that association's members. He used the rhetorical device of posing a set of objections to DSM-III and of answering his own challenges; this is a common tactic used by campaigners. He restated some carefully reformulated criticisms made by psychologists and responded to them. He claimed that "what follows is an attempt to clarify the most common misunderstandings about DSM-III, many of which have been disseminated in psychology journals" (p. 3). He addressed eight objections, which he pointedly characterized as non-medical myths. "Nonsense" was his response to the criticism that DSM-III was published to give psychiatrists "hegemony over the mental health professions because of the diminishing mental health dollar" (p. 3). He claimed that the board of trustees had developed a policy in the 1960s that revisions of DSM were to be made compatible with the ICD. For this reason, DSM-III's publication was timed to coincide with the publication of ICD-9. This often reasserted rationale was contradicted, not only by the policy formulated by the psychiatric association's board of trustees in 1973 (see Chapter 4), which his audience could not have known, but also by public statements about the manual including the following observation in DSM-III: "In a number of instances, the conceptual reclassification of disorders is unique to DSM-III and does not conform to the classification of these disorders in ICD-9" (Spitzer, Hyler, & Williams, 1980:371). His audience was unlikely to know that a crisis had occurred subsequent to the publication of DSM-III and that a member of the APA's staff had to formulate a postpublication system to relate the two manuals, DSM-III and ICD-9, to each other.

Another objection that Spitzer countered was that scientific values were sacrificed for economic considerations, particularly to ensure that the manual could be used to facilitate payment from the government and insurance companies. Spitzer responded that the criticism was "absurd." He asserted that "one would have to know the over 100 members of the Task Force and the various advisory committees (primarily academic and research psychiatrists and several distinguished psychologists) to know how unlikely it was that economic motives could have distorted their decisions" (p. 3). This implied that the DSM-III Task Force or the subcommittees had the final decision-making authority in these matters, and that the APA's organizational hierarchy was not influenced by the economic consequences of these decisions. He did acknowledge that in one minor case a diagnosis was dropped because a group of clinicians feared that insurance companies would not reimburse it. We know that economic considerations often had an impact on the way that decisions were made about a number of disorders, such as homosexuality, tobacco addiction, and post–traumatic stress disorder (Scott, 1990). Furthermore, there were financial influences over other aspects of the manual's design and production in addition to the formulation of specific diagnoses.

Spitzer discussed a number of the other major controversies in the same fashion. His response to the claim that DSM-III promotes a medical model was to ask, "What is the medical model?" He then reviewed the aborted attempt to include the statement that medical disorders are a subset of mental disorders in the manual. He claimed that the motivation for proposing it was to convince the followers of Thomas Szasz that psychiatry was a legitimate branch of medicine, but the idea was dropped when he and his colleagues realized that they "wouldn't convince any Szaszians . . . and that we would only alienate our psychology colleagues who had made so many important contributions to the field of psychopathology" (p. 33). The tone and substance of this response was very different from the belligerent statements he and the leadership of the APA used in its communications with the president of the American Psychological Association during the controversy. Of course, the objectives were different. Then the psychiatrists were trying to establish their dominance over the process of defining diagnosis; now they were trying to convince psychologists to accept their handiwork.

Spitzer answered the criticism that DSM-III contributed to negative labelling by asserting that the manual only identified disorders, not people, e.g., it used the term *schizophrenia*, not *schizophrenics*. He acknowledged that it could be used inappropriately to stigmatize people, but he asserted that "it is difficult to see how mental health professionals can function without using a standardized nomenclature" (p. 33).

He countered another complaint that only psychiatrists were competent to use the manual by pointing out that the word *psychiatrist* was never used in the manual. Instead the terms *clinician* and *mental health professional* were employed.

The charges that there had been an expansion in the concept of mental disorder and that there were no scientific bases to justify the increased number of diagnoses was dismissed as "not true." But Spitzer subsequently justified the expansion by saying that "The larger number of diagnostic categories in DSM-III as compared with DSM-II reflects the clinical and research need for greater specificity in describing behavioral syndromes" (p. 33).

His answer to another challenge was magnanimous. He responded to the threat by some psychologists to adopt an alternative diagnostic system and to boycott DSM-III by asserting that "Psychologists . . . need not be content with DSM-III and may profitably explore other approaches" (p. 33), but he warned that "to ignore DSM-III is to ignore one of the most important developments within the last decade in psychopathology" (p. 33).

He squelched criticisms with such emphatic reactions as "absurd," "nonsense," and "not true," while simultaneously acknowledging them and justifying his position. If there were other facts that contradicted his explanation, he did not have to worry about being challenged, since he was both critic and defender; his was the last word. He even addressed the reliability problem, repeating verbatim a complaint by Rosenhan that no proper study of reliability or validity had been published. Spitzer responded that validity studies will take time, although DSM-III was based on information from numerous prior studies, which were listed in a bibliography in the manual. As for reliability, he pointed out that the largest study ever undertaken was completed prior to the publication of DSM-III. Furthermore he reported, "The published results indicate far better reliability than has been previously reported for official classifications of mental disorders" (p. 33).

Although the format of Spitzer's editorial foreordained the outcome of the discussion that he conducted with himself, psychologists were not ready to concede just yet. A debate was arranged between Spitzer (1985a, 1985b) and Schacht (1985), a frequent critic during the period when DSM-III was being formulated.

Schacht argued that the controversy over DSM-III had been hopelessly muddled because of confusion about the relationship between science and politics. Schacht observed that the general perception was that the two are mutually exclusive and, as a consequence, "any mention of the political dimension is seen as an attack upon the scientific integrity of the taxonomy" (p. 522). He contended that the integral aspects of science and politics should be acknowledged, because the failure to do so "cause[s] many communications about DSM-III to become mired in double-talk, in which the disavowal of DSM-III's politics often serves to affirm what is being denied" (p. 522). In order to illustrate his point, he reviewed some of the controversies that occurred during the development of DSM-III, but he focused most of his attention on Spitzer's editorial in the *Monitor*. Schacht's argument was that Spitzer's attempts backfired when he tried to rebut charges that many decisions about DSM-III were not scientific but political. To illustrate his point he made a careful analysis of many of Spitzer's responses. We report one example completely in order to illustrate the tenor of Schacht's argument:

> Critic's claim: DSM-III adheres to a medical model that is inappropriate for psychologists as exemplified by abandoned plans to include a statement that mental disorders are a subset of medical disorders.
>
> Spitzer's defense: In discussing the rationale for excluding the medical disorders statement from the final DSM-III, Spitzer cited no scientific arguments, but rather noted a task force consensus that exclusion of the statement "would not convince any Szaszians that psychiatry was a legitimate branch of medicine (our motivation for having such a statement), and . . . would alienate our psychology colleagues.
>
> [Schacht's] Analysis: Here again, in an article attempting to deny charges that political considerations influenced the creation and structure

of the DSM-III, Spitzer named only political and not scientific advantages among the reasons for the statements ultimate exclusion. (Schacht, 1985b:519)

This was the tenor of Schacht's arguments. He responded to the explanation that DSM-III's publication was timed to coincide with ICD-9, not to assert political hegemony over the mental health field, by observing:

> Because the World Health Organization [which published the ICD] is a "bigger" authority than the American Psychiatric Association, to link DSM-III to the ICD-9 is to acquire more "authority" and hence more validity and more social power by sheer strength of political bedfellowship. . . . This denial ironically reinforces the very political implications it seeks to disavow. (p. 519)

Spitzer's assertions that there had been reliability studies, which involved over 800 clinicians, "many of them psychologists," met with this response from Schacht:

> Although the citation of data is laudable, the reference to the professional affiliation of the clinicians appears to have no relevance to the scientific quality of the studies. Instead this phrase seems clearly cast in the "who says?" metaphor of an authority-epistemology (i.e., psychologists should have faith in the data because their colleagues participated in its collection.) Spitzer's subtly political point invites psychologists to emphasize an inter-professional perspective on DSM-III and to feel free to count themselves among "who's who" in "who says." (p. 520)

Spitzer responded to Schacht's article by trumping his critique. Although Spitzer objected that the definition of politics was overly broad, he agreed to accept it and listed a number of political and economic aspects of the manual that Schacht had overlooked. For example, he boasted that the manual had advanced the careers and increased the publications of many participants including himself, as well as of many critics. He observed that "appeals to objective data for resolving controversies were relatively rare" (Spitzer, 1985:523) and that "rhetoric" played an important role in resolving controversies. Because he was the chair, "This was particularly true in my case" (p. 523). As for the economic value of the manual, it was a surprising runaway best-seller, primarily because of sales to nonpsychiatrists. He boasted that the profits were used to initiate the APA Press, and they also made it possible to avoid an increase in the association's dues.

Having acknowledged these and other gains, Spitzer playfully suggested a new mental disorder—PSDS (Politics-Science Dichotomy Disorder)—and he also proposed to evaluate himself to see if he suffered from it. He went through the list of objections to DSM-III again, and of his responses and Schacht's counterclaims. He acknowledged that there were political and economic motives, but he insisted that there were also sound scientific arguments that had influenced the critical decisions. He asserted that the question was not whether there were political motives involved in the creation of DSM-III but whether the blend of politics and science was professionally responsible or not. This, of course, had been Schacht's basic point, but Spitzer was unwilling to concede even this to his antagonist. He concluded that he did not suffer from PSDS because all of his actions were not prompted by political considerations; there were sound scientific justifications as well.

What was the outcome of this debate? In an indirect manner, Spitzer was able to acknowledge the criticisms of his adversaries and, by the time of his interchange with Schacht in 1985, use them to his advantage. He could boast about the success of DSM-III and about his political craftiness. Since the manual was an overwhelming triumph by then, even the complaints about the economic profits to the psychiatric profession were reinterpreted as signs of the widespread acceptance of the manual by those outside the psychiatric profession.

This ended the debate over DSM-III with Schacht and many of his colleagues among the psychologists, but not because the issues were resolved. Schacht later claimed that Spitzer had largely missed or muddled his major points (Schacht, 1985b). The debate ended because the APA decided to publish another edition; Spitzer and his colleagues were well along the way to completion of DSM-III-R. A new group of critics would come to the fore in the next few years. In fact, in 1985, the year of the exchange between Spitzer and Schacht, a brand new controversy erupted with greater intensity and publicity than any controversy that had occurred in almost a decade. This time the objection was over the proposed inclusion in DSM-III-R of three new diagnoses, Premenstrual Dysphoric Disorder, Paraphilac Rapism, and Masochistic Personality Disorder. Feminist Psychotherapists, led principally by psychologists, mounted a well-publicized and partially successful campaign to prevent the adoption of these diagnoses, which they believed discriminated against women.

The issue was not a new one. Spitzer and his colleagues (Spitzer et al., 1983) had published an exchange with Kaplan (1983) in the *American Psychologist* about sexism in DSM-III. Nothing had been resolved as a result of the earlier exchange. Feminists were not satisfied with Spitzer's responses, and he and his colleagues were intransigent in their unwillingness to work with them. When *The New York Times* published the

complaints of feminist psychotherapists in 1985, they were better tar-
geted, and the protesters did not confine their complaints to academic
journals.

Even though the feminist psychotherapists were able to prevent the
adoption of the three diagnoses (modified versions were included in an
appendix to DSM- III-R for further study), DSM-III-R received the same
public acclaim as its predecessor. The complaints that Schacht or the
feminist psychotherapists had made were not resolved. But they did not
have a serious impact on the public or professional perception of DSM-
III as a scientifically constructed nosological system. Spitzer's indefatig-
able attention to all the details in the construction of the manual, and his
willingness to respond to all critics with great intensity, lead to its unde-
niable preeminence as the Bible of psychiatric diagnosis.

Managing Believers

Like most professionals, psychotherapists believe in what they do.
They see people in pain and, as best they can, try to help them. It is
uncertain work. Their clients' suffering is often diffuse, connected in so
many intricate ways to their past lives, their personalities, and their
current social relationships and social circumstances. Their problems
seldom can be quickly understood or crisply described. In offering help,
there are few certainties about what interventions will be most effective,
who should administer them or for how long. Both client and therapist
enter a relationship that may be immensely intimate and long-lasting,
brief and bureaucratic, or something in between.

The uncertainties of psychotherapeutic work are frequently the butt of
jokes in the popular media. Since questions about the border between
sanity and madness are enduring ones for every society, those who
work on the boundaries and try to retrieve those lost to insanity are
under constant public scrutiny. It is not a visibility that they enjoy, for
often their trade is criticized or dismissed. This is part of the public
background for the emergence of the reliability problem as a threat to
the integrity of the psychiatric profession. Efforts to shore up its scientific respectability would enhance the public reputation of psychiatrists
and other mental health professionals and would be welcome indeed.

Mental health practitioners who are not physicians are often the most
impressed by diagnostic nomenclature. Psychologists and social workers labor on the periphery of medicine and being able to make psychiatric diagnoses gives them a sense of medical legitimacy and power.
Being able to use diagnostic jargon, particularly jargon dressed in new
scientific respectability, was welcomed. The developers of DSM-III were

clearly aware of this nonmedical market and deliberately made no mention of physicians in the text of the manual. Furthermore, an array of accessories was developed to make the manual easy to use: various casebooks, tape cassettes, minimanuals, workshops, interview protocols, and computer programs—self-help for diagnosticians.

While the developers of DSM-III were aware that a new diagnostic system, particularly one that deviated so substantially from its predecessor, would encounter resistance, if for no other reason than institutional inertia, they also must have known that any system that claimed to remedy a problem for which the whole profession had been repeatedly and publicly criticized—that of distinguishing reliably the sane from the insane and the types of insanity—would be difficult to resist. Mental health practitioners wanted to believe in the scientific merit of their trade. The rosy pronouncements about DSM-III told them what they wanted to hear. They were easy converts, eager believers.

Good news is always more quickly embraced. But good news must be simple. Reliability studies, with their methodological complexities, accompanied by kappa coefficients that control for chance agreement, are not digestible good news. Good news loses its impact if it is embedded in too much technical jargon. Laypersons do not want a complicated lesson about nuclear physics; they want to hear about cold fusion and how it may solve the energy problem. They do not want biochemistry; they want announcements that cancers can be cured. They do not want a treatise on econometrics; they want to know that the economy is improving, inflation is under control, and their jobs are not in jeopardy. What psychiatrists wanted to hear about DSM-III, they heard over and over again, in brief, clear language: Diagnostic reliability was much better than before and so much better than expected. As far as they needed to be concerned, the problem was solved.

It was not only that they were predisposed to believe, but that the problem had been sufficiently mystified so that they could no longer seriously question whether the simple good news matched the methods and statistics on which it was based. Why should they have any doubts, anyway? They were hearing from some of the most respected research psychiatrists in the country. Their work was sponsored by their APA, partially funded by the National Institute of Mental Health, and hailed by many of the leaders in the field. It was very convincing publicity. It is known from social psychology, for example, that communications are more persuasive if they come from sources that are credible, trustworthy, and attractive. The claims about DSM-III came from those with positions in outstanding universities and in prestigious journals. They were imbued with respectability (Lipton & Hershaft, 1985).

The manual itself, quickly purchased by nearly everyone in the mental health business, also testified to its own importance. It was big, complex, detailed, and long awaited. Whatever their discomfort with its innovations, whatever their disappointment that some old familiar categories had been replaced by awkward new ones, practitioners saw that the manual was something that they must come to terms with. This was not a reference book to be stuck away on a crowded shelf. This was a book that intended to change the way they thought about their clinical work.

8

SECURING DIAGNOSTIC TURF

Although members of Congress serve only two-year terms, they usually enjoy a very long tenure. While the federal system was not designed to encourage such stability, aspects of the current political environment ensure that a congressional seat once won is hard to lose. This state of affairs is related to the increasing costs of mounting a campaign, the political advantages enjoyed by officeholders and the comforts of old ties to special interest groups who have considerable funds to contribute to familiar politicians.

What would happen, we might fantasize, if incumbents continued to be virtually unbeatable, but new seats in the House of Representatives were made available to congressional aspirants if they at least ran a decent campaign? Instead of allowing only 435 congressional seats, new ones could be added if they had proper justification. Three developments would be very likely: First, new seats would be quickly added. Second, incumbents would have even less opposition and would become politically more secure. Third, since as the number of congressional seats grew, the proportional influence of each one would inevitably decrease, there would come a time when incumbents would tighten up the standards for allowing new seats to be created in order to prevent further dilution of their prominence.

Something like this has happened with psychiatric diagnoses. Diagnoses have rapidly expanded in number to cover broader areas of social behavior and to slice narrower disorders out of broader established ones. Newer categories of disorder contend for territory with established ones, as each revision of the diagnostic manual proclaims the latest nosological redistricting. Since DSM-III, incumbent diagnoses are increasingly hard to unseat. Although there are few limits to the number of new diagnoses that can be added, the standards for adding new diagnoses have been raised, lest the number of disorders become so vast as to undermine the integrity of the entire enterprise. DSM-I (1952) contained 106 different diagnostic categories; DSM-II (1968) had 182; DSM-III (1980) offered 265; and its revision, DSM-III-R (1987), raised it to 292 (Blashfield, Sprock & Fuller, 1990; Frances, Pincus, Widiger, Davis,

& First, 1990). DSM-IV is undergoing redistricting now and proponents are clamoring for the inclusion of new disorders such as "maladaptive denial of physical illness" (Strauss, Spitzer & Muskin, 1990); Delusional Dominating Personality Disorder, feminists' proposal for defining men's beliefs about themselves and women (Albee, Canetto, & Sefa-Dedeh, 1991); *Koro*, anxiety associated with the fear of penis retraction causing death, found among Asian cultures (Bernstein & Gaw, 1990); and many more.

One reason for the seemingly endless proposals for new disorders is the fact that diagnostic criteria for many of them involve behaviors or experiences that are fairly common among the general population. Creating a "mental disorder" involves specifying the features of these experiences and then demarcating where normality shades into abnormality. Splitting one disorder from another requires only that all the features of one disorder not be shared by another, even though they may share some criteria (i.e., overlapping symptoms). Determining when relatively common experiences such as anxiety or sadness or memory lapses should be considered evidence of some disorder requires the setting of arbitrary boundaries. Where those boundaries are set determines how prevalent that disorder is in the population (cf. Liptzin et al., 1991; Robins & Regier, 1991). If the threshold for the disorder is set too low, making many common experiences evidence of mental disorder, the diagnosis may be ridiculed. Making the criteria stringent makes it politically easier to create a new disorder, since its defined statistical rarity buttresses its "abnormality," but it may render the disorder too rare to be of any practical interest to clinicians or researchers.

The lumping and splitting of behaviors and personal experiences into categories of disorder involves more than technical decisions. It also involves negotiations among contending interest groups of theoreticians, researchers, clinicians, and, at times, potential patients. Changing the psychiatric nosology involves struggles among constituencies and balancing conflicting interests. Over time, the process of changing DSM has become much more elaborate. The last four revisions of the nomenclature of the APA illustrate this growing complexity.

Changing DSM-I

DSM-I, published in 1952, marked a triumph of psychodynamic perspectives over the older, organic, institutionally based nosology (Grob, 1991). Developing its successor, DSM-II, was justified primarily by the need to keep the United States's nosology in rough alignment with the World Health Organization's (WHO) International Classification of Diseases (ICD), a list of diseases that included mental diseases and that was revised periodically in consultation with health officials from many countries. The eighth edition of the ICD was approved in 1966 and became effective in 1968. American psychiatrists who had been directly involved in working with ICD committees during the early and mid-1960s played key roles in the APA's Committee on Nomenclature and Statistics, which produced DSM-II in 1968 (APA, 1968). Thus, the international manual exerted some direct control over the revision of DSM-I.

By contemporary standards, changing DSM-I was a relatively private and simple process, more like changing rules and regulations within one organization than negotiating treaties among many rival factions each with very different objectives. In 1965, the APA assigned the task of preparing a new manual to its Committee on Nomenclature and Statistics, chaired by Ernest Gruenberg, who had been involved in preparing ICD-8. By February 1967 a draft manual was circulated to 120 psychiatrists. After being revised, it was approved by the APA in December 1967 and it became effective on July 1, 1968. The process was short and simple.

There is very little information about the process of changing DSM-I in DSM-II or in an accompanying promotional article published in AJP in June 1968 (Spitzer & Wilson, 1968). The presentations avoided highlighting any controversies or bitter disputes that may have arisen in the revision, and instead simply reported how the new manual differed from the former version. Mention was made that the term *reaction*, as in *schizophrenic reaction*, had been dropped, but that this should not be read as endorsement for a Kraepelinian way of thinking. Rather, the intent of the APA committee was to avoid terms that suggested etiology where it was still in doubt. The presentation of DSM-II to the mental health community was couched in language that suggested that nothing substantive had been done. And yet, new categories of disorder were added, the nomenclature was organized in a different way, the recording of multiple psychiatric diagnoses and associated physical conditions was explicitly encouraged, qualifying phrases were changed, and there were numerous revisions in the definitions of disorders (Spitzer & Wilson, 1968).

What is striking about these first reports about DSM-II is that they were presented as matter-of-fact updates and reorganizations of categories, rather than as changes that represent major rethinking or new decision-making standards. The changes were explained simply, sometimes with, but most often without any explanation or rationale for the change. Almost completely absent was any attempt to justify the many changes on the basis of scientific evidence.

Changing DSM-I was a process that involved a small committee of experts (eight members and two consultants), who worked privately and quickly to make many changes in the manual. They apparently never felt compelled to justify their decisions on scientific grounds. In the words of the chairman, "The Committee has attempted to put down what it judges to be generally agreed upon by well-informed psychiatrists today" (APA, 1968:viii). DSM-II was designed to reflect psychiatric opinion, not to produce it. It was not an instrument for change.

Spitzer and Wilson (1969), in what may have constituted the first—and only—defense of DSM-II, recommended that a small group be in charge of producing DSM-III and that the committee be supplemented by subcommittees of experts, that a draft version of DSM-III be distributed more widely, that the next manual be given an adequate clinical trial, and that a multidimensional approach be considered. This was written at least six years before Spitzer was appointed to head the DSM-III Task Force, but foreshadowed by a decade exactly what was eventually done.

Changing DSM-II

DSM-II may have had a relatively easy birth, but by 1975, congenital defects were apparent. DSM-II came quickly under attack, because it was a convenient scapegoat for the weaknesses of American psychiatry. By using unreliability of DSM-II, the work of the developers of the next version of the nosology was made considerably easier. Although DSM-II had been used for a decade, it was vague, inconsistent, theoretically clumsy (despite earlier claims that it eschewed theory), and empirically weak in terms of both the validity and reliability of its diagnostic categories. Nevertheless, for psychodynamic therapists who emerged after World War II as the dominant group in American psychiatry, DSM-II served as a comforting and familiar small desk manual. Many clinicians appreciated its modest administrative uses; few viewed it as a treatise on psychiatric philosophy or treatment (Grob, 1991; Wilson, 1990). As a minor desk reference, DSM-II was neither prominent nor controversial among practicing clinicians. It did not impose on their treatment plans or restrict their professional judgment. DSM-II had few defenders or spokespersons because no one sensed a need to protect it.

For psychiatric researchers, however, DSM-II was nearly useless as a scientific guidebook. This problem, in conjunction with the high ambitions of the DSM-III Task Force, composed of researchers, led to the extensive revision of the manual that has been characterized as transforming American psychiatry in this century (Wilson, 1990). The revolution in nosology that was represented by DSM-III can be attributed in part to the lack of scholars ready to defend the scientific validity of DSM-II, the control and influence exercised by the original DSM-III Task Force, and the spirit of inclusion and innovation that characterized the orientation of those most deeply committed to changing DSM-II. The first two of these factors have been discussed in earlier chapters. The third deserves comment.

Millon (1986), one of the original members of the DSM-III Task Force and, by his own estimate, one of those most responsible for encouraging the APA to undertake a major revision of the manual, has offered a detailed and revealing account of the early development of DSM-III. It is apparent from his account that the DSM-III Task Force was eager to capitalize on a political opportunity presented by a unique historical moment in American psychiatry. From the beginning, members of the DSM-III Task Force wanted to make a radical change in psychiatric nosology. They had no interest in a cosmetic updating of the antiquated manual or in merely tidying up differences between it and the ICD-9. The DSM-III Task Force recognized the inherent difficulties of developing a classification system. American psychiatry and the field of mental health were more fragmented and diverse than they had been in 1960. The developers knew that it was impossible to organize a classification system that would satisfy multiple constituencies with different views about etiology, prognosis, structure, severity, or relevant dimensions (axes).

One advantage of the DSM-III Task Force was that it was chaired by someone who had been intimately involved with DSM-II, and who had signed an "imprimatur" page in DSM-II personally approving the manual and who became the public defender of DSM-II when it was published. Thus, few would suspect that within five years, such a key actor in DSM-II would spearhead its complete demise.

While attempting to weed out theoretical biases from the manual, the DSM-III Task Force was predisposed to include many new diagnostic categories. Millon admitted that their intentions were to "embrace as many conditions as are commonly seen by practicing clinicians" in order to maximize the research opportunities in the future "to evaluate the character of each condition as a valid syndromal entity" (1986:39). While initially requiring that any potentially new category be specified by diagnostic criteria and distinctness, the ultimate inclusion test was in part political: whether the diagnosis was used with reasonable frequency, whether interested professionals and patient representatives offered positive comments about it, and whether the new condition maximized its utility for outpatient populations (Millon, 1986:39–40). This philosophy of change that welcomed new diagnoses was very different from that adopted fifteen years later by the DSM-IV Task Force (Frances, 1990a, 1990b).

The guiding philosophy of the DSM-III Task Force during its first year when the groundwork and structure for DSM-III were firmly planted, was to err on the side of inclusion of new categories. One motivation was to make the new manual reflective of the array of conditions that practitioners confronted, particularly in outpatient settings where psychiatric treatment increasingly took place. Understandably, many practitioners wanted to see an expanded array of disorders to reflect the diversity of patients that they were treating. A second motivation was that the expansion of psychiatric turf might capture more fiscal coverage from third party reimbursements, which had become so much more important to the financing of mental health care.

A third motivation, and one very compatible with the empirical research orientation of the developers, was to cast the diagnostic net wide so that data could be routinely gathered via the manual about the merits of various psychiatric conditions. Those who supported this direction argued that only by including new categories and diagnostic criteria would clinical and, more importantly, research attention be focused on them. This strategy of inclusion was in keeping with the more global effort to fit a practicing profession into an ongoing empirical research agenda.

Changing DSM-III

DSM-III was published in February 1980, and almost immediately planning began on its revision. The APA appointed a Committee to Evaluate DSM-III. Robert Spitzer was appointed "to aid the committee in its work," although in his words, "it is difficult to be objective about the strengths and limitations of one's own offspring" (Spitzer & Williams, 1987:425). The Committee to Evaluate DSM-III recommended in March 1983 that a new group be created to "fine-tune" DSM-III. In May 1983, with DSM-III barely three years old, the formal revision process began with the appointment by the APA of the Work Group to Revise DSM-III, composed of eight psychiatrists and chaired by—the parent—Robert Spitzer (Millon, 1986; Work Group, 1985).

The DSM-III-R Work Group, like its predecessor, used 25 advisory committees and involved over 230 consultants (Work Group, 1985). Two drafts of the revision were made available to the public, one in October 1985 and a final draft in August 1986. The revised manual, the *Diagnostic and Statistical Manual of Mental Disorders, Third Edition, Revised* (DSM-III-R) was published in May 1987.

This move to revise DSM-III almost as soon as it was published was quite different from the path taken with DSM-II. The quick move to revise had strategic advantages. For one, DSM-III became a moving target, unlike DSM-II, which sat still in the water for 12 years, becoming a dead duck long before it was replaced. Talk of the revision of DSM-III began even before DSM-III was published, a tactically brilliant way of deflecting criticism during the controversial approval process. The new manual could be presented as "a still frame" in a moving picture, an imperfect attempt that would be continually improved as time went on. Serious questions could be deferred for the next time around; criticisms could be accommodated by pledging that experience with the new manual would guide its revision; imperfections could be tolerated since the DSM-III was only temporary. By presenting the manual as provisional, not final, as one important step in an ongoing scientific process, the force of criticism was muted and opponents were offered future opportunities for change. Doors appeared to be left opened.

Developing a manual that was in perpetual motion was a strategic advantage in deflecting opposition, but it was also a potential disadvantage to those who wanted to maintain the structure of the new system and secure the many changes that had been made. With victory still fresh, the developers of DSM-III now had to open the door for modifications. The reappointment of Spitzer to the key leadership position was one early signal that backsliding was not contemplated. Another signal that the Work Group was not inviting serious challenges to DSM-III was its charge "to recommend modifications in the DSM-III text and criteria that would clarify ambiguities, resolve inconsistencies, and incorporate factual changes based on data that had accumulated since the publication of DSM-III in 1980" (Work Group, 1985:5). These explicit objectives are examples of what Kuhn (1970) calls "normal science," mopping up activities to strengthen and elaborate a reigning paradigm. Since DSM-IV was already scheduled to appear in the early 1990s, the revision of DSM-III could be presented as a minor, technical update, once again appearing to defer substantive changes for yet another time, place, and process.

Although participation in the revision process was encouraged, the Work Group tried to control controversy. Members of subcommittees were nominated by Work Group members and letters were sent to these resource people asking them to note ways they wanted to participate in the revision. Most simply agreed to review drafts of the revision. Spitzer selected specialists for the many subcommittees and they, in turn, recommended other members (Franklin, 1987). Spitzer and his wife, Janet B. W. Williams, were once again members of every subcommittee.

Even the process of making minor changes was tightly controlled.

Letters that announced the planned revision were sent to major psychiatric journals, asking those who wished to make suggestions to complete a new page for each category or general topic they proposed to change. When the first draft of the new manual, *DSM-III-R in Development*, was published, readers were invited to participate in the revision process but were asked to remember "the Critical Cs" in preparing their criticisms:

> Correct: Are the criteria useful for correctly identifying individuals with the disorder . . . ?
> Clinical: Can you provide better clinical examples . . . ?
> Clarity: Can you improve on clumsy, awkward, or obscure phraseology . . . ?
> Compassion: The most important C. Please show it by following these guidelines. (Work Group, 1985:7)

All this guidance suggested that criticisms should be limited to improving the existing description of disorders. Clearly, lengthy discourses about their validity or extended debates about larger issues were discouraged. To interested professionals, the Work Group maintained the guise of pursuing minor, technical improvements, and these within rigid parameters. Instead of publicly displaying the spirit of innovation and inclusion of new ideas that marked the development of DSM-III, the Work Group portrayed itself as a maid less interested in the rearrangement of furniture than in making certain that it was dusted and in place.

In fact, much more substantial changes were in process, but were not broadcast. In the end, four of the five axes that are the basic dimensions of the DSM-III diagnostic system were refashioned. Over a third of the more than 200 diagnostic categories were changed, many in extensive ways. And significantly, more than 30 new diagnostic categories were added, according to APA advertisements for DSM-III-R paraphernalia. One researcher has claimed that because of the extensiveness of the changes, this version should have been called DSM-IV (Zimmerman, 1988). Most of this passed without controversy, until feminist psychotherapists confronted the APA about the proposed inclusion of three new psychiatric disorders that they viewed as having serious negative consequences for women: Paraphilac Rapism, Premenstrual Dysphoric Disorder, and Masochistic Personality Disorder (for a discussion of this controversy, see Kutchins & Kirk, 1989). A media bonanza flowed from that conflict, resolved in the end by relegating the revised controversial diagnoses to the appendix of DSM-III-R.

The process of changing DSM-III was designed so that the Work Group enjoyed multiple advantages. DSM-III being in what seemed like perpetual revision, critics had difficulty taking aim at it. Even when striking a target they learned that the target was already moribund, cast off during the last revision. By soliciting suggestions for minor clarification, the Work Group discouraged serious confrontations and invited only editorial assistance. Moreover, by suggesting to outsiders that changes should be based on empirical evidence, the Work Group limited the kind of suggestions that would be entertained, while, in fact, decisions were not usually made on those grounds (Kendler, Spitzer, & Williams, 1989). Meanwhile, they made hundreds of alterations, some very substantial. Furthermore, by appearing to be just tinkering with the old system, they avoided any demands that their revisions undergo systematic tests for reliability. No new reliability studies were conducted and the reliability appendix symbolically included in DSM-III was dropped when DSM-III-R was published. In changing DSM-III, research psychiatrists tightened their grip on psychiatric nomenclature, while they attempted to present to outsiders the illusion that nothing of much significance had taken place.

Changing DSM-III-R

Only four months after DSM-III-R was published, at a time when most clinicians and researchers had not had time to review or become familiar with the new version, the APA Committee on Psychiatric Diagnosis and Assessment met to explore possible timetables for the publication of DSM-IV. In May 1988, the board of trustees of the APA proceeded to appoint another task force to begin work on the fourth edition of the DSM. The first draft was scheduled to be completed in 1990 (*Psychiatric News*, April 15, 1988, p. 13) and final publication was to be in December 1992 (see Frances, 1990a:1), but this was quickly moved to 1993 (Frances, Widiger, & Pincus, 1989) and then slid tentatively to 1993–1994 (E. Benedek, president of APA, remarks in APA session May 16, 1990; Frances, 1990b). Allen Frances, who served on the Work Group to Revise DSM-III and had participated on the Personality Disorders subcommittee of the DSM-III Task Force, was appointed as chairman of the DSM-IV Task Force. Spitzer was appointed as a member of the new group, but his title was changed to special consultant. Before copies of DSM-III-R made their way into the offices of clinicians, the APA nosologists had already focused their attention on what needed to be changed. Clearly before clinicians could develop informed judgments about the new manual or before any empirical research could begin, a new manual was entering the design phase. Planned obsolescence, long a dominant theme of the American auto industry, was adopted by the APA for the business of psychiatric diagnosis.

But the process of changing DSM-III-R and producing DSM-IV—or at least how it was initially presented to the APA membership—was quite different than earlier revisions of the manual. One difference was that it was initiated amid controversy about whether a new revision was even needed. This controversy, surprisingly, came not from practitioners scrambling to keep track of the flow of new diagnostic categories and criteria, but from researchers whose work was very much in keeping with the new empirical, criterion-oriented diagnostic system.

Mark Zimmerman, a prominent psychiatric researcher who had participated in one of the Work Group subcommittees producing DSM-III-R, published a stinging brief article questioning the usefulness of proceeding with DSM-IV (Zimmerman, 1988) and another even stronger statement in response to his critics (Zimmerman, 1990). It prompted a revealing rejoinder from the new leadership of the DSM-IV Task Force (Frances et al., 1989), first defensively titled "Why Work Has Begun on DSM-IV," but later published under the less assertive title "The Development of DSM-IV." The exchange sheds light on the role of empirical research in the process of revising the diagnostic manual. Zimmerman pointed out the frequency of manual revisions, and questioned whether the rapidity of changes allowed time for the findings of empirical research to be used as a basis for decisions. He argued:

> I envision the following timetable: much of the initial research on the validity of the new DSM-III-R criteria will have begun in the fall of 1987, a few months after the publication of DSM-III-R. Allowing a year for data collection; six months for data entry, data analysis, and writing of the manuscript; and another year until the report appears in print, we should not expect to read even the first of these results until 1990. . . . the first draft [of DSM-IV] is scheduled to be completed in 1990. Thus, only limited data will be available to guide the revisers, and more importantly, there will be no time to replicate those results that suggest that changes are needed. . . . I am skeptical that the DSM-IV committee(s) will be able to limit themselves to changes based on replicated research. Instead, we will have groups of experts making changes (on the basis of clinical experience). (1988:1135)

He directly challenged the proposition that frequent revisions improve the manual scientifically. He questioned whether constant revisions have really improved diagnostic reliability or validity, the ability of researchers to study these matters, or the quality of psychiatric care provided to patients. He asked whether the constant revisions might have more to do with financial considerations of the APA, hinting, for example, that new manuals lead to new sales and profits for the APA and perhaps for others who develop after-market paraphernalia. Other researchers raised similar questions about the need for a new revision (Ellis & Mellsop, 1990; Blashfield et al., 1990).

The sting in these criticisms comes from their well-aimed point that the timing of the revisions impedes the careful development and testing of the knowledge required to advance the scientific foundation of psychiatric nosology. This concern was raised about the prior revision of the manual as well (Regier, 1987). Zimmerman went further. He and associates surveyed four groups of psychiatrists about their opinion regarding the appropriate interval before publishing DSM-IV (Zimmerman, Jampala, Sierles, & Taylor, 1991). A majority of their national sample of practicing psychiatrists, residency directors, researchers, and residents believed that DSM-IV is being published prematurely. More revealing is that fact that this opinion was strongest among the researchers (two out of three agreed). Since the major ostensible rationale for revision is to incorporate new scientific findings, when respected researchers such as Zimmerman and others show how the revision process undercuts the very activity that is suppose to justify the changes, the APA feels a understandable chill from the icy breeze.

The response to Zimmerman from those responsible for the DSM-IV Task Force is revealing because they argue that "the most compelling reason for beginning work on DSM-IV" is not scientific, but political, an obscure treaty obligation the United States has with the World Health Organization to maintain terminological consistency with the ICD, which is undergoing its tenth revision (ICD-10). They maintain that revising the DSM and the ICD, although they are different nosologies that have never been completely consistent, should be coordinated in some fashion. Frances et al. (1989) argue that DSM-II and DSM-III were revised when ICD was. They are silent on the rationale for DSM-III-R, since that revision did not coincide with any ICD edition and the new DSM-III Task Force chairman admitted that he thought it was a mistake to have produced DSM-III-R (Frances, 1990b).

Basing the rationale for DSM-IV on ICD-10 has struck some observers as disingenuous (Kendell, 1991). ICD-10 was in an advanced state of preparation *before* the DSM-IV Task Force ever met. The first formal meetings to plan ICD-10 took place in 1983, a first draft was produced in 1986, a comprehensive version was circulated for field trials in 1987, and by 1989 formal approvals were obtained. Although both DSM-IV and ICD-10 may appear in 1993, suggestions that they are being developed simultaneously are very misleading (Kendell, 1991). Kendell suggests that one explanation for the APA's increasingly frequent revisions of DSM is not to coordinate work with the ICD, but to reap the "huge and unexpected profit" that DSM-III and subsequent editions generated.

Against this backdrop of criticism, the DSM-IV Task Force has gone to great lengths to assure mental health professionals that changes incorporated into DSM-IV would not be arbitrary or whimsical. In fact, the process of changing DSM-III-R is quite elaborate (Frances, First, Pincus,

Widiger, & Davis, 1990). The president of the APA appointed 16 members to the DSM-IV Task Force, one of whom chaired each of the 13 work groups to develop revisions. Each work group drew on the expertise of between 50 and 100 consultants and advisors (*DSM-IV Update*, January 1989). This elaboration of committees and experts is matched by an elaboration of conferences and processes designed to control decision-making. Two conferences to discuss methodological issues in the construction of DSM-IV were held early. Elaborate outlines were developed for the review and synthesis of available empirical data (Widiger, 1988a, 1988b) which were scheduled to be published as a DSM-IV source book, providing explicit documentation of the evidential bases for the DSM-IV text and criteria sets (Frances et al., 1989). Later, plans for field trials were developed (*DSM-IV Update*, January/February 1990).

But most revealing is the way in which the developers of DSM-IV characterized the processes used to develop DSM-III and DSM-III-R in contrast to their own approach to DSM-IV. In responding to Zimmerman, they acknowledged that they have noticed the temptation for a task force or work group member to argue for the inclusion of changes that express his or her theoretical or empirical perspective, rather than changes based on the totality of the research evidence (Frances et al., 1989). They also acknowledged that:

> It must be recognized that DSM-III and DSM-III-R were, by necessity, the result of expert group consensus subject to the limitations of group process. Although the recommendations of the members of the DSM advisory groups were based on their knowledge and understanding of the research literature, the lack of any systematic review of this literature before decisions were made and the lack of documentation of the empirical and/or conceptual bases for the revisions sometimes led to at least the appearance of arbitrariness. (p. 374)

The principles that guide DSM-IV were supposed to be different. To sooth the concerns of a potential hostile audience, Frances et al. (1989) asserted that:

> we have developed criteria for including changes in DSM-IV that are much more conservative than was the case for DSM-III and DSM-III-R. It is in fact possible that the major innovation of DSM-IV will not be in its having surprising new content but rather will reside in the systematic and explicit method by which DSM-IV will be constructed and documented. (p. 375)

They attempted to reassure the psychiatric community that they will be guided by the following perspective:

Nothing in DSM-III-R is sacred but revisions should not be based simply on expert opinion. Decisions should be substantiated by explicit statements of rationale and an explicit, systematic review of the evidential basis. Consideration should be given to clinical utility, user friendliness, and the impact on other diagnoses or criteria within the DSM. It is very important to achieve greater compatibility with ICD-10 but this should not be at the cost of sacrificing important clinical concepts or distinctions. It is recognized that revisions can be disruptive to research programs, and that some revisions are more disruptive than others. . . . The intent will be to find the optimal balance among historical tradition as embodied in DSM-III and DSM-III-R, compatibility with ICD-10, evidence from the current reviews of the literature and analysis of unpublished data sets, and widely established expert consensus. The requirements for evidence to support change in DSM-IV will be set much higher than was demanded in DSM-III and DSM-III-R, but the evidential requirements will also vary across disorders since the quantity and quality of data available to DSM-III and DSM-III-R were themselves not consistent across disorders. (p. 374)

Here is an exquisitely crafted political shuffle. Under the guise of making explicit the decision rules that will be used to make changes in the manual, they wrote a carefully balanced statement that no one could possibly disagree with because it indicated that everything will be taken into account when tough decisions have to be made. Expert opinion will not be enough, but expert consensus will be considered. Systematic reviews of evidence will be required, except where it is limited or not available. Nothing is sacred, but historical tradition is to be respected.

This early rhetoric about the development of DSM-IV is significant, independent of what will actually transpire in the process of creating the revised manual. First, there is an explicit attempt to emphasize scientific merit, rigor and values over personal whim, preference, and bias. "We now have an opportunity in DSM-IV," they claim, "to provide the first well-documented psychiatric nosology" (Frances et al., 1989:374). As late as November 1990, they claimed that the "major methodological innovation of DSM-IV will be its effort to move beyond expert consensus by placing greater emphasis on the careful, objective accumulation of empirical evidence" (Frances, Pincus, Widiger, Davis, & First, 1990:1446). They strive to be psychiatric pioneers, carrying diagnosis into the rock-solid land of scientific evidence and leaving a well-marked trail so everyone can understand how they traversed the difficult topography. Of course, these were the claims of the developers of DSM-III a decade before. Science and evidence are always unassailable justification for tinkering with a technical reference manual.

The other significant element in the rhetoric is the sharp, but respectful, contrast they made between the standards and processes used to create both DSM-III and DSM-III-R and those being used for IV. Frances et al. (1989) paint a portrait of the earlier revisions as depending too much on opinion and group process and not enough on systematic and rigorous review of existing evidence. At the 1990 annual meeting of the APA, Frances claimed that his DSM-III Task Force was trying to "reduce the politics of the articulate spokesman" that had influenced earlier revisions (Frances, 1990a). Moreover, Frances et al. imply that there was a too liberal, inclusionary ethic at play in the past. By contrast, "the requirements for evidence to support changes in DSM-IV will be set much higher than was demanded in DSM-III and DSM-III-R" (Frances et al, 1989:374) and the "criteria for including changes in DSM-IV . . . are much more conservative than was the case for DSM-III and DSM-III-R" (p. 375).

Rhetorically, this language accomplishes two things. First, by implication it undercuts the scientific integrity of the processes used in earlier revisions, very much as the integrity of DSM-II was destroyed by the negatively biased interpretations of the early reliability studies. By questioning the processes of revisions in the past, Frances et al. strengthen indirectly their claim that another revision is required. If the former processes were flawed—too liberal, too personal—then, by implication, the final product must be flawed as well. Second, by playing on these weaknesses, they can present their own revision as scientifically more rigorous and credible, thereby setting the stage for what will undoubtedly be later claims that the newest version is much improved and fully worthy of the effort.

There has been a steady and concerted effort by the developers of DSM-IV to get the word out about why DSM-IV is necessary and how it will be better than previous versions. The process of revision is described as both rigorous and open (cf. Widiger, Frances, Pincus, Davis, & First, 1991), a claim that some find strained. Responding to one description of the DSM-IV development process, one psychiatrist thought that desire to base the new manual on empirical data was going to be compromised by other issues:

> These include the "crucial" need to incorporate the suggestions of hundreds of work group advisors and *over* 65 organizations; the need for an "optimal balance" with regard to literature reviews, tradition, ICD-10, and "common sense"; and applicability to the "widest diversity of settings," ranging from clinical work and research to disability determinations and insurance reimbursement.
>
> I submit that the task force has set itself two mutually contradictory goals. One is the formulation of a data-based nomenclature; the other is a consensus-based system acceptable to a hodgepodge of committees and organizations, attorneys, and insurance companies.

> If history is any guide, the consensus-based system will prevail. (Dean, 1991:1426)

To this and other letters criticizing aspects of DSM-IV, the developers usually respond very respectfully, by emphasizing how different their development process is from the development of DSM-III and III-R and how faithful they will be to data (Frances, Pincus, Widiger, Davis, & First, 1991). Their responses so far have little of the combative tone that characterized the responses to critics of DSM-III, but final decisions about DSM-IV have not been unveiled. Certainly the energy devoted to these public relations activities appears to far exceed what was expended on any prior revision of DSM. A periodic newsletter, *DSM-IV Update*, is mailed to interested professionals, informing them about the work of the DSM-IV Task Force. A regular column, "DSM-IV in Progress," appears in the APA journal, *Hospital and Community Psychiatry*, usually summarizing the work of one or another of the DSM-IV Task Force subcommittees or work groups. Informational sessions are held at the annual meetings of the APA. In addition, articles from various work groups have been appearing regularly in the professional literature.

By the end of 1991, however, most of these communications described the processes of review, emphasized the attempts to be systematic and unbiased and reviewed the issues or dilemmas that the DSM-IV Task Force or its work groups faced. The bulk of the material emphasized the decisions that still lay ahead, rather than the decisions that had already been made. Indeed, rather than a draft of DSM-IV, as had been anticipated earlier, the first official publication of the DSM-IV Task Force was a book of "options" (Task Force on DSM-IV, 1991). Presenting options had the benefit of not staking out territory that has to be defended against critics and at the same time it presented the process as wide open to everyone. The options book made the DSM-IV Task Force relatively impervious to direct criticism since it presented no decisions. Furthermore, the empirical grounding for these options—extensive literature reviews and data reanalyses—were not scheduled for publication until sometime in 1992, four years after the revision process began and a year after the options were identified. As 1992 arrived, it was difficult for an observer of DSM-IV to link any decisions or directions with "empirical data." The links come later, the DSM-IV Task Force has promised.

The Change Process

In a 25-year period (1968–1993), American psychiatry will have adopted at least four substantially different official diagnostic nosologies. Furthermore, within only 14 years (1979–1993) all four will have been operative. With each change, diagnoses disappear, others are created, and almost all of those with tenure are redefined. Four observations can be made about these processes of nosological change in American psychiatry.

First, none of the revisions has been stimulated by clinical practitioners demanding a new classification system. Since DSM is ostensibly a clinical tool, outsiders may find this lack of clinician demand a curious fact. The explanation of this peculiarity has to do with the fact that DSM is a very different type of tool to clinicians than to either psychiatric researchers or to the developers of DSM.

Second, the process of decision-making has become more elaborate. With each revision, the approval of changes in the manual moves through increasing layers of advisors, work groups, task forces, governance committees, and boards. In this process, and by open invitations for advice and comment, more and more participants play some minor role in the revision. Many of their names and titles are prominently displayed in the published manual, lending superficial legitimacy to the product through the number of hands that have touched it. But just as important, the involvement of larger groups of individuals has made the task of revising the nosology much more politically complex. Since available scientific data will not provide definitive answers to many questions, the remaining issues must be handled through complicated rounds of negotiation.

Third, new diagnostic categories are frequently added and old ones are split into two or more. Diagnostic criteria, both inclusion and exclusion criteria, are continually churned, resorted, and redefined. With each shuffle, the claim is made that the outcome is greater validity and more precision in the diagnostic system. The unmistakable implication is that reliability will be improved through this painstaking process. Mistakes are corrected, ambiguities are clarified, and new knowledge is incorporated. Thus, every change, even ones that will be abandoned within a few months, are presented as scientifically grounded. And since the final product, incorporating hundreds of minor and major changes, has not been explicitly tied (e.g., through citations to research articles) to the body of knowledge on which it is presumably based, the claims of science at work are usually sufficient persuasion.

Fourth, the process of revising each version of the DSM begins with the first official questioning of the scientific status of the current nosology, proceeds to tout the superior process being used for the version being developed, moves to proclaim that the brand-new version represents vast improvements over the old, encourages everyone to purchase the new publication with its paraphernalia (casebooks, tapes, instructional aids, etc.), and ends with a new task force questioning the scientific status of the latest version. The cycle of denigration, enthusiasm, and denigration is recognizable in many claims of scientific achievement, where breakthroughs make an old system appear antiquated and a new system necessary.

Although this is the underlying justification for the continual revisions in the diagnostic manual, the evidence for breakthroughs is not self-evident. In fact, the leaders of the DSM-IV Task Force did not even try to argue that scientific knowledge had increased so much since the issuing of DSM-III-R in 1987 that another revision was necessary. Had they attempted to, their claims would have been viewed incredulously. Hence, the DSM-IV Task Force appealed to distant, vague treaty obligations that do not obligate the APA as justification where scientific evidence was absent.

Securing Turf for Normal Science

Zimmerman's (1988, 1990) critical point, however, was more profound. He not only argued that there was not an accumulation of new knowledge that needed to be incorporated, but that the increasing rapidity of change actively disrupted the ability of researchers effectively to test the current system in time to have the scientific findings replicated and then considered in the next revision of the manual. Not only was change not justified, it would inevitably not be guided by the accumulation of replicated scientific findings. He argued that the frequency of changing the nosology had become an impediment to psychiatric research and knowledge development, not its finest expression.

The issue of diagnostic reliability serves as the most prominent example of this tendency to begin with significant scientific questions and end by clutching onto cherished beliefs regardless of their scientific standing. We have already described how DSM-III, having been proposed as the solution to the problem of diagnostic reliability, distorted the interpretation of the available evidence on the way to becoming a smashing success. After a few other studies failed to confirm the reliability of DSM-III, attention turned increasingly to the reliability of specific narrow diagnostic categories, rather than to the nosology itself. Shortly thereafter the question of the reliability of DSM-III was made obsolete by the activity to produce DSM-III-R. The reliability of DSM-III was both taken for granted and made irrelevant in a matter of a few years. Having successfully solved the reliability problem, DSM-III was put to rest and never fully scrutinized.

DSM-III-R became the heir to the reliability claims made successfully about its predecessor. DSM-III-R's reliability was never questioned, no field trials were conducted to study interrater agreement, and no evidence of its ability to produce consistent diagnostic judgments was offered. No one even called for such tests to be done. The child of DSM-III inherited the widely acclaimed scientific status of the parent without any effort on its own.

What tests of diagnostic reliability have appeared in the literature, and there has been a small trickle, are specialized studies of particular diagnoses, of particular populations, or of different diagnostic criteria (Mannuzza et al., 1989). For example, Vitiello, Malone, Buschle, Delaney, & Behar (1990) studied the diagnoses of 46 hospitalized children using three methods and concluded that the reliability of child psychiatric diagnoses remain problematic. But these studies are largely irrelevant to the current nosology, suggesting only that criteria need to be tidied up in one particular section of the system. In this way, all counterevidence is easily co-opted and defused. The passage of time serves to cloud the professional memory of the exaggerated claims made about reliability during the birth of the new system.

After lying dormant for almost a decade, the issue of diagnostic reliability re-emerged somewhat belatedly in the DSM-IV Task Force. In early 1990 the APA (Office of Research, 1990) announced that a grant from the MacArthur Foundation would support:

> the development of an extensive series of videotapes representing typical and not-so-typical presentations of common DSM disorders. The videotapes will be shown to clinicians to help determine the range of reliability achieved by selected diagnoses under different conditions of patient prototypicality, clinician experience and evaluation method. (p. 1)

In a later publication (Widiger et al., 1991), the developers of DSM-IV provided some additional information about how they regard the reliability studies that were planned on the eve of the publication of DSM-IV. They placed the new reliability studies in the historical context of the DSM-III field trials, which to them "demonstrated good to excellent interrater reliability for many of the major classes of disorders, a finding of considerable importance" (p. 284). They conceded that some reliability studies of DSM-III were disappointing, but they did not fault the manual. Instead, they blamed the way that practitioners use or misuse it. They made the argument that reliability levels are artifacts of research methodology (e.g., the simplicity of clinical cases used, the training of diagnosticians, the degree of adherence to a structured interview, and the rigid use of the diagnostic criteria), a view, of course, articulated 30 years ago by Beck (1962). The focus of the DSM-IV reliability field trials will be to document the extent to which some of these methodological factors affect reliability levels (Widiger et al., 1991).

Although by late 1990, the exact details of the field trial had not been finalized, the plan called for the development of five videotaped interviews for each of ten DSM-IV diagnoses. The prototypicality (i.e., the extent to which they illustrate clearly a particular disorder) of the five interviews would vary. The interviewers on the videotapes will use a modified version of the Structured Clinical Interview. The videotapes will be viewed by three thousand clinicians from a wide variety of settings who will be asked to record diagnoses. Reliability levels will be assessed in relation to case prototypicality, level of training, and various demographic factors (Widiger et al., 1991).

From this preliminary information about DSM-IV's proposals, there are several clues about how the reliability issue is viewed. First, there is absolutely no indication that reliability is seen as a major problem for DSM-IV—it is simply one of the details that must be checked out. Second, since videotapes cannot be developed for every disorder, a prior decision will be made about which disorders will be studied, limiting the potential impact of any unexpected bad news. Third, by using videotapes and structured interviews, rather than live interviews, the developers will control information variance much more rigidly than in the DSM-III field trials, thus eliminating one of the common sources of interrater disagreement. Fourth, reliability levels themselves will be of secondary importance as other aspects of the diagnostic process are studied. Fifth, how reliably clinicians use DSM-IV in their regular practice has been defined as an irrelevant question. The reliability of DSM-IV as a technical innovation has been almost completely separated from how it is actually used in real circumstances. If its actual use is later found to be unreliable, the fault will be in practitioner mistakes, not in the instrument itself.

The reliability studies of DSM-IV will be carefully controlled and removed from the realities of normal practice. That is, cases will be canned (artificially created and scripted), clinicians will be selected and perhaps trained, and information variance will be minimized. More importantly, the guiding research question will not be the overall reliability of the new diagnostic system, but second-order questions regarding prototypicality. This approach should maximize the reliability results and minimize the potential for negative or embarrassing findings. Even Robert Spitzer, writing now as an outsider, has questioned the utility of the new reliability studies and suggested that in the end professional consensus, not empirical data will be needed to make decisions (Spitzer, 1991).

The announced timing of the reliability studies will prevent any scrutiny, not to mention replication, of their results by outsiders before final decisions about DSM-IV are made. Although the first draft of DSM-IV that was scheduled to be completed in 1990 (*Psychiatric News*, April 15, 1988, p. 13) never materialized and was apparently replaced by the publication of the options book in the fall of 1991, neither could possibly benefit from the videotaped reliability studies, which were not yet underway in 1990. Since no timetable has been announced for the completion and publication of the videotaped studies, it is uncertain what role if any they are likely to play in the development of the next version of DSM. Attention to reliability in the development of DSM-IV may once again play a symbolic role at the end of a long struggle.

There is a paradox in the development of DSM-IV. The DSM-IV Task Force emphasized that its procedures and standards were more rigorously scientific than either of its predecessors. Yet, by making it more difficult to change the diagnostic system, they are implicitly institutionalizing the current nosology. Using conservative criteria for changes, as opposed to the more liberal "let all flowers bloom" philosophy of the DSM-III, makes it appear that radical change is unlikely. Rather than requiring higher standards of scientific evidence for what is already in the manual, DSM-IV has higher standards only *for changing* what is already in the manual. Instead of stripping the manual of whimsical criteria or questionable diagnostic categories, a stance that would narrow the psychiatric domain, the APA chose a strategy of institutionalizing what already exists and placing the burden of proof on those who want things differently. DSM-III's ultimate success can be measured by the extent to which DSM-IV makes it difficult to introduce new or remove old content.

Like the Congress with unlimited seats that we initially described, the APA is slowly tightening (or at least claims to be tightening) the eligibility criteria for aspiring candidates. Better to gain respect by proclaiming the rigor and high admissions standards of the Congress today, than to reveal the questionable competence of the old-timers who enjoy the power of incumbency.

9

THE SOCIAL CONTEXT
OF DIAGNOSTIC ERROR

Scientists do not debunk only to cleanse and purge. They refute older ideas *in the light of* a different view about the nature of things.

Stephen Jay Gould, *The Mismeasure of Man*

One of the things a scientific community acquires with a paradigm is a criterion for choosing problems that, while the paradigm is taken for granted, can be assumed to have solutions. To a great extent these are the only problems that the community will admit as scientific or encourage its members to undertake. Other problems, including many that had previously been standard, are rejected as metaphysical, as the concern of another discipline, or sometimes as just too problematic to be worth the time. A paradigm can, for that matter, even insulate the community from those socially important problems that are not reducible to the puzzle form, because they cannot be stated in terms of the conceptual and instrumental tools the paradigm supplies.

Thomas S. Kuhn, *The Structure of Scientific Revolutions*

The issues raised about the reliability of psychiatric diagnosis in the 1950s and 1960s went to the heart of the scientific basis of psychiatry. The ability to label illness accurately was a fundamental first step for psychiatrists. A classification system of mental disorders that was scientifically respectable, however, was more than a scientific and professional imperative; it had become a public relations necessity. If psychiatrists could not agree on what the disorder was for an individual client, how could they agree on prognosis or treatment, and how could they maintain social legitimacy? The desire to name disorders reliably was the reasonable first step in developing knowledge and keeping skeptics at bay.

Diagnosis as Technical Rationality

In Chapter 2, we indicated that many professions claim that they provide service in specific circumstances through the application of general scientific knowledge and principles. This belief in what has been called "technical rationality" is used by mental health professionals and the organizations in which they work to explain many of their decisions and behaviors. They purport to apply specialized scientific knowledge consciously and carefully to specific cases and circumstances in order to solve particular problems. A well-known psychiatrist, Robert Jay Lifton, has analyzed therapeutic activity in similar terms:

> The technicist model in psychiatry works something like this: A machine, the mind-body function of the patient, has broken down; another machine, more scientifically sophisticated, is called upon to "treat" the first machine; and the treatment process itself, being technical, has nothing to do with place, time or individual idiosyncrasy. It is merely a matter of being a technical-medical antagonist of a "syndrome" or "disease." Nor is this medical-technical model limited to physicians—non-medical psychoanalysts and psychotherapists can be significantly affected by it. (Lifton, 1973:423)

Diagnosis is the presumed, crucial starting point of the technical-rational system that is used by mental health workers. The very concept of diagnosis connotes systematic problem-solving. In medicine, clinicians develop a hypothesis about the nature of a person's disease after observing the patient or being told about the symptoms or interpreting biological tests about a person's health. Facts are objectively gathered and, based on the clinician's expert knowledge, a disease or disorder is inferred. This inferred disease is then treated, with the assumption that the symptoms will disappear if the disease is effectively treated. Beyond what the physician can see and feel, diagnosis is increasingly aided by high-technology probes into heretofore unobservable phenomena: biological tests of urine and blood samples, X-rays, electrocardiogram (EKG), electroencephalogram (EEG), various genetic screening tests, computer-assisted tomography (CAT), magnetic resonance imaging (MRI), and positron emission tomography (PET) (Nelkin & Tancredi, 1989).

Judging by the vast expansion of diagnostic tests and procedures in American life, identifying "abnormalities" has become big business. A *New Yorker* cartoon (reprinted in Nelkin & Tancredi, 1989) shows cars lined up at Joe's Drive-Thru Testing Center, where customers can be quickly checked for emissions, drugs, intelligence, cholesterol, polygraph, blood pressure, soil and water, steering and brakes, stress, and loyalty. Although testing and diagnostic practices are always presented as grounded in science and technology, they are frequently inaccurate and often meaningless. Moreover, there are many chilling stories about the way that evidence for the validity of such tests is fabricated and how they are used to promote ideological and racist perspectives (Gould, 1981). The significant and growing role of diagnosis and testing in American society suggests that we should be attentive both to their purpose as well as to how they are actually used by organizations and interest groups. The practice of psychiatric diagnosis is no exception.

Psychiatric disorders are inferred by clinicians, who are supposed to adhere to objective diagnostic criteria and to prescribed decision rules. For example, for children who are "argumentative with adults, frequently lose their temper, swear, and are often angry, resentful, and easily annoyed by others" the current psychiatric nomenclature provides a diagnosis of Oppositional Defiant Disorder. To use that diagnosis, clinicians are instructed to apply a series of inclusion and exclusion criteria (see Table 9.1).

The language used to present these criteria and procedures exudes the spirit of technical rationality. The diagnosis comes with its unique code number; references to other complex concepts, e.g., mental age; specifications about precise duration (six months) and the number of symptoms needed; vague references to unspecified research about "discriminating power" and national field trials; and defined levels of severity. Through these criteria, describing common, everyday behaviors of children, the rhetoric of science transforms them into what are purported to be objective symptoms of mental disorder.

On closer inspection, however, there is little that is objective about the diagnostic criteria. For example, the first criterion, "often loses temper," consists of three ambiguous concepts. How often is often? Hourly? Once a week? What is temper? Webster's dictionary defines it as "calmness of mind." How are we to gauge when an eight-year-old "loses" his or her calmness of mind "considerably more frequent[ly] than that of most people of the same mental age"? Questions such as these could be raised about all the diagnostic criteria in Table 9.1. It would be easy to show that each depends on broad social context, particular circumstances, and subjective judgment. The point is not that these specific diagnostic criteria contain flaws or lack precision. The point is that almost all the diagnostic criteria for all the disorders require considerable subjectivity and inference. Thus, while diagnostic criteria were viewed as the major innovation of DSM-III—making diagnosis more objective and technically rational—they fail to eliminate subjectivity from psychiatric diagnosis. Instead of subjectivity influencing global diagnostic judgments, as with

Table 9.1.   Example of Diagnostic Criteria

DIAGNOSTIC CRITERIA FOR 313.81
OPPOSITIONAL DEFIANT DISORDER

Note: Consider a criterion met only if the behavior is considerably more frequent than that of most people of the same mental age.

A.   A disturbance of at least six months during which at least five of the following are present:
   (1)   often loses temper
   (2)   often argues with adults
   (3)   often actively defies or refuses adult requests or rules, e.g., refuses to do chores at home
   (4)   often deliberately does things that annoy other people, e.g., grabs other children's hats
   (5)   often blames others for his or her own mistakes
   (6)   is often touchy or easily annoyed by others
   (7)   is often angry and resentful
   (8)   is often spiteful and vindictive
   (9)   often swears or uses obscene language
   Note: The above items are listed in descending order of discriminating power based on data from a national field trial of DSM-III-R criteria for Disruptive Behavior Disorders.
B.   Does not meet the criteria for Conduct Disorder, and does not occur exclusively during the course of a psychotic disorder, Dysthymas, or a Major Depressive, Hypomanic, or Manic Episode.

Criteria for severity of Oppositional Defiant Disorder:
Mild: Few, if any, symptoms in excess of those required to make the diagnosis and only minimal or no impairment in school and social functioning.
Moderate: Symptoms or functional impairment intermediate between "mild" and "severe."
Severe: Many symptoms in excess of those required to make the diagnosis and significant and pervasive impairment in functioning at home and school and with other adults and peers.

Source: From American Psychiatric Association. Copyright © 1987. *Diagnostic and Statistical Manual of Mental Disorders, Third Edition, Revised.* Washington, D.C. Reprinted with permission.

DSM-II, subjectivity in DSM-III has been moved into many smaller subdecisions revolving around diagnostic criteria.

Regardless of the degree of subjectivity or inference involved, diagnosis is the first step in the technological process of transforming a person with an ambiguous complaint into a client with a defined mental disorder. It was precisely because of the pivotal role that diagnosis presumably plays in mental health practice that it had been for many decades the target of pointed criticism. The development of DSM-III by the APA was a major public effort to defend psychiatry by making diagnosis appear to conform more closely with the image of technical rationality. The APA's objective is understandable. How could treatment planning for clients, the development of new services, the assessment of the prevalence of mental disorder in communities, or claims on the allocation of scarce resources be made rationally, if there is substantial disagreement about the definition, nature, or procedures to be used to identify mental health problems? Improving the diagnostic classification system was one approach to making professional decision-making appear to be less haphazard and more the application of science.

The APA's efforts were also consistent with the efforts of all professions to exert control over their domains and over public policy (Abbott, 1988). By making claims about specialized knowledge and expertise, professions seize control of a problem area. They exert their right to exclusive jurisdiction and they secure autonomy and privilege in dealing with it. Through extensive education, examination, accreditation, and licensing, professions attempt to control the entrance and the process of the socialization into the occupation. Through professional associations and by having their members occupy positions in key governmental agencies, they try to influence the allocation of resources and the conditions of practice.

Maintaining or restoring credibility regarding the meaning, revision, and use of psychiatric nomenclature was the foundation for psychiatric influence and power. Fundamental problems with the integrity of diagnostic practices were unwelcome. Once recognized, they had to be politely excused as insignificant, as nothing out of the ordinary, or resolved. One tack would have been to argue that diagnosis in the medical mode was premature for the mental health professions, that knowledge about human problems, about the interaction of the mind and body and about the person and the environment were too elementary, too unrefined to fit into a rigid classification of discrete disorders. Further, the argument could be extended to suggest that knowledge of effective treatment was much too loosely tied to diagnostic categories to provide much help for treatment planning. Therefore, the argument would go, diagnostic imprecision was neither troubling nor particularly harmful to therapeutic activity at its current stage of development. The reliability problem could have been discarded as trivial.

This was not the favored interpretation. Instead, unreliability was interpreted as profoundly troubling. It was troubling because the ideology of technical rationality suggested that there was supposed to be an enormously important relationship among diagnosis, clinical reasoning, and therapeutic intervention. If diagnoses were inaccurate, the entire therapeutic enterprise was vulnerable. Thus, unreliability was something that needed to be explained and then remedied.

Meanings of Diagnostic Error

The favored explanation, as discussed in Chapter 2, was that unreliability was a result of error—errors in gathering information, errors in organizing information, errors in using information to reach decisions, errors prompted by ambiguities in nomenclature, and so forth. Diagnostic error was due to the failure of clinicians and the psychiatric nosology to conform to the full agenda of technical rationality. These assumptions about the nature and sources of diagnostic error were fundamental to the entire strategy and rationale for developing DSM-III, because they suggested that these errors were remediable through technical solutions.

Concern about clinical errors is well founded (cf. Paget, 1990). There is an extensive literature on the myriad ways in which clinical perception, reasoning, and judgment may waver from the ideal of technical rationality (Gambrill, 1990; Nurius & Gibson, 1990; Kahneman, Slovic, & Tversky, 1982). Formulating a diagnosis is dependent on complex perceptual, cognitive, and interpersonal processes. These processes are easily distorted by the clinician's past personal experiences, expectations, emotions, and by illogical thinking, unfounded inferences, selective attention, stereotypes, and all sorts of other subtle biases (cf. Loring & Powell, 1988). When these ambiguities were tied to the use of a nonspecific psychiatric nosology, like DSM-II, it was not surprising that inconsistencies in judgment were commonplace.

No one could object to any effort that attempted to reduce such errors. Errors are by definition things that are incorrectly done through ignorance or carelessness. Mental health practice, like other endeavors, is not immune to error. An incorrect diagnosis may be made, the wrong treatment may be employed, or the patient may be neglected; the clinician may be ignorant of readily available knowledge, possess unrefined skills, or have poor professional judgment. The constantly changing psychiatric nomenclature and coding can lead to additional confusion and error (Perr, 1984). Even among researchers deliberately trying to use the same diagnostic criteria, subtle variations in personal interpretations occur (Helzer & Coryell, 1983). Thus, under the best circumstances, mistakes are made because knowledge is incomplete or intervention technology is too crude to achieve the desired objectives. Mistakes and failures in these situations are regrettable, but inevitable when dealing with the uncertainty and ambiguity of individual cases. Mistakes vary in their forgivability and keep lawyers and insurance companies busy processing claims of malpractice (Besharov, 1985; Kutchins & Kirk, 1987b; Kutchins, 1991).

A second type of error is not really a mistake in the same sense as used above. It is an act that is deliberately inaccurate. Such acts may be legal and ethical transgressions involving deceit, fraud, or abuse. Charges made for services not provided, money collected for services to fictitious patients, or patients encouraged to remain in treatment longer than necessary are examples of intentional inaccuracy (Sharfstein, Gutheil, & Stoddard, 1983; Geis, Jesilow, Pontell, & O'Brien, 1985; Kerr, 1991a, 1991b; Goleman, 1991b; Freudenheim, 1991). These activities are more likely to be reported by journalists than by the professionals who may abhor such practices, but believe that they occur too rarely to be consequential. Very little has been written about these kinds of legal and ethical misdeeds in the mental health field.

The impetus for revising the diagnostic nomenclature stemmed largely from the serious concern among mental health professionals about *unintentional* errors made in diagnosis, rather than about fraud or deceit. Diagnostic errors, while unfortunate, were approached by the APA as remediable through increased knowledge, better training, higher standards for practice, and, of course, a bigger and better classification system. This approach arises naturally out of the scientific model of psychiatric practice in which technical experts are better trained to apply technical procedures. The quest for improved diagnostic reliability through the development of DSM-III rested on a technological view of clinical practice that was, in some measure, unstated. It was also, in some measure, inaccurate. The practice of psychiatric diagnosis by clinicians, working outside closely supervised research settings, is not nearly as technically rational as the medical model has suggested.

Uncertainty and Mental Health Practice

During the last three decades, the mental health industry in America has expanded and diversified. There has been a vast expansion in the number of mental health professionals (Goleman, 1990), the number of caregiving episodes (Schulberg & Manderscheid, 1989), the number of mental health organizations providing services, and, not surprisingly, the costs of mental health care (Mechanic, 1980). Services that were once delivered within the state hospitals are now scattered among a diverse array of facilities and professionals. From a system in which most psychiatric patients were in public institutions of last resort, mental health care is now provided in many settings and to people who voluntarily seek help. Mental health care has evolved into a much more complex system of services in which mental health clinicians face increasing uncertainties. Within any societal sector, rapid growth, by itself, can create instability. Within the mental health enterprise, uncertainties stem from other factors as well.

For starters, mental health agencies are founded on a concept that many think is of dubious merit: that there are discrete "disorders" that are "mental." There is little agreement among mental health experts that disorders can be easily or clearly separated from nondisorders. Even more divisive among scholars is the notion that the mental can be separated clearly from the physical, behavioral, social, or moral. The fundamental concepts of mental health and mental illness and how well they actually apply to those receiving help from therapists have been hotly contested for decades. Mental health organizations operate despite or—some might argue—because of these fundamental ambiguities.

The primary tasks of mental health organizations involve working with people as the "raw materials." Clients follow many routes in arriving at a mental health agency, come at times and in numbers that may not conform to the clinician's or the organization's capacities or work flow, present a bewildering array of personal and interpersonal troubles, and possess all manner of idiosyncratic personal histories. The work of clinicians is made more difficult because clients are also simultaneously the consumers of and active participants in the therapeutic process. Clients have a major role in determining what the desired outcome should be and how the goal will be accomplished. Despite the clients' active role, they frequently do not know what they want or how to get it. They are in emotional pain for which they seek relief, but are not certain about the proper remedy. Their confusion is often shared by the clinic's staff. The precise nature of a client's trouble is frequently ambiguous, its causes obscured by a lifetime of personal experiences, environmental stresses, and psychological confusion.

The services that may be offered to the client consist largely of a special relationship with a clinician, making the relationship itself a primary part of the service technology. Given the uniqueness of both client and clinician and the ambiguities surrounding the nature of the problem, the intervention itself introduces additional uncertainties into the helping process. This is particularly so because there may be no widely shared or scientifically established best method of effectively helping the disturbed client. Finally, there are different perspectives about what would actually constitute the desired client outcome. For example, the client, the family, the neighbors, the mental health professionals, and the health insurance companies might have different preferred treatments or outcomes for a client with a serious and persistent disturbance.

Despite these inherent difficulties, mental health professionals and the organizations in which they work strive to present their efforts as carefully coordinated and efficient activities in pursuit of some established, legitimate purpose. In other terms, they want to make their organizations "rational" or to appear to be rational. Whatever the agency goals, the activities of the organization should appear to contribute in some way to those objectives. By establishing objectives, structuring production or service procedures, developing rules and procedures, allocating resources, hiring and training staff, and monitoring outcomes, organizations attempt to make their actions purposeful and effective. Developing successful plans and courses of action is much easier when there are few uncertainties within the organization or in its external environment.

All organizations abhor environmental uncertainty and devise ways of minimizing it or buffering themselves from its currents (Thompson, 1967). Uncertainty is endemic for mental health organizations and a common enemy for those who work in them. Mental health organizations use many methods to reduce the external uncertainties they face. For example, they create boundary units, like screening, intake and referral services, to buffer their organizations from fluctuating client demand. Waiting lists are developed because they are flexible devices for stockpiling raw material. Information and referral procedures are established to send clients elsewhere, which eliminates excess pressure for service. When there are shortages of clients, agencies advertise their services and increase their service domain to cover more geography, clients or problems. Through active lobbying, grantsmanship, and fund-raising, managers attempt to diversify their fiscal base, maintain a steady source of funds, and buffer themselves from unpredictable budget cuts.

Within mental health organizations, uncertainties are usually more easily, and less visibly, managed. Trained professionals are hired because they are supposed to know what to do with clients and how to do it, usually behind closed doors. Even if they do not know how to resolve the problems that clients present, they will at least act in a predictable way, usually by making diagnoses and providing medication or the talking cure; the predictability of the therapist's responses reduces uncertainty. Furthermore, internal organizational structures and procedures are created to clarify who is responsible for what tasks so there will be a minimum of confusion and conflict. Intake units monitor the nature of the "raw material" and make decisions about which clients to assign to which clinicians or programs. Clients are enrolled, given service, and discharged, often without demonstrable change in their condition. And all these activities are accompanied by a blizzard of paperwork explaining, justifying, and certifying what was done.

Although environmental uncertainties are always troublesome, internal uncertainties about clients and the services they need, i.e., technological ambiguities, frequently present opportunities. Paradoxically, uncertainty within mental health organizations can be very useful to them. If uncertainty is great, organizational discretion increases. To be sure, not every organization can benefit as much from uncertainty. For example, NASA has clearly defined and visible goals to get a shuttle into space and back again without damage or injury. If there is too much uncertainty about how to achieve this objective successfully or if their attempts end in observable failure, the agency will have to submit to greater oversight by other organizations such as Congress or presidential commissions.

But since the goals of mental health organizations are not as clear or visible as those of the space agency, uncertainty over how or whether the objectives are achieved is a basis for greater organizational latitude. If there is ambiguity about what they should do in regard to clients, then there is also room for creativity and negotiation. If there are few specific organizational actions that will predictably produce specific outcomes for clients, then many organizational actions are permissible. Uncertainty for mental health organizations has the advantage of allowing wide latitude in internal decision-making. Nowhere is this more apparent than in the first step of client processing—in the diagnosis of mental disorder.

Diagnosis as Rationalization of Action

Psychiatric diagnosis as an expression of technical rationality conforms closely to the conventional views of both professions and bureaucratic organizations. With each there is an emphasis on goal-directed behavior. An explicit organizational mission is established, specific goals that will achieve that mission are set, objective information is gathered, alternative courses of action are considered, rational decisions are made, action is carried out, and progress is evaluated.

There are other strikingly different views of organizational behavior, however, that have special salience for human service organizations, particularly those that provide mental health care. These alternative views question conventional wisdom about the nature of organizational goals (Perrow, 1978, 1986; Lipsky, 1980) and the underlying assumption that goals are rationally pursued as part of some generic problem-solving method. Organizational goals, instead of serving as the focus of action, may be the least important explanation of organizational behavior (Perrow, 1978). Instead, human service organizations can be analyzed as collections of individuals and groups that are in a never-ending struggle for survival, security, power, discretion, and autonomy. Moreover, the publicly espoused goals are often highly ambiguous and may obscure a myriad of objectives that are disparate or in conflict. Organizational behavior, it has been suggested, is more accurately described as a struggle for power among contending interests than as a cooperative endeavor among those striving for a shared, cherished objective (see, for example, Morgan, 1986; Perrow, 1986; Hasenfeld, 1983; Lipsky, 1980). One has merely to point to the resistance shown by staff of state mental hospitals (and their employee unions) to the transfer or discharge of patients to illustrate the multiple and often conflicting objectives of members of such facilities.

Furthermore, if goals are multiple, ambiguous, and in conflict, decision-making discretion among organizational members is greatly broadened. If no precise goal is established, if there is incomplete understanding of how to achieve vague objectives, and if there are few systematic methods of monitoring organizational outcomes, then staff and managers have considerable leeway in explaining what they do. Some organizational theorists have proposed that instead of viewing organizational behavior as an attempt to develop solutions to problems, that it may be more informative to view staff as having available a drawer full of solutions that they use to scan a large pool of potential problems in search of one that will justify their course of action (Cyert & March, 1963; Cohen, March, & Olsen, 1972). This "garbage can model" of organizational behavior views decision-making as attempts to rationalize past actions, actions that are stimulated by a host of private, personal, and technical developments, rather than by a collective desire rationally to pursue some overarching explicit goal.

If one recognizes the ambiguities involved in organizational life, then one more easily recognizes the latitude enjoyed by mental health organizations. Mental health practitioners and the organizations that employ them have considerable discretion in selecting, defining, and processing their clients (Lipsky, 1980). Moreover, mental health clients arrive at agencies with problems that are undifferentiated. Professionals can define clients' problems in a variety of ways: on the basis of presenting complaint, observed symptoms, inferred causes, or prognosis. These ambiguities allow mental health staff considerable discretion in the type of diagnosis they can impose on the client (see, for example Scott, 1969; Lipsky, 1980; Greenley & Kirk, 1973; Freidson, 1960).

It was, in fact, a major purpose of the development of DSM-III to restrict just such discretion among clinicians, to bind them to criteria-based decisions. The developers of DSM-III wanted to ensure that as a result of the use of the new manual, diagnosis would be more scientific or at least more consistent. The central assumption of the view of diagnosis as technical rationality is that mental health professionals will arrive at the same diagnostic conclusion when assessing the same client. To promote this, DSM- III went to great length in offering explicit criteria and formal decision-making rules for diagnoses. When using these criteria and rules, clinicians were supposed to reach the same conclusion; evidence of reliability was to be the proof of the success of technical rationality in psychiatric diagnosis.

But various problems in conceptual clarity, reliability, and actual use of DSM-III undermine the claims of psychiatry that diagnosis is now an expression of the application of scientific procedures. While some of the unreliability of diagnosis and some of the departures from the established diagnostic criteria can be dismissed as simple, random error that exists in all measurement or classification efforts, there is evidence that the problems are more profound. For example, in one national survey of clinical social workers, 55% indicated that DSM-III diagnoses did not, in their opinion, accurately reflect clients' problems, 45% said it obscures individual differences, and only a third felt it was very helpful for treatment planning, one of the major tenets of the technical rationality view of diagnosis. Only half (49%) of the respondents thought that DSM-III served the purposes of their profession. More revealing, perhaps, were the views of 57% who described DSM-III more as a management than a clinical tool (Kutchins & Kirk, 1988a, 1988b). What they appeared to be suggesting is that the use of official diagnoses as provided in DSM-III is frequently not determined by the clinical needs of the client or the treatment planning activities of the therapist, but by the organization's need to manage service delivery.

If clinicians have or take considerable latitude in decision-making, particularly in diagnosis, for what purposes is discretion used? Five such purposes will be described. With each, we will indicate how diagnosis is used to help fulfill these purposes. These purposes, although by no means unique to mental health organizations, have special expressions within them. The five purposes are to regulate client flow, to protect clients from harm, to acquire fiscal resources, to rationalize decision-making, and to advance a broader political agenda.

Regulating Client Flow

Clients can be a source of resources or a burden to psychiatric facilities. Clients bring legitimacy as indicators of the community's need for the agency's services. They also bring financial resources through fees paid by themselves, government agencies, or insurance companies. On the other hand, they consume agency resources by using staff time and scarce facilities (Rhodes, 1991). Consequently, mental health organizations must balance serving clients and protecting the resources of the organization.

Psychiatric diagnosis plays a pivotal role in allowing mental health organizations to choose the number and type of clients they serve. The ambiguities involved in using (or ignoring) DSM diagnostic criteria allow agencies discretion and a rationale for accepting, rejecting, or referring an applicant for service. A clinic offering a special program for people with "mood disorders" may need operationally to liberalize their interpretation of the criteria when in need of clients and narrow it when their caseloads are full. Since the specific diagnostic criteria depend on subjective judgments, this is accomplished easily. For example, the criteria for Major Depressive Episode include depressed mood, markedly diminished interest in all activities, psychomotor agitation, loss of energy, and diminished ability to think. Although the purpose of DSM-III is to reduce flexibility in applying these criteria, they all permit considerable subjective judgment on the part of the clinician. Clinicians can narrow diagnostic requirements to restrict their service domains when there is an excess demand for service and broaden them when they need more clients (Greenley & Kirk, 1973; Lipsky, 1980).

When an applicant is accepted for services, diagnostic labeling is a way of defining the client's problem in the most favorable manner for the organization. For example, one mental hospital observed by the authors sometimes uses Axis V—the global assessment of functioning (GAF)—to determine whether a client requires emergency, involuntary hospitalization. This hospital adopted the policy of only admitting clients who received GAF scores of 40 or less (on a 99-point scale), indicating relatively low functioning. When emergency room personnel wanted to admit someone to this facility, they made certain that the patient was given a rating of 40 or less, even though the score they should have given was higher. Conversely, some hospitals require evidence of improvement before a client is discharged. Knowing this, clinicians who want to discharge a patient may add 20 points or more to the admitting GAF score, whether or not this rating is merited. Other studies of emergency units found that a psychiatric diagnosis was "malleable and ambiguous, often valued more for its strategic than its medical purposes" (Rhodes, 1991). Among these strategic purposes were meeting minimum administrative requirements ("whatever takes less writing") and getting the patient discharged to some other facility. In these ways, the diagnostic system introduced by DSM-III, while appearing to provide a technically rational way of assessing clients, is easily manipulated by staff to control client flow into and out of facilities.

Protecting Clients From Harm

Ironically, in making diagnoses, clinicians frequently want to use "the least noxious diagnosis," acknowledging the well-recognized negative effects of psychiatric labeling (Link, 1987; Link, Cullen, Struening, Shrout, & Dohrenwend, 1989; Link, Mirotznick, & Cullen, 1991). Clinicians do this to minimize communicating damaging, confidential information to insurance companies and others, to avoid the labeling effects of more severe diagnoses, and to limit the adverse impact on the client's self-esteem if the client becomes aware of the diagnosis. Such under-diagnosing is very common among clinicians. Eighty-seven percent of a national sample of clinical social workers indicated that a less serious diagnosis than is clinically indicated was used sometimes to avoid labeling (Kirk & Kutchins, 1988) and the majority of those who were aware that this occurred said that it happened frequently. Seventy-eight percent said that on some occasions only the least serious of several appropriate diagnoses were used on official records, and more than half of the respondents who acknowledged this practice indicated that it happened frequently. Eighty-two percent admitted that Adjustment Disorder is sometimes used when a more serious diagnosis might be more accurate, and more than a third of them reported that this practice occurred frequently. Only a small fraction of respondents were unaware of any occurrence of these types of deliberate misdiagnoses. Brown (1987) made similar observations of underdiagnosis in a community mental health center. He documented a variety of ways in which clinicians coped with the demands to make diagnoses "on paper" in the face of a variety of clinical uncertainties. Organizational and interorganizational factors were often decisive in choosing diagnoses.

In a major study of the accuracy of diagnostic information submitted to insurance companies by psychiatrists, investigators found that diagnostic information sent to insurance companies was considerably different from information provided in an anonymous survey (Sharfstein, Towery, & Milowe, 1980). Diagnoses of neuroses were submitted three times more frequently to insurance companies than the more serious disorders reported in other independent surveys. Clinicians appear to distort official diagnoses frequently to protect clients. Undoubtedly, the concerns of clinicians are genuine; they do not want to harm in the act of trying to help.

Nevertheless, such protectiveness may not always benefit clients. False diagnoses create their own problems. They establish a written record of professional "scientific" judgments that affirms that clients meet criteria for disorders that they, in fact, do not have. Whatever the disadvantages of more severe, but accurate diagnoses, they at least have the benefit of someone's best judgment about a clinical condition. A deliberately false diagnosis, whatever the merits of the motivation behind it, officially labels a client as suffering from a mental disorder that he or she in fact does not have. A chain of such false diagnoses over the years hardly enhances the meaningfulness of a person's dossier or an organization's official medical records.

Deliberately underdiagnosing, however, does indirectly serve some organizational interests. To the extent that people are aware of the potentially stigmatizing labels that clinicians can affix to personal medical records, they may be appropriately reluctant to seek service voluntarily from those facilities (Link, 1987). By practicing underdiagnosis on a broad scale, agencies signal to clients that the stigmatization will be minimized; that they are there only to help. By thus encouraging clients to seek help when they might otherwise be reluctant, mental health practitioners reduce one barrier for clients and thereby promote a demand for mental health services. Diagnosis in these circumstances represents the application of a political calculation about the negative effects of diagnosis within some ambiguous technical constraints. These widespread practices depart significantly from the conventional view that psychiatric diagnosis is an objective, scientific decision.

Acquiring Fiscal Resources

All human service organizations need resources, particularly money, which can be used flexibly in exchange for other things. In mental health, fiscal resources are increasingly coming from fees paid by clients or, more commonly, by their private insurance companies or government programs, such as Medicaid. In addition to their scientific and clinical uses, diagnoses also have fiscal implications (Nelson, 1986). A formal clinical label is frequently required for reimbursement by third-party insurance companies and government programs. Recently adopted diagnostic related groups (DRGs) have made medical diagnosis the foundation for the financing of health care. Consequently, diagnostic practices have direct fiscal consequences. Diagnosis in mental health, now more than ever before, is a business act, as well as a clinical one. And the business of mental health is getting more competitive (Chodoff, 1987; Goleman, 1985; Greenberg, 1980). Diagnosis increasingly provides a mechanism for clinicians to be reimbursed and for clients who cannot afford treatment to get the service they need.

But not all personal troubles are equally reimbursable. Reimbursement directly to the client or the agency is tied to particular psychiatric diagnoses, often the more serious ones. Personality disorders, family problems, or routine adjustment difficulties may not be reimbursable. Thus, the acquisition of fiscal resources depends directly on the clinician's decision about the nature of the client's mental disorder.

Mental health practitioners and their agencies are very aware of this connection. More importantly, they admit that it affects their use of diagnosis. In the survey mentioned above (Kirk & Kutchins, 1988), there is evidence of widespread overdiagnosis, in which clinicians use more serious diagnosis than warranted in order to qualify the client or the agency for reimbursement from third parties. For example, 72% believed that there were occasions when a more serious diagnosis was used than was warranted clinically in order to help clients qualify for reimbursement for treatment. Over half of the respondents who acknowledged the existence of these practices felt that they occurred frequently. Since reimbursement is rarely available for family problems, 86% admitted that a diagnosis for an individual was used even when the primary problem was in the family system. Over half said this was done frequently.

Another study of clinicians (Brown, 1987) found that they coped with these diagnostic dilemmas by using humor and sarcasm to express their dissatisfaction with the requirement to make official diagnoses in order to fulfill external organizational requirements. Frequently the requirements of the referring agency or the client's social needs dominated the diagnostic outcome. One staff member quipped that a client's DSM-III diagnosis was an "insurance claim."

Such jokes reveal the close ties that can exist between reimbursement and clinical judgments. These matters have become more than clinical humor. In the fall of 1991, *The New York Times* ran a series of articles, "Psychiatry for Profit: Private Hospitals under Fire," detailing investigations by law enforcement agencies in several states into charges that private psychiatric hospitals systematically misdiagnosed, mistreated, and abused patients to increase their profits from insurance claims (Kerr, 1991a, 1991b; Goleman, 1991b; Freudenheim, 1991).

The prospects for reimbursement or, more pointedly, the prospects for the denial of reimbursement have profoundly affected the practice of inpatient psychiatry in other ways as well. Gabbard, Takahashi, Davidson, Bauman-Bork, & Ensroth (1991) argue that the insurance review process can have deleterious effects on patients, treatment staff, and families. These review processes and the threat that treatment reimbursement may be discontinued have been known to be themselves major stressors for patients. In fact, in some cases psychiatrists have included the insurance review process itself as a new problem on the patient's problem list in the medical record (Gabbard et al., 1991).

Rationalizing Decision-Making

The ostensible clinical purpose for making a formal psychiatric diagnosis is to guide the choice of therapeutic intervention. Pneumonia, take penicillin. Infection, take an antibiotic. Manic-depressive psychosis (bipolar affective disorder in the DSM-III-R technical-rational lexicon), take lithium. In these cases the diagnosis precedes and determines the choice of treatment. In mental health, under- and overdiagnoses suggest that diagnoses are sometimes determined by considerations other than the clinical condition of the client and often by factors external but important to the organization.

Nevertheless, it could be argued that despite a deceptive official diagnosis, the treatment used was based on the "real, " if unofficial, diagnosis. For example, a family with communication problems may receive family therapy, although the problem had been diagnosed officially as if the mother alone had a disorder. Thus, it could be said that the diagnosis (the unofficial, not the official one) led to treatment. However, many third-party payers insist that treatment conform to the diagnosis. In the example just given, once a diagnosis is made on the mother, an insurer might refuse to pay for family therapy, and reimburse only individual treatment.

There are also circumstances in mental health organizations where the treatment determines diagnosis; the diagnosis is made only after a particular treatment has been found to be effective. If the patient got better with lithium, the diagnosis should be bipolar affective disorder. In this case diagnosis provides the rationale for treatment that has already occurred. Social workers in one agency told the authors that with some clients the consulting psychiatrist was unable to figure out what the diagnosis was, but would sequentially prescribe different medications until one seemed to work. The diagnosis would then be changed to reflect the clinical condition that the particular drug is supposed to treat. If it was pounded by a hammer, it must have been a nail.

Sometimes diagnoses are simply irrelevant. The staff at one agency explained that diagnosis was the art of "making distinctions without differences." Psychiatrists would frequently debate the fine points about the correct diagnosis for a disturbed client, but always would prescribe Haldol regardless of the outcome of the diagnostic debate. In cases like these, precise diagnostic classification, instead of leading to specific differential actions, is largely irrelevant.

Using diagnoses that are largely irrelevant to subsequent decisions is not unique to mental health organizations. Ritualistic use of diagnosis occurs regularly in other institutions. For example, almost all the nation's colleges require high school students to take the SAT given by the Educational Testing Service (ETS), under the assumption that the assessment of "scholastic aptitude" will make a difference in their admissions decisions. For elite institutions, this may be the case. However, many of the less selective colleges must accept virtually all their applicants, regardless of their SAT scores, in order to obtain a sufficiently large student body (Owen, 1985). Although these colleges may require SAT scores, the economics of higher education and the relative shortage of eligible college-age students force these institutions to have a de facto open-door policy. For them, the ETS provides scholastic information that they do not really need. This type of unnecessary testing, however, does serve an important symbolic function for these colleges, which can present themselves as basing decisions on standardized, objective, scientific information. This permits both the accepted and rejected applicants to believe that their fate is tied directly to some empirical database.

Sometimes diagnoses are simply ignored or concealed when they interfere with the agency functions. In one mental health agency, known to the authors, the staff tries to find shelter for the homeless mentally ill. The staff knows that some available housing facilities will not admit mentally ill clients who have problems with substance abuse. Consequently, the staff will occasionally make a diagnosis, but avoid making the warranted diagnosis of substance abuse when doing so would jeopardize the client's chance for admission to housing. Consequently, an incomplete and inaccurate formal diagnosis is used to describe the client. In situations like these, the inaccurate official diagnosis becomes the instrumentally appropriate label that can be used to achieve the clinician's objective—getting housing for clients.

At times, an organization's objective may be to protect itself in litigation. In the famous *Osheroff* case briefly mentioned in Chapter 1, the patient had received various diagnoses and the litigation revolved around whether the treatment he received was appropriately consistent with the diagnoses or negligent. The case divided the psychiatric profession and a decade later is still the topic of acrimonious debate. One of the antagonists in this ongoing argument suggested in an exchange of letters in the *American Journal of Psychiatry* that the staff of the treatment facility (Chestnut Lodge) emphasized the diagnosis of narcissistic personality disorder in a post hoc manner in order to legitimate the treatment given (Klerman, 1991). Had the psychotic depression diagnosis remained salient, Chestnut Lodge would have been more legally vulnerable for malpractice. That one of psychiatry's leading spokespersons was so quick to accuse the staff of one of the profession's most famous treatment facilities of misusing diagnoses to rationalize action taken is a testament to how familiar practitioners are with the alternative uses of diagnoses.

Advancing a Political Agenda

Diagnosis marks the boundaries of psychiatry and the other mental health professions that use the psychiatric diagnostic system; it is, to some extent, a political claim. A narrow definition of mental disorder, strict diagnostic criteria, and fewer diagnostic categories would greatly limit the scope of the mental health field, would encourage fewer people to seek services, would provide reimbursement for fewer human troubles, and would require fewer clinicians to be trained and employed. A broad, flexible approach has the opposite effects. Thus, what is included or not included in the diagnostic manual has implications beyond those pertaining to the clinical condition of any individual client or the functioning of any one agency. It reflects what the society is willing to designate as mental illness. The shape of the diagnostic manual and the use that is made of it involve strategic choices for psychiatry, some of them very controversial.

In the last 15 years, the APA has battled groups who wanted certain conditions withdrawn from the DSM list of mental disorders. Homosexuality is the most celebrated case of a controversial diagnosis, which psychiatrists were forced to discard in 1974 (Bayer, 1981). More recently, in 1985, several diagnoses pertaining specifically to women created another major political flap during the revision of DSM-III. The women argued, less successfully than gay activists did a decade earlier, that such diagnoses as self-defeating personality disorder would be used against abused women (Kutchins & Kirk, 1989). As a political compromise, these controversial diagnoses were placed in the appendix of the revised manual.

Publicized instances of attempts to remove diagnostic categories are in stark contrast to the relatively quiet way in which most diagnostic categories are revised, split, combined, or created for the official psychiatric manual. It would be a mistake to believe that all potentially affected groups try to keep their conditions out of the diagnostic manual. After years of work, Vietnam veterans and their advocates succeeded in inserting a new Post–Traumatic Stress Disorder into DSM-III (Scott, 1990). And many mental health clinicians and some clients would like to see diagnoses expanded to exclude marital and family problems, so that a broader array of therapeutic services would be reimbursable. In fact, the expansion of the psychiatric domain is limited by nothing except the political judgment of the APA.

The expanding scope of mental health, advanced through an ever-growing list of official diagnoses of mental disorders, produces two important political gains for psychiatry: First, if increasing numbers of people have definable mental disorders, the mental health professions can argue that increasing funds should be allocated to conduct research and provide treatment for them. An expanded scope allows more claims on society for legitimation and support. Second, an expanding list of mental disorders that contains everything, including low intelligence, tobacco dependence, antisocial personality, schizophrenia, caffeine intoxication, and childhood misconduct, offers an ideology for understanding a potpourri of dysfunctional or devalued behaviors as medical disorders rather than as diverse forms of social deviance. This trend to medicalize deviance has a long history (Conrad & Schneider, 1980). Diagnostic decisions routinely made in mental health organizations for reimbursement purposes institutionalize this medicalization in a way that cannot be easily reversed.

Social Context of Deliberate Misdiagnosis

All of these uses of diagnosis depart radically from the view that technical rationality alone guides diagnostic practices or that diagnostic errors are simply failures of technical procedures. Instead, the apparently widespread use of deliberate misdiagnosis in the mental health professions suggests that clinicians use diagnosis for other instrumental purposes, not at all remedied by the technical revisions of the DSM. If misdiagnosis is as widespread as is suggested, it is puzzling that it has hardly been recognized in the literature on DSM and on diagnostic errors. Even when it is discussed, as by Sharfstein et al. (1980), neither those who report it nor their audience in the helping professions argue that it is a serious problem. For example, one study found that psychiatrists constitute a disproportionately large number of those physicians suspended from the Medicare and Medicaid programs for fraud, but the actual number of those involved in fraud was small. The reason offered for the higher rate of fraud among psychiatrists was that they were an easy target for prosecutors (Geis et al., 1985). To our knowledge, only investigating journalists and law enforcement agencies claim that deliberate misdiagnoses are a problem that requires attention. These types of "errors" have attracted little attention, funding, or problem-making rhetoric within the mental health professions.

Rationales of Clinicians
for Misdiagnosis

One explanation for the apparent indifference to deliberate misdiagnosis is that both under- and overdiagnosing are justified as either harmless or in the client's best interest; the client is helped to avoid a stigmatizing label or to obtain needed services. The DSM-III code may be viewed by clinicians as a fiscal formality unrelated to treatment, a white lie for a good purpose. In fact, only a third of the respondents in our study found DSM helpful in planning treatment (Kutchins & Kirk, 1988a). Because there is no professional consensus about the appropriate treatment for specific disorders, the importance of misdiagnosis is often discounted. The widespread practice of underdiagnosis or using the least serious diagnosis even when it is not the most accurate appears, ironically, to be an attempt to shield the client from the recognized negative consequences that come from the diagnostic process itself.

The situation of overdiagnosis is different, but also apparently prevalent. It also seems to be done for the client's benefit, but the rationale is economic rather than therapeutic. The manifest function of underdiagnosis is to protect clients; with overdiagnosis, the accurate diagnosis is replaced by a deliberately inaccurate one to deceive others. In particular, misdiagnosis is used so that the therapist's services will qualify for third-party reimbursement. Here the rationale is also nonclinical, but the argument that the therapist is acting only for the client's benefit is strained. The rationale that it is being done so that the client can obtain needed service is colored by the obvious self-interest of the therapist. Agencies, both public and private, also benefit when they obtain reimbursement as a result of such diagnostic practices.

Finally, the rationale for overdiagnosis directly contradicts the justification for underdiagnosis. To the extent that there are negative effects of psychiatric labeling, overdiagnosis may unnecessarily harm the client. The practice of overdiagnosis, however, can be rationalized. Altering a diagnosis by substituting one that is plausible for a fully accurate one is an example of the creative management and selective presentation of information that occurs in many large bureaucratic organizations. In fact, doing so well, is often the mark of an effective bureaucrat. And when such practices are justified as placing the client's welfare ahead of that of the agency, the rationalization will find substantial support among professionals.

Are there acceptable or nonharmful levels of overdiagnosis? Acceptable or nonharmful to whom? Misdiagnosis has consequences not only for clients, but for practitioners, professions, government policymakers, insurance companies, and taxpayers. By focusing only on the presumed benefits to clients, clinicians avoid the broad ethical implications that emanate from the practice of misdiagnosis.

Conditions for Misdiagnosis

Diagnostic practices that are common and patterned, but incorrect, cannot be dismissed as simply due to individual malfeasance or lack of proper training. Explanations must be sought in the social context of clinical work. Professionals, especially mental health clinicians, enjoy considerable freedom in their work. Certainly in private practice, but even when employed in agencies, they have substantial discretion in conducting their activities. The conditions for this autonomy derive from the nature of the human services and the conditions of clinical work within them (Smith, 1965; Lipsky, 1980). Clients are, or at least often perceive themselves to be, dependent and powerless. Clinical work is not easily supervised or easily evaluated. It is very easy to make incorrect decisions, whether or not they are intended to deceive, without being detected.

In mental health practice, diagnostic latitude is particularly great because of the unreliability of DSM-III and earlier classification systems, even when clinicians are trying hard to be precise and accurate. Under conditions where mistakes or disagreements are commonplace, deliberate misdiagnoses are hard to detect. Furthermore, when the nature of the disorder is itself ambiguous, controversial, unverifiable, and subject to extraclinical influences, intentional falsification may merge with unconscious distortion.

Clients themselves provide few obstacles to misdiagnosis, since they often are not told about their diagnoses. Even if they are informed, it is reasonable to expect them to accept these diagnostic practices. They have sought help from others with greater wisdom, knowledge, and skill. Their dependence in the relationship is part of the bargain. Disgruntled clients are unlikely to complain about under-diagnosis, although there are risks of suit for malpractice if it results in inappropriate treatment (Kutchins & Kirk, 1987b).

Overdiagnosis, on the other hand, might lead to angry reactions from clients. Nonetheless, clients are not generally able to detect overdiagnosis when it occurs, because of the technical expertise needed for psychiatric assessment. Even when they are aware of deliberate overdiagnoses, clients may accept them in order to obtain reimbursement. They may join the clinician in a covert action against "the bureaucracy" that might otherwise deny them the help they seek (Michels, 1986; Gabbard et al., 1991). Thus clients may have good reasons to believe that misdiagnoses are in their best interests. We know of one clinician who negotiates a diagnosis with each client, after explaining the possible consequences of each diagnosis for reimbursement, legal status, treatment modes, and stigma.

Reimbursement systems have changed markedly in recent years and these changes have altered the consequences of diagnoses. In the past, outpatient psychiatric care was financed on the basis of patient fees for those who could afford private care or on the basis of third-party reimbursement to service providers. State hospitals were financed on a per capita or per bed basis. It mattered little whether a patient had a borderline personality or was schizophrenic. The increase in third-party reimbursement from government programs and private insurance companies for mental health care, in tandem with the general trend of contracting out services to nonprofit and profit agencies, have altered the consequences of diagnosis. DRGs and case-by-case reimbursement schemes have given diagnosis a special new status. In the related field of alcoholism, such changes in financing eventually had significant effects on treatment ideology and clients served (Weisner & Room, 1984).

The sensitivity of clinicians to the potential negative effects of psychiatric labeling, which may encourage the practice of underdiagnosis, does not completely counteract the financial pressure to overdiagnose. Reimbursement systems, which have become increasingly important for psychiatric treatment in the last decade, are undoubtedly a major factor in encouraging overdiagnosis. Not only do government programs like Medicaid and private health insurance policies now cover treatment for psychiatric disorders, but they are diagnosis based. Although DSM-III has greatly expanded the number of mental disorders, not all categories qualify for reimbursement for treatment. Garfield (1986) has speculated that the influence of third party payers might lead to "some peculiar practices" for reimbursement purposes. In a critical review of DSM-III, he asked, What purposes are served if diagnosis is not linked in important respects to prognosis and treatment or to etiology? Some of those purposes seem to have now emerged.

Certainly the introduction of DSM-III into mental health practice has not been the sole, or even the primary, cause of deliberate misdiagnoses. Undoubtedly, it occurred previously, as is suggested by the earlier study of insurance claims filed by clinicians using DSM-II (Sharfstein et al., 1980). Nevertheless, DSM-III may have served to facilitate misdiagnosis. When the manual was introduced it was advertised as a major scientific advance that improved the accuracy of diagnosis. Data published in the manual were used to claim its reliability and provide a greater air of scientific respectability to psychiatric diagnosis, so long the whipping boy of mental health critics. These scientific claims continue to be made, even though recent surveys of psychiatrists report that diagnoses are frequently inaccurate (Jampala, Sierles, & Taylor, 1986; Lipkowitz & Idupugnati, 1985), and the original data, as we have seen, are hardly supportive of such bold claims. Nevertheless, the rapid adoption of DSM-III by the mental health professions and by government and private insurance companies has institutionalized its influence. As the compendium of legitimate psychiatric diagnoses, it served as the technological instrument for the allocation of resources and for control over the mental health business.

Consequences of Misdiagnosis

DSM-III and a variety of other remedial efforts have been undertaken to reduce diagnostic errors that are made unintentionally. Whatever the eventual success of these efforts, they may not address a more common source of diagnostic mistake in mental health, those errors that are deliberate. While the extent and pattern of deliberate misdiagnosis are only suggested by some of the evidence reviewed, the implications could be profound.

Policy and program development in mental health frequently rely on reported rates of treated disorder. Are depression, alcoholism, and schizophrenia becoming more or less prevalent? Uncharted and unrecognized distortion of diagnostic practices could lead to invalid conclusions and misguided intervention efforts. Deliberate misdiagnosis to avoid stigma or to obtain reimbursement for treatment for individual clients cannot be justified ethically or legally, but such practices, in the aggregate, present even greater problems for mental health planners.

Considerable scientific effort has been devoted to improving the accuracy of psychiatric diagnosis through structured interview schedules and revised diagnostic classification systems. Any progress that has been made is relevant primarily to research arenas, where diagnostic practices are carefully controlled and where there are minimal incentives for distortion. Clinical practice in the real world may be governed by a different set of influences that are not well recognized or fully understood. Research on psychiatric diagnosis as it is actually practiced would be quite different in focus and methodology than research now appearing in the literature or planned for DSM-IV.

Finally, there are subtle consequences for the mental health professions. The bargain struck between clients and professionals is that clients will entrust their care to professionals who are obligated to use their best knowledge and skills to help clients. Professionals have a fiduciary duty to their clients. The professional is expected to perform in a "disinterested" or selfless fashion, putting the needs of the client above his or her own feelings and prejudices. To ensure disinterested service, physicians do not care for their own families, lawyers do not represent both parties in a dispute, and decision-makers remove themselves from decisions where they may have a conflict of interest. Their intent is to remove themselves from circumstances where they might not be able to provide objective service of high quality to the client (Kutchins, 1991).

Professional practice may be distorted to the extent that deliberate misdiagnosis involves the deception or manipulation of clients. Clients are given diagnoses that are not clinically accurate and they are encouraged to go along with misdiagnoses that qualify for reimbursement. In both cases, their trust in the professional relationship is violated. Second, deliberate misdiagnosis may violate professionals' obligation to their profession to use their knowledge and skill in an ethical manner. Truthfulness is an obligation of practice. Third, deliberate misdiagnosis may violate the agreement all professions have with society. Professions enjoy special privileges and entitlements, not given to all occupations. Professionals historically are allowed to govern themselves, to control entrance into their ranks, to prescribe required training, and to set their own standards of practice, somewhat free of the supervision and control of nonmembers. Some are even protected from divulging confidences in court under many circumstances. In return, professions agree to abide by their codes of ethics, to protect the interests of their clients, to practice in a disinterested manner, and to use their substantial knowledge for the betterment of the society. Deliberate misdiagnosis may violate these agreements and, in so doing, corrupt the mental health professions.

Diagnoses in mental health serve many functions. Sometimes they conform to the conventional view by classifying people and their problems so that they can be properly treated or studied by researchers. At other times and in other situations, diagnoses provide the rationalization for organizational processing decisions already made or dispositions that are readily available. When the goal of diagnosis is to support organizational needs rather than to determine what treatment clients need, the process is often distorted and frequently involves intentional misdiagnoses. Diagnoses in situations where deliberate misdiagnosis occurs are rarely recognized in the literature on diagnostic "errors." In fact, even viewing these occurrences as errors imposes on the situation a model of diagnostic rationality that fails to recognize that clinicians often deliberately use diagnosis for organizational purposes, not primarily for clinical ones. Even when the goal is to place a homeless person who abuses drugs into housing, then a diagnosis that conveniently overlooks a significant clinical reality reveals the many instrumental uses of psychiatric assessment. The goal may be laudable, but the process distorts diagnostic activity and calls into question its scientific assumptions.

Diagnostic practices function to screen clients into and out of organizations, to sort clients into programs and services that are available, and to label prospective clients in such a way as to make the referral decision appear to be clinically, rather than organizationally motivated. The inherent uncertainties involved in assessing clients' problems and determining what to do about them allows organizations to buffer themselves against fluctuating client demands and to keep or dispose of them as desired. In so doing, mental health organizations are merely practicing what has been widely recognized as processes of "creaming," "dumping," and "typifying" clients. Moreover, because of the structure of third-party reimbursement for certain psychiatric diagnoses, the clinical ambiguities involved present mental health organizations with irresistible opportunities to gain fiscal resources by merely labeling and mislabeling clinical conditions. These organizational maneuvers can be accomplished while the agency appears, through the use of the much acclaimed diagnostic manual, to be applying technical rationality to the assessment of human pain.

There is much about these processes that is still not well understood. Because psychiatric diagnosis has been narrowly viewed as the application of scientific procedures, most attention has been given to developing technical procedures and criteria that will constrain the behavior of clinicians in making diagnoses. Comparatively little attention has been given to how diagnosis is actually accomplished by clinicians working within the constraints and demands of mental health organizations. Broadening the analysis of diagnosis to include the organizational context in which it occurs points to an unexplored topic that can have major consequences for the mental health industry.

Diagnostic Conclusions

[W]e need to guard against exaggerating the potential impact of science on our nosology. Many important nosologic questions in psychiatry are *fundamentally* nonempirical.

As psychiatry takes up the "banner" of a scientific nosology, we must take care not to promise more than we can deliver. While enthusiasm in support of an empirical nosology is certainly appropriate . . . , we should not in our enthusiasm overlook the inherent limitations of the empirical methods. There is a danger that this process will degenerate into pseudoscience, in which we pretend to be "objective" and "empirical" when, in reality, we are making informed value judgments.

The fundamental problem is that the scientific method can only answer "little" questions. . . . In many cases, obtaining answers to the little questions will not provide unambiguous answers to the big questions. (Kenneth S. Kendler, 1990:972)

In a recently published study, some of the principal participants in the development of DSM-III and its revision—DSM-III-R (Williams et al., in press)—reported on a major reliability study that was conducted in 1985–1986. Six sites in the United States and one in Germany participated. The study was part of the revision of one of the major structured interview protocols: the Structured Clinical Interview for DSM (SCID). The SCID, originally developed for DSM-III, was being updated to reflect the revised diagnostic criteria being incorporated into DSM-III-R (Spitzer, Williams, Gibbon, & First, in press).

Experienced mental health professionals at the seven sites were selected to be interviewers. There were several rounds of training provided by the senior project staff, including the use of audiotaped interviews, monthly conference calls, on-site training, and a two-day plenary training session of interviewers from all of the sites. In addition, interviewers conducted a series of pilot interviews that were audiotaped and sent to the project headquarters for feedback. After this training and practice, 592 people were interviewed by pairs of these trained staff. The subjects consisted of 390 psychiatric patients and 202 people from a nonpatient population.

This study used all of the major elements that had been developed over two decades to improve the reliability of psychiatric diagnosis: a finely tuned classification system (DSM-III-R) developed and revised over a ten-year period by outstanding psychiatric researchers; specific diagnostic criteria for each diagnostic category to guide clinical decisions; carefully developed interview protocols designed specifically for use with this particular diagnostic system; deliberate and careful selection and training of experienced professional interviewers; and the competent oversight by a research team that is perhaps the most experienced and able at conducting diagnostic studies in the world. Such a study is the envy of many psychiatric researchers who have attempted the difficult tasks of conducting methodologically rigorous studies in actual clinical settings. The care and competence of those conducting this study should be expected to produce the highest diagnostic reliability that is possible in supervised research settings in which the clinicians have few motivations other than to produce accurate diagnoses.

The findings of this reliability study were apparently disappointing to the investigators, who "had expected higher reliability values" (Williams et al., in press:16). The findings, however, are familiar. Among the patient sample, aggregated across the five sites, the kappas ranged from .40 to .86 and averaged .61. Among the nonpatient community sample at two sites, the kappas ranged from .19 to .59 and averaged .37. Figure 9.1 displays these results in relation to the findings from the early studies of the 1950s and 1960s. There are 37 kappas for various diagnostic categories for the patient sample reported by the five patient sites. If one examines these kappas, only 1 is above .90, 21 are in the *only satisfactory* range, 27 are in the *no better than fair* range, and 21 lie in the *poor* range. These ranges, of course, overlap. Among the 6 kappas reported for the nonpatient sample, 1 is *only satisfactory*, 5 are *no better than fair*, and all 6 fall within the *poor* range.

Can we determine from this latest study whether the reliability of psychiatric diagnosis has improved by any significant amount in three decades? Have diagnostic criteria and structured interviews transformed the reliability of clinical judgments? Does kappa really provide a metric for easy comparisons among diverse studies?

For years, these questions appeared to have relatively simple answers.

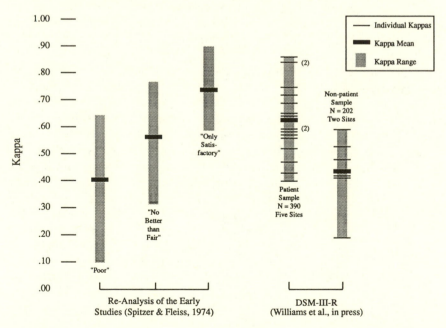

Figure 9.1.   Comparison of kappas from the early studies and DSM-III-R.

Today, many observers still think that the answer to all of them is yes. To us, the answers are much more ambiguous. More importantly, the methodological problems have become so complex that the generalizability of the findings is questionable. With every reliability study, contextual issues arise: what about variations in the training of clinicians, their motivation and commitment to diagnostic accuracy, their prior skill, the homogeneity of the clinical setting in regard to patient mix and base rates, the theoretical orientation and collaborative style of clinicians, and the degree of methodological rigor achieved by the investigators, and so on? The reliability problem, once thought of as a simple matter of diagnostic consistency, is now a different series of research problems, far removed from the everyday world of most clinicians (cf. Nelson-Gray, 1991).

In studies where these methodological problems can be adequately addressed through controlled research procedures, a host of other questions arise about the extent to which diagnostic consistency in specialized research settings has any bearing on the actual diagnostic decisions of clinicians in normal, uncontrolled clinical settings, where external bureaucratic demands, reimbursement probabilities and potential stigma influence the judgments of practitioners. What should we conclude if we found that under some very special circumstances a research instrument could be used accurately, but under most normal circumstances it was not? Diagnosis in research settings for research purposes may constitute a very different social activity than diagnosis in clinical settings for practical purposes. If so, do not different questions need to be asked and different methodological approaches used?

These questions do not have easy answers. Perhaps they are not even the right questions. But even if one addresses the question, Is reliability now good or better than before? the answer cannot be found in the numbers usually provided in most reliability studies, however revealing the numbers may be for some purposes. The numbers presented in reliability studies, by themselves, often tell us very little. On the other hand, what people claim the numbers mean and the effects of those claims on shaping professional consciousness tell us a great deal about how problems get defined, how approaches to solving them are developed, and how solutions come to be accepted. Tracking the numbers and the corresponding rhetoric of reliability provides a glimpse of the interplay of science and the politics of professions. Science and the images of science are used by contending factions in their struggle for influence, position, and advantage. Science and the images of science are used by professions to present themselves and their expertise to a wider public to gain legitimacy and prominence.

The story of reliability is not the full story of DSM-III's development or its success—far from it. The reliability story, as a case study, illuminates some of the processes involved in the emergence and resolution of one professional problem. The problem of reliability provided an important core theme for the renovation of psychiatric nosology during the 1970s. A full explanation of DSM-III's development would require a much broader examination of American psychiatry and would include an analysis of many issues and events barely touched in this book. Undoubtedly, however, the interplay of scientific claims and political positioning would offer an important perspective in analyzing many other issues and developments in the mental health field.

Although we have suggested that attention to reliability as a problem waned following the appearance of DSM-III, reliability may be an interminable issue. The symbolic uses of reliability will probably continue to engage the APA and the various subgroups that vie for influence. Reliability problems, while quiescent during the late 1980s, could emerge again around DSM-IV, perhaps defined as a different kind of problem with a different role to play. One only has to listen to the current APA leaders to suspect that the struggles over psychiatric diagnoses are far from over. Melvin Sabshin, the medical director of the APA, in his annual report to the association last year, praised the work of the DSM-IV Task Force: "The DSM process has been pivotal in documenting the scientific credibility and reliability of psychiatric diagnosis and has done much to improve psychiatry's image" (Sabshin, 1991:1447).

At about the same time that the medical director was applauding DSM's scientific credibility, Lawrence Hartmann, the new president of the APA, was raising dormant concerns about it (Hartmann, 1991). At his address to the annual meeting of the APA, Hartmann stated:

> Psychiatry remains at some risk as a science and as an insurable medical specialty, partly because its complexity makes it a major example of a general problem in the accumulation of scientific knowledge: what is easiest to measure tends to get measured, published, and called "real" or "important"; what is harder to measure, even if as important or more important, gets measured far less and valued far less.
>
> DSM-III and III-R and IV are part of the movement toward reliable categorization and measurement. They have helped many aspects of psychiatry, but they have harmed others, partly by oversimplifying. They emphasize clarity and reliability but, many clinicians think, sacrifice validity and the whole person. (p. 1132)

Indeed, the diagnostic manuals emphasize and use reliability, measurement, oversimplification, and publication to make a case for what is important. But the developers of these manuals have done it in ways and with consequences that even the president of the APA does not fully recognize. This book explained why that should be no surprise.

REFERENCES

Abbott, A. (1988). *The system of professions: An essay on the division of expert labor.* Chicago: University of Chicago Press.

Albee, G., Canetto, S., & Sefa-Dedeh, A. (1991). Naming a syndrome is the first step. *Canadian Psychology, 32*(2), 154–160.

Alexander, F. G., & Selesnick, S. T. (1966). *The history of psychiatry.* New York: Harper & Row.

American Psychiatric Association. (1952). *Diagnostic and statistical manual of mental disorders* (2nd ed.). Washington, DC: Author.

American Psychiatric Association. (1968). *Diagnostic and statistical manual of mental disorders* (2nd ed.). Washington, DC: Author.

American Psychiatric Association. (1977). Revised response to request for proposal for field test of DSM-III submitted to the National Institute of Mental Health by the American Psychiatric Association, July 18, 1977. NIMH DB 77-0022.

American Psychiatric Association. (1978a). NIMH-sponsored field trial procedure manual—Phase One. Washington, DC: Author.

American Psychiatric Association. (1978b). Field trial questionnaire no. 1. Unpublished report, Washington, DC.

American Psychiatric Association. (1980). *Diagnostic and statistical manual of mental disorders* (3rd ed.). Washington, DC: Author.

American Psychiatric Association. (1987). *Diagnostic and statistical manual of mental disorders* (3rd. ed., revised). Washington, DC: Author.

Andreasen, N. C. (1989). The American concept of schizophrenia. *Schizophrenia Bulletin, 15,* 519–531.

Anthony, J., Fostein, M., Romanoski, A., et al. (1985). Comparison of the lay Diagnostic Interview Schedule and a standardized psychiatric diagnosis: Experience in Eastern Baltimore. *Archives of General Psychiatry, 42,* 667–675.

Arnstein, R. (1977). *DSM-III on trial in a college mental health service.* Paper presented at the Annual Meeting of the American Psychiatric Association, Toronto, May.

Ash, P. (1949). The reliability of psychiatric diagnosis. *Journal of Abnormal and Social Psychology, 44,* 272–277.

Barlow, D. H. (Ed.). (1991). Diagnosis, dimensions, and DSM-IV: The science of classification [Special issue]. *Journal of Abnormal Psychology, 100*(3), August.

Barrett, J. (1987). DSM-III in evolution. In G. Tischler (Ed.), *Diagnosis and classifi-*

cation in psychiatry: A critical appraisal of DSM-III (pp. 435–442). New York: Cambridge University Press.

Bassett, A. S., & Beiser, M. (1991). DSM-III: Use of the multiaxial diagnostic system in clinical practice. *Canadian Journal of Psychiatry, 36*(May), 270–274.

Bayer, R. (1981). *Homosexuality and American psychiatry: The politics of diagnosis.* New York: Basic Books.

Bayer, R., & Spitzer, R. L. (1982). Edited correspondence on the status of homosexuality in DSM-III. *Journal of the History of the Behavioral Sciences, 18,* 32-52.

Bayer R., & Spitzer, R. L. (1985). Neurosis, psychodynamics, and DSM-III: A history of the controversy. *Archives of General Psychiatry, 42,* 187–195.

Bazerman, C. (1981). What written knowledge does: Three examples of academic discourse. *Philosophy of Social Science, 11,* 361–387.

Beck, A. T. (1962). Reliability of psychiatric diagnoses: 1. A critique of systematic studies. *American Journal of Psychiatry, 119,* 210–216.

Beck, A. T., Ward, C., Mendelson, M., Mock, J., & Erbaugh, J. (1962). Reliability of psychiatric diagnoses: 2. A study of consistency of clinical judgments and ratings. *American Journal of Psychiatry, 119,* 351–357.

Bemporad, J. R., & Schwab, M. E. (1986). The DSM-III and clinical child psychiatry. In T. Millon & G. L. Klerman (Eds.), *Contemporary directions in psychopathology: Toward the DSM-IV* (pp. 135–150). New York: Guilford Press.

Berk, H. (1977a). Letter to the editor. *Psychiatric News,* March 30.

Berk, H. (1977b). DSM-III, comments. Unpublished statement, New York.

Berk, H., & Jaso, H. (1976). Comments on the conference, DSM-III in Midstream. Unpublished manuscript, New York, June 11.

Bernstein, R. L., & Gaw, A. C. (1990). Koro: Proposed classification for DSM-IV. *American Journal of Psychiatry, 147,*(12), 1670–1674.

Besharov, D. (1985). *The vulnerable social worker: Liability for serving children and families.* Silver Spring, MD: National Association of Social Workers.

Best, J. (1989). *Images of issues: Typifying contemporary social problems.* Hawthorne, NY: Aldine de Gruyter.

Blashfield, R. K. (1982). Feighner et al., invisible colleges, and the Matthew effect. *Schizophrenia Bulletin, 8*(1), 1–6.

Blashfield, R. K., Sprock, J., & Fuller, A. K. (1990). Suggested guidelines for including or excluding categories in the DSM-IV. *Comprehensive Psychiatry, 31,* 15–19.

Brodeur, P. (1989). *Currents of death.* New York: Simon & Schuster.

Brookes, C. (1982). Toward a meaningful coordination of etiology, nosology and therapy in psychoanalysis. *Journal of the American Academy of Psychoanalysis, 10,* 351–368.

Brown, P. (1987). Diagnostic conflict and contradiction in psychiatry. *Journal of Health and Social Behavior, 28,* 37–50.

Byalin, K. (1980). DSM-III. *Catalyst, 7,* 67–69.

Cantwell, D., Russell, A., Mattison, R., & Will, L. (1979). A comparison of DSM-II and DSM-III in the Diagnosis of childhood psychiatric disorders. *Archives of General Psychiatry, 36,* 1208–1222.

Carey, G., & Gottesman, I. I. (1978). Reliability and validity in binary ratings. *Archives of General Psychiatry, 35,* 1454–1459.

Carson, R. C. (1991). Dilemmas in the pathway of the DSM-IV. *Journal of Abnormal Psychology, 100*(3), 302–307.

Castel, R., Castel, F., & Lovell, A. (1982). *The psychiatric society.* New York: Columbia University Press.

Chodoff, P. (1987). Effects of the new economic climate on psychotherapeutic practice. *American Journal of Psychiatry, 144*(10, October), 1293–1297.

Chu, F. D., & Trotter, S. (1974). *The madness establishment.* New York: Grossman.

Clancy, R., & Noyes, J. (1977). *DSM-III field trial psychiatric consultant service.* Paper presented at the annual meeting of the American Psychiatric Association, Toronto.

Cleary, P. D. (1989). The need and demand for mental health services. In C. A. Taube & D. Mechanic (Eds.), *The future of mental health services research* (pp. 161–184). Washington, DC: U.S. Department of Health and Human Services.

Cohen, D. (Ed.). (1990). Challenging the therapeutic state [Special issue]. *Journal of Mind and Behavior, 11*(3/4).

Cohen, J. (1960). A coefficient of agreement for nominal scales. *Educational and Psychological Measurement, 20,* 37–46.

Cohen, M. D., March, J. C., & Olsen, J. P. (1972). A garbage can model of organizational choice. *Administrative Science Quarterly, 17,* 1–25.

Conrad, P., & Schneider, J. W. (1980). Deviance and medicalization: From badness to sickness. St. Louis, MO: Mosby.

Cooper, J., Kendell, R., Gurland, B., Sharpe, L., Copeland, J., & Simon, R. (1972). *Psychiatric diagnosis in New York and London.* London: Oxford University Press.

Cyert, R. M., & March, J. C. (1963). *A behavioral theory of the firm.* Englewood Cliffs, NJ: Prentice-Hall.

Dean, C. E. (1991). *Development of DSM-IV.* Letter to the editor. *American Journal of Psychiatry, 148,* 10.

D'Ercole, A., Skodal, A., Struening, E., Curtis, J., & Millman, J. (1991). Diagnosis of physical illness in psychiatric patients using axis III and a standardized medical history. *Hospital and Community Psychiatry, 42*(4), 395–400.

DeVault, S., & Dambrot, F. (1983). Sex of a case history and the DSM-III diagnosis of depression. *Journal of Clinical Psychology, 39,* 824–828.

DSM-III Assembly Liaison Committee (1976). Report to the assembly. October 29–30.

Dumont, M. (1984). The nonspecificity of mental illness. *American Journal of Orthopsychiatry, 53,* 326–334.

Ellis, P., & Mellsop, G. (1990). Development of DSM-IV. Letter to the editor. *Archives of General Psychiatry, 47,* 92.

Endicott, J., & Spitzer, R. L. (1978). A diagnostic interview. *Archives of General Psychiatry, 35,* 837–844.

Eysenck, H. J. (1952). The effects of psychotherapy: An evaluation. *Journal of Consulting Psychology, 16,* 319–323.

Eysenck, H. (1986). A critique of contemporary classification and diagnosis. In T. Millon & G. L. Klerman (Eds.), *Contemporary directions in psychopathology: Toward the DSM-IV* (pp. 73–98). New York: Guilford Press.

Eysenck, H., Wakefield, J., & Friedman, A. (1983). Diagnosis and clinical assessment: The DSM-III. *Annual Review of Psychology, 34*, 167–193.

Faust, D., & Miner, R. A. (1986). The empiricist and his new clothes: DSM-III in perspective. *American Journal of Psychiatry, 143* (8), 962–967.

Faust, D., & Ziskin, J. (1988). The expert witness in psychology and psychiatry. *Science, 241* (July 1), 31–35.

Feighner, J. P., Robins, E., Guze, S. B., Woodruff, R. A., Winokur, G., & Munoz, R. (1972). Diagnostic criteria for use in psychiatric research. *Archives of General Psychiatry, 26*, 57–63.

Foucault, M. (1965). *Madness and civilization: A history of insanity in the age of reason.* New York: Random House.

Frances, A. J. (1990a). *DSM-IV update.* Presentation at the annual meeting of the APA, New York, May 16.

Frances, A. (1990b). *DSM-IV: Works in progress.* Presentation at the Annual Meeting of the American Orthopsychiatric Association, Miami, May.

Frances, A., First, M., Pincus, H., Widiger, T. A., & Davis, W. (1990). An introduction to DSM-IV. *Hospital and Community Psychiatry, 41*, 493–494.

Frances, A., Pincus, H. A., Widiger, T. A., Davis, W. W., & First, M. B. (1990). DSM-IV: Work in progress. *American Journal of Psychiatry, 147*(11), 1439–1448.

Frances, A., Pincus, H., Widiger, T. A., Davis, W., & First, M. (1991). Dr. Frances and associates reply. Letter to the editor. *American Journal of Psychiatry, 148*(10), 1426–1427.

Frances, A. J., Widiger, T. A., & Pincus, H. A. (1989). The development of DSM-IV. *Archives of General Psychiatry, 46*, 373–375.

Franklin, D. (1987). The politics of masochism. *Psychology Today, 2*, 52–57.

Freidson, E. (1960). Client control and medical practice. *American Journal of Sociology, 65*, 374–382.

Freudenheim, M. (1991). The squeeze on psychiatric chains. *The New York Times*, October 26.

Gabbard, G. O., Takahashi, T., Davidson, J., Bauman-Bork, M., & Ensroth, K. (1991). A psychodynamic perspective on the clinical impact of insurance review. *American Journal of Psychiatry, 148*(3), 318–323.

Gambrill, E. (1990). *Critical thinking in clinical practice.* San Francisco: Jossey-Bass.

Garfield, S. L. (1986). Problems in diagnostic classification. In T. Millon & G. L. Klerman (Eds.), *Contemporary directions in psychopathology: Toward the DSM-IV* (pp. 99–114). New York, Guilford Press.

Garmenzy, N. (1978). Never mind the psychologists; Is it good for children? *Clinical Psychologist 31*(Spring), 1.

Geis, G., Jesilow, P., Pontell, H., & O'Brien, M. (1985). Fraud and abuse of government medical benefit programs by psychiatrists. *American Journal of Psychiatry, 142*(2, February), 231–234.

Goffman, E. (1961). *Asylums: Essays on the social situation of mental patients and other inmates.* Garden City, NY: Anchor Books.

Goleman, D. (1985). Social workers vault into leading role in psychotherapy. *The New York Times*, April 30, C1 and C9.

Goleman, D. (1990). New paths to mental health put strains on some healers. *The New York Times*, May 17, A1, B12.

Goleman, D. (1991a). Feeling unreal? Many others feel the same. *The New York Times,* January 8, C1, C8.

Goleman, D. (1991b). Battle of insurers vs. therapists: Cost control pitted against proper care. *The New York Times,* October 24, D1.

Gould, S. J. (1981). *The mismeasure of man.* New York: Norton.

Greenberg, D. S. (1980). Reimbursement wars. *New England Journal of Medicine* (August 28), 538–540.

Greenley, J. R., & Kirk, S. A. (1973). Organizational characteristics of agencies and the distribution of services to applicants. *Journal of Health and Social Behavior, 14,* 70–79.

Grob, G. N. (1991). Origins of DSM-I: A study in appearance and reality. *American Journal of Psychiatry, 148*(4), 421–431.

Grove, W. M. (1987). The reliability of psychiatric diagnosis. In C. G. Last & M. Hersen (Eds.), *Issues in diagnostic research* (pp. 99–119). New York: Plenum.

Grove, W. M., Andreasen, N. C., McDonald-Scott, P., Keller, M. B., & Shapiro, R. W. (1981). Reliability studies of psychiatric diagnosis: Theory and practice. *Archives of General Psychiatry, 38,* 408–413.

Guze, S. B. (1982). Comment on Blashfield's article. *Schizophrenia Bulletin, 8*(1), 6–7.

Gusfield, J. R. (1981). *The culture of public problems: Drinking-driving and the symbolic order.* Chicago: University of Chicago Press.

Halpern, A. (1986). Paraphilac coercive disorder: Old sewage in new pipes. Unpublished manuscript.

Hanada, K., & Takahashi, S. (1983). Multiaxial-institutional collaborative studies of diagnostic reliability of DSM-III. In R. Spitzer, J. Williams, & A. Skodal (Eds.), *International Perspectives on DSM-III* (pp. 273–290). Washington, DC: American Psychiatric Press.

Hartmann, L. (1991). Response to the presidential address: Humane values and biopsychosocial integration. *American Journal of Psychiatry, 148*(9), 1130–1134.

Hasenfeld, Y. (1983). *Human service organizations.* Englewood Cliffs, NJ: Prentice-Hall.

Hazen, R. M. (1988). *The break-through: The race for the superconductor.* New York: Summit Books.

Helzer, J. E., & Coryell, W. (1983). More on DSM-III: How consistent are precise criteria? *Biological Psychiatry, 18*(11), 1201–1203.

Helzer, J. E., Clayton, P. J., Pambakian, R., Reich, T., Woodruff, R. A., & Reveley, M. A. (1977b). Reliability of psychiatric diagnosis: II. The test/retest reliability of diagnostic classification. *Archives of General Psychiatry, 34,* 136–141.

Helzer, J. E., Robins, L. N., Croughan, J. L., & Welner (1981). Renard diagnostic interview. *Archives of General Psychiatry, 38,* 393–398.

Helzer, J. E., Robins, L. N., Taibleson, M., Woodruff, R. A., Reich, T., & Wish, E. D. (1977a). Reliability of psychiatric diagnosis: I. A methodological review. *Archives of General Psychiatry, 34,* 129–133.

Hinds, M. (1990). DuPont millions at issue in an heir's sanity case. *The New York Times,* January, 29, p. A16.

Huxley, P. (1986). Statistical errors in the British Journal of Social Work, Volumes 1–14. *British Journal of Social Work, 16*, 645–658.

Huxley, P. (1988). "Quantitative-descriptive" articles in the British Journal of Social Work. *British Journal of Social Work, 18*, 189–199.

Hyler, S., Williams, J. B. W., & Spitzer, R. L. (1982). Reliability in the DSM-III field trials. *Archives of General Psychiatry, 39*, 1275–1278.

Illich, I. (1975). *Medical nemesis.* New York: Pantheon.

Jampala, V. C., Sierles, F. S., & Taylor, M. A. (1986). Consumers' views of DSM-III: Attitudes and practices of U.S. psychiatrists and 1984 graduating psychiatric residents. *American Journal of Psychiatry, 143*, 148–153.

Johnson, A. B. (1990). *Out of Bedlam: The truth about deinstitutionalization.* New York: Basic Books.

Joint Commission on Mental Health and Illness. (1961). *Action for mental health.* New York: Basic Books.

Kachigan, S. (1986). *Statistical Analysis.* New York: Radius.

Kahneman, D., Slovic, P., & Tversky, A. (Eds.) (1982). *Judgment under uncertainty: Heuristics and biases.* Cambridge: Cambridge University Press.

Kanfer, F. H., & Saslow G. (1965). Behavioral diagnosis. *Archives of General Psychiatry, 12*, 529–538.

Kaplan, M. (1983). A woman's view of DSM-III. *American Psychologist, 38*, 786–792.

Katz, M. M. (1982). Comments on Blashfield's article. *Schizophrenia Bulletin, 8*(1), 9–11.

Kendell, R. E. (1975). *The role of diagnosis in psychiatry.* Oxford: Blackwell Scientific Publications.

Kendell, R. E. (1982). Comments on Blashfield's article. *Schizophrenia Bulletin, 8*(1), 11–12.

Kendell, R. E. (1991). Relationship between the DSM-IV and the ICD-10. *Journal of Abnormal Psychology, 100*(3), 297–301.

Kendell, R. E., Cooper, J. E., & Gourlay, A. G. (1971). Diagnostic criteria of American and British psychiatrists. *Archives of General Psychiatry, 25*, 123–130.

Kendler, K. S. (1990). Toward a scientific psychiatric nosology: Strengths and limitations. *Archives of General Psychiatry, 47*(October), 969–973.

Kendler, K. S., Spitzer, R. L., & Williams, J. B. W. (1989). Psychotic disorders in DSM-III-R. *American Journal of Psychiatry, 146*(8), 953–962.

Kerlinger, F. N. (1986). *Foundations of behavioral research.* New York: Holt, Rinehart and Winston.

Kerr, P. (1991a). Chain of mental hospitals faces inquiry in 4 states. *The New York Times,* October 22, A1.

Kerr, P. (1991b). Mental hospital chains accused of much cheating on insurance. *The New York Times,* November 24, A1.

Kiesler, C. A., & Sibulkin, A. (1987). *Mental hospitalization: Myths and facts about a national crisis.* Newbury Park, CA: Sage.

Kirk, S. A., & Kutchins, H. (1992). Diagnosis and uncertainty in mental health organizations. In Y. Hasenfeld (Ed.), *Human services as complex organizations* (pp. 163–183). Newbury Park, CA: Sage.

Kirk, S. A., & Kutchins, H. (1988). Deliberate misdiagnosis in mental health practice. *Social Service Review, 62*, 225–237.

Kittrie, N. (1972). *The right to be different*. Baltimore: Johns Hopkins University Press.

Kleinman, A. (1988). *Rethinking psychiatry: From cultural category to personal experience*. New York: Free Press.

Klerman, G. L. (1978). The evolution of a scientific nosology. In J. C. Shershow (Ed.), *Schizophrenia: Science and practice* (pp. 99–121). Cambridge, MA: Harvard University Press.

Klerman, G. L. (1984). The advantages of DSM-III. *American Journal of Psychiatry, 141*, 539–542.

Klerman, G. L. (1985). Diagnosis of psychiatric disorders in epidemiologic field studies. *Archives of General Psychiatry, 42*(July), 723–724.

Klerman, G. L. (1986). Historical perspectives on contemporary schools of psychopathology. In T. Millon & G. L. Klerman (Eds.), *Contemporary directions in psychopathology: Toward the DSM-IV* (pp. 3–28). New York: Guilford Press.

Klerman, G. L. (1987). Is the reliability of DSM-III a scientific or a political question? *Social Work Research & Abstracts, 23*, 3.

Klerman, G. L. (1990). The psychiatric patient's right to effective treatment: Implications of Osheroff v. Chestnut Lodge. *American Journal of Psychiatry, 147*, 409–418.

Klerman, G. L. (1991). The Osheroff debate: Finale. Letter to the editor. *American Journal of Psychiatry, 148*(3), 387–388.

Kraemer, H. C. (1987). Charlie Brown and statistics: An exchange. *Archives of General Psychiatry, 44*, 192–195.

Kreitman, N. (1961). The reliability of psychiatric diagnosis. *Journal of Mental Science, 107*, 876–886.

Kreitman, N., Sainsbury, P., Morrissey, J., Towers, J., & Scrivener, J. (1961). The reliability of psychiatric assessment: An analysis. *Journal of Mental Science, 107*, 887–908.

Kuhn, T. S. (1970). *The structure of scientific revolutions* (2nd ed.). Chicago: University of Chicago Press.

Kutchins, H. (1991). The fiduciary relationship. *Social Work, 36*, 106–113.

Kutchins, H., & Kirk, S. A. (1986). The reliability of DSM-III: A critical review. *Social Work Research & Abstracts, 22*(4), 3–12.

Kutchins, H., & Kirk, S. A. (1987a). Is the reliability of DSM-III a scientific or a political question: A response to Gerald Klerman. *Social Work Research & Abstracts, 23*, 3–5.

Kutchins, H., & Kirk, S. A. (1987b). DSM-III and social work malpractice. *Social Work, 32*(2), 205–212.

Kutchins, H., & Kirk, S. A. (1988a). The business of diagnosis: DSM-III and clinical social work. *Social Work, 33*, 215–220.

Kutchins, H., & Kirk, S. A. (1988b). The future of DSM: Scientific and professional issues. *Harvard Medical School Mental Health Letter, 5*(3), 4–6.

Kutchins, H., & Kirk, S. A. (1989). DSM-III-R: The conflict over new psychiatric diagnoses. *Health and Social Work, 34*(4), 91–103.

Laing, R. D. (1967). *The politics of experience*. Baltimore: Penguin Books.

Latour, B. (1987). *Science in action: How to follow scientists and engineers through society*. Cambridge, MA: Harvard University Press.

Latour, B. (1988). *The Pasteurization of France*. Cambridge, MA: Harvard University Press.

Latour, B., & Woolgar, S. (1986). *Laboratory life: The construction of scientific facts.* Princeton, NJ: Princeton University Press.

Lieberman, P., & Baker, F. (1985). The reliability of psychiatric diagnosis in the emergency room. *Hospital and Community Psychiatry, 36,* 291–293.

Lifton, R. J. (1973). *Home from the war.* New York: Simon and Schuster.

Link, B. (1987). Understanding labeling effects in the area of mental disorders: An assessment of the effects of expectations of rejection. *American Sociological Review, 52,* 96–112.

Link, B., Cullen, F., Struening, E., Shrout, P., & Dohrenwend, B. (1989). A modified labeling theory approach to mental disorders: An empirical assessment. *American Sociological Review, 54,* 400–423.

Link, B., Mirotznik, J., & Cullen, F. (1991). The effectiveness of stigma coping orientations: Can negative consequences of mental illness labeling be avoided? *Journal of Health and Social Behavior, 32,* 302–320.

Lipkowitz, M. H., & Idupugnati, S. (1983). Diagnosing schizophrenia in 1980: A survey of U.S. psychiatrists. *American Journal of Psychiatry, 140,* 52–55.

Lipkowitz, M. H., & Idupugnati, S. (1985). Diagnosing schizophrenia in 1982: The effect of DSM-III. *American Journal of Psychiatry, 142,* 634–637.

Lipsky, M. (1980). *Street-level bureaucracy: Dilemmas of the individual in public services.* New York: Russell Sage Foundation.

Lipton, A., & Simon, F. (1985). Psychiatric diagnosis in a state hospital. *Hospital and Community Psychiatry, 36,* 368–373.

Lipton, J. P., & Hershaft, A. M. (1985). On the widespread acceptance of dubious medical findings. *Journal of Health and Social Behavior, 26*(December), 336–351.

Liptzin, B., Levfoff, S. E., Cleary, P. D., Pilgrim, D., Reilly, C., Albert, M., & Wetle, T. (1991). An empirical study of diagnostic criteria for delirium. *American Journal of Psychiatry, 148*(4), 454–457.

Loring, M., & Powell, B. (1988). Gender, race, and DSM-III: A study of the objectivity of psychiatric diagnostic behavior. *Journal of Health and Social Behavior, 29,* 1–22.

Mannuzza, S., Fyer, A. J., Martin, L. Y., Gallops, M., Endicott, J., Gorman, J., Liebowitz, M., & Klein, D. (1989). Reliability of anxiety assessment: I. Diagnostic agreement. *Archives of General Psychiatry, 46,* 1093–1101.

Maricle, R., Leung, P., & Bloom, J. (1987). The use of DSM-III axis III in recording physical illness in psychiatric patients. *American Journal of Psychiatry, 144,* 1484–1486.

Matarazzo, J. D. (1983). The reliability of psychiatric and psychological diagnosis. *Clinical Psychology Review, 3,* 103–145.

Maxmen, J. (1985). *The new psychiatrists.* New York: New American Library.

McCloskey, D. N. (1983). The rhetoric of economics. *Journal of Economic Literature, 21,* 481–517.

McLemore, C., & Benjamin, L. (1979). Whatever happened to interpersonal diagnosis? A psychosocial alternative to DSM-III. *American Psychologist, 34,* 17–34.

Mechanic, D. (1980). *Mental health and social policy* (2nd ed.). Englewood Cliffs, NJ: Prentice-Hall.

Mellsop, G., & Varghese, F. (1983). An Australian study reflecting on the reliability and validity of Axis II. In R. Spitzer, J. Williams, and A. Skodal (Eds.), *International Perspectives on DSM-III* (pp. 259–272). Washington, DC: American Psychiatric Press.

Mellsop, G., Varghese, F., Joshua, S., & Hicks, A. (1982). The reliability of Axis II of DSM-III. *American Journal of Psychiatry, 139,* 1360–1361.

Merton, R. K. (1973). The normative structure of science. In R. K. Merton (Ed.), *The sociology of science* (pp. 267–278). Chicago: University of Chicago Press. (Originally published in 1942.)

Michels, R. (1984a). First rebuttal. *American Journal of Psychiatry, 141,* 548–551.

Michels, R. (1984b). Second Rebuttal. *American Journal of Psychiatry, 141,* 553.

Michels, R. (1986). Comments in A. M. Freedman, R. Brotman, I. Silverman, & D. Hutson (Eds.), *Issues in psychiatric classification: Science, practice and social policy* (pp. 184–185). New York: Human Science Press.

Millon, T. (1983). The DSM-III: An insider's account. *American Psychologist, 38,* 804–815.

Millon, T. (1986). On the past and future of the DSM-III: Personal recollections and projections. In T. Millon and G. L. Klerman (Eds.), *Contemporary Directions in Psychopathology: Toward the DSM-IV* (pp. 29–70). New York, Guilford Press.

Mintzberg, H. (1981). Organization design: Fashion or fit? *Harvard Business Review* (January–February), 103–116.

Mirowsky, J., & Ross, C. (1989a). Psychiatric diagnosis as reified measurement. *Journal of Health and Social Behavior, 30,* 11–25.

Mirowsky, J., & Ross, C. (1989b). *Social causes of psychological distress.* Hawthorne, NY: Aldine de Gruyter.

Morgan, G. (1986). *Images of organizations.* Newbury Park, CA: Sage.

National Institute of Mental Illness (1991). *Caring for people with severe mental disorders: A national plan of research to improve services.* DHHS Publ. No. (ADM) 91-1762. Washington, DC: USGPO.

Nelkin, D., & Tancredi, L. (1989). *Dangerous diagnostics: The social power of biological information.* New York: Basic Books.

Nelson, K. M. (1986). Economic considerations of diagnosis. In A. Freedman, R. Brotman, I. Silverman, & D. Hutson (Eds.), *Issues in psychiatric classification: Science, practice and social policy* (pp. 160–163). New York: Human Sciences Press.

Nelson-Gray, R. O. (1991). DSM-IV: Empirical guidelines from psychometrics. *Journal of Abnormal Psychology, 100*(3), 308–315.

New York Times. (1990). Sex assault case may get new trial. December 19.

Nunnally, J. C. (1978). *Psychometric theory.* New York: McGraw-Hill.

Nurius, P. S., & Gibson, J. W. (1990). Clinical observation, inference, reasoning, and judgment in social work: An update. *Social Work Research & Abstracts,* 26(2), 18–25.

Office of Research (1990). DSM-IV update. Washington, D.C.: American Psychiatric Association (January/February, mimeo).

Owen, D. (1985). *None of the above: Behind the myth of scholastic aptitude.* Boston: Houghton Mifflin.

Paget, M. A. (1990). Life mirrors work mirrors text mirrors life . . . *Social Problems, 37*(2), 137–148.

Perr, I. N. (1984). Medical and legal problems in psychiatric coding under the DSM and ICD systems. *American Journal of Psychiatry, 141*(3, March), 418–420.

Perrow, C. (1978). Demystifying organizations. In R. C. Sarri & Y. Hasenfeld (Eds.), *The management of human services* (pp. 105–120). New York: Columbia University Press.

Perrow, C. (1986). *Complex organizations: A critical essay* (3rd ed.). New York: Random House.

Regier, D. (1987). Overview. In G. Tischler (Ed.), *Diagnosis and classification in psychiatry: A critical appraisal of DSM-III* (pp. 443–445). New York: Cambridge University Press.

Rey, J. M., Plapp, J. M., Stewart, G., Richard, I., & Bashir, M. (1987). Reliability of the psychosocial axes of DSM-III in an adolescent population. *British Journal of Psychiatry, 150*, 228–234.

Rey, J., Stewart, G., Plapp, J., Bashir, M., & Richards, I. (1988). DSM-III Axis IV revisited. *American Journal of Psychiatry, 145*, 286–292.

Rhodes, L. A. (1991). *Emptying beds: The work of an emergency psychiatric unit.* Berkeley: University of California Press.

Robins, L. N., Helzer, J. E., Croughan, J., & Ratcliff, K. S. (1981). National Institute of Mental Health diagnostic interview schedule. *Archives of General Psychiatry, 38*, 381–389.

Robins, L. N., & Regier, D. A. (1991). *Psychiatric disorders in America: The epidemiologic catchment area studies.* New York: Free Press.

Rosenhan, D. L. (1973). On being sane in insane places. *Science, 179*(January 19), 250–258.

Rothblum, E. D., Solomon, L. J., & Albee, G. W. (1986). A sociopolitical perspective of DSM-III. In T. Millon & G. L. Klerman (Eds.), *Contemporary directions in psychopathology: Toward the DSM-IV* (pp. 167–189). New York: Guilford Press.

Rothman, D. J. (1971). *The discovery of the asylum: Social order and disorder in the new republic.* Boston: Little, Brown.

Rutter, M., & Shaffer, D. (1980). DSM-III: A step forward or back in terms of the classification of child psychiatric disorders? *Journal of the American Academy of Child Psychiatry, 19*, 371–394.

Sabshin, M., Diesenhaus, H., & Wilkerson, R. (1970). Dimensions of institutional racism in psychiatry. *American Journal of Psychiatry, 127*, 787–793.

Sabshin, M. (1990). Turning points in twentieth-century American psychiatry. *American Journal of Psychiatry, 147*(10), 1267–1274.

Sabshin, M. (1991). Report of the medical director. *American Journal of Psychiatry, 148*(10), 1444–1447.

Salzinger, K. (1977). *But is it good for the patient?* Paper presented at the symposium, Psychological Taxonomy: An Alternative to DSM, at the annual meeting of the American Psychological Association, San Francisco.

Salzinger, K. (1986). Diagnosis: Distinguishing among behaviors. In T. Millon & G. L. Klerman (Eds.), *Contemporary directions in psychopathology: Toward the DSM-IV* (pp. 115–134). New York: Guilford Press.

Sandifer, M., Hordern, A., Timbury, G., & Green, L. (1968). Psychiatric diagnosis: A comparative study in North Carolina, London and Glasgow. *British Journal of Psychiatry, 114*, 1–9.

Sandifer, M., Pettus, B., & Quade, D. (1964). A study of psychiatric diagnosis. *Journal of Nervous and Mental Disease, 139*(4), 350–356.

Sartorius, N. (1990). Introduction. In N. Sartorius, A. Jablensky, D. Regier, J. Burke, & R. Hirschfield (Eds.), *Sources and traditions of classification in psychiatry* (pp. 1–6). Lewiston, NY: Hogrefe & Huber.

Schacht, T., & Nathan, P. (1977). But is it good for psychologists? Appraisal and status of DSM-III. *American Psychologist, 32*, 1017–1025.

Schacht, T. (1985a). DSM-III and the politics of truth. *American Psychologist, 40*(5), 513–521.

Schacht, T. (1985b). Reply to Spitzer's "Politics-science dichotomy syndrome." *American Psychologist, 40*, 562–563.

Scheff, T. J. (1966). *Being mentally ill: A sociological theory.* Chicago: Aldine.

Scheff, T. J. (1986). Accountability in psychiatric diagnosis: A proposal. In T. Millon & G. L. Klerman (Eds.), *Contemporary directions in psychopathology: Toward the DSM-IV* (pp. 265–278). New York: Guilford Press.

Schmidt, H., & Fonda, C. (1956). The reliability of psychiatric diagnosis: A new look. *Journal of Abnormal and Social Psychology, 52*, 262–267.

Schofield, W. (1964). *Psychotherapy: The purchase of friendship.* Englewood Cliffs, NJ: Prentice-Hall.

Schon, D. A. (1983). *The reflective practitioner: How professionals think in action.* New York: Basic Books.

Schulberg, H. C., & Manderscheid, R. W. (1989). The changing network of mental health service delivery. In C. A. Taube & D. Mechanic (Eds.), *The future of mental health services research* (pp. 11–22). Washington, DC: U.S. Department of Health and Human Services.

Scott, R. A. (1969). *The making of blind men: A study in adult socialization.* New York: Russell Sage Foundation.

Scott, W. J. (1990). PTSD in DSM-III: A case in the politics of diagnosis and disease. *Social Problems, 37*(3), 294–310.

Sharfstein, S. S., Gutheil, T. G., & Stoddard, F. J. (1983). Money and character disorders: Or how to get the recalcitrant third party and the impossible patient to pay your bills. In M. Zales (Ed.), *Character pathology: Theory and treatment* (pp. 196–215). New York: Brunner Mazel.

Sharfstein, S., Towery, O., & Milowe, I. (1980). Accuracy of diagnostic information submitted to an insurance company. *American Journal of Psychiatry, 137*(1), 70–73.

Shrout, P. E., Spitzer, R. L., & Fleiss, J. L. (1987). Quantification of agreement in psychiatric diagnosis revisited. *Archives of General Psychiatry, 44*, 172–177.

Shuchman, M., & Wilkes, M. S. (1990). Dramatic progress against depression. *The New York Times Magazine*, Part 2, October 7, 12–32.

Shulruff, L. (1990). In sex case, focus is on multiple personalities. *The New York Times*, August 10.

Skodal, A. E. (1989). *Problems in differential diagnosis.* Washington, D.C.: American Psychiatric Press.

Skodal, A., Williams, J. B. W., & Spitzer, R. L. (1984). Identifying common errors in the use of DSM-III through diagnostic supervision. *Hospital and Community Psychiatry, 35,* 251–255.

Smith, D. E. (1965). Front-line organization of the state mental hospital. *Administrative Science Quarterly, 10*(December), 381–399.

Specht, H. (1990). Social work and the popular psychotherapies. *Social Service Review, 64*(3), 345–357.

Spector, M. (1977). Legitimizing homosexuality. *Society, 14*(July/August), 52–56.

Spector, M., & Kitsuse, J. I. (1987). *Constructing social problems.* Hawthorne, NY: Aldine de Gruyter.

Spitzer, R. L. (1973). A proposal about homosexuality and the APA nomenclature: Homosexuality as an irregular form of sexual behavior and sexual orientation disturbance as a psychiatric disorder. *American Journal of Psychiatry, 130,*(11), 1214–1216.

Spitzer, R. L. (1975). On pseudoscience in science, logic in remission, and psychiatric diagnosis: A critique of Rosenhan's "On being sane in insane places." *Journal of Abnormal Psychology, 84,* 442–452.

Spitzer, R. L. (1980). *Introduction to diagnostic and statistical manual of mental disorders.* Washington, D.C.: American Psychiatric Association.

Spitzer, R. L. (1981a). The diagnostic status of homosexuality in DSM-III: A reformulation of the issues. *American Journal of Psychiatry, 148,* 210–215.

Spitzer, R. L. (1981b). Nonmedical myths and the DSM-III. *American Psychological Association Monitor* (October), 3.

Spitzer, R. L. (1984). A debate on DSM-III: Second rebuttal. *American Journal of Psychiatry, 141*(4), 551–552.

Spitzer, R. L. (1985). DSM-III and the politics-science dichotomy syndrome. *American Psychologist, 40*(5), 522–526.

Spitzer, R. L. (1989). The development of diagnostic criteria in psychiatry. *Current Contents, 19*(May 8), 20.

Spitzer, R. L. (1991). An outsider-insider's views about revising the DSMs. *Journal of Abnormal Psychology, 100*(3), 294–296.

Spitzer, R. L., Cohen, J., Fleiss, J., & Endicott, J. (1967). Quantification of agreement in psychiatric diagnosis. *Archives of General Psychiatry, 17,* 83–87.

Spitzer, R. L., & Endicott, J. (1976). *Proposed definition of medical and psychiatric disorders for DSM-III.* Paper presented at the annual meeting of the American Psychiatric Association.

Spitzer, R. L., Endicott, J., & Robins, E. (1974). *Research diagnostic criteria.* New York: Biometrics Research, New York Department of Mental Hygiene.

Spitzer, R. L., Endicott, J., & Robins, E. (1975). Clinical criteria for psychiatric diagnosis and DSM-III. *American Journal of Psychiatry, 132*(11), 1187–1192.

Spitzer, R. L., Endicott, J., & Robins, E. (1978). Research Diagnostic Criteria. *Archives of General Psychiatry, 35,* 773–782.

Spitzer, R. L., & Fleiss, J. L. (1974). A re-analysis of the reliability of psychiatric diagnosis. *British Journal of Psychiatry, 125,* 341–347.

Spitzer, R. L., & Forman, J. (1979). DSM-III field trials: II. Initial experience with the multiaxial system. *American Journal of Psychiatry 136,* 818–820.

Spitzer, R. L., Forman, J., & Nee, J. (1979). DSM-III field trials: I. Initial interrater diagnostic reliability. *American Journal of Psychiatry, 136,* 815–817.

Spitzer, R. L., Hyler, J., & Williams, J. B. W. (1980). Appendix C: Annotated comparative listing of DSM-II and DSM-III. In American Psychiatric Association, *Diagnostic and statistical manual of mental disorders (3rd ed.)*. Washington, DC: Author.

Spitzer, R. L., Sheehy, M., & Endicott, J. (1977). DSM-III: Guiding principles. In V. Rakoff, H. Stancer, & H. Kedward (Eds.), *Psychiatric diagnosis* (pp. 1–24). New York: Brunner/Mazel.

Spitzer, R. L., & Williams, J. B. W. (1983). Classification in psychiatry. In H. I. Kaplan & B. J. Sadock (Eds.), *Comprehensive textbook of psychiatry* (pp. 591–613). Baltimore: Williams & Wilkins.

Spitzer, R. L., & Williams, J. B. W. (1987). Revising DSM-III: The process and major issues. In G. Tischler (Ed.), *Diagnosis and classification in psychiatry: A critical appraisal of DSM-III* (pp. 425–433). New York: Cambridge University Press.

Spitzer, R. L., & Williams, J. B. W. (1988). Having a dream: A research strategy of DSM-IV. *Archives of General Psychiatry, 45*, 871–874.

Spitzer, R. L., Williams, J. B. W., Gibbon, M., & First, M. (in press). The structured clinical interview for DSM-III-R (SCID) I.: History, rationale and description. *Archives of General Psychiatry.*

Spitzer, R. L., Williams, J. B. W., Kass, F., & Davies, M. (1989). National field trial of the DSM-III-R diagnostic criteria for self-defeating personality disorder. *American Journal of Psychiatry, 146*(12), 1561–1567.

Spitzer, R. L., Williams, J. B. W., & Skodal, A. (1980). DSM-III: The major achievements and an overview. *American Journal of Psychiatry, 137*, 151–164.

Spitzer, R. L., & Wilson, P. T. (1968). A guide to the American Psychiatric Association's new diagnostic nomenclature. *American Journal of Psychiatry, 124*, 1616–1629.

Spitzer, R. L., & Wilson, P. T. (1969). DSM-II revisited: A reply. *International Journal of Psychiatry, 7*, 421–426.

Spitzer, S. P., & Denzin, N. K. (Eds.). (1968). *The mental patient: Studies in the sociology of deviance.* New York: McGraw-Hill.

Spitznagel, E. L., & Helzer, J. E. (1985). A proposed solution to the base rate problem in the kappa statistic. *Archives of General Psychiatry, 42*, 725–728.

Spitznagel, E. L., & Helzer, J. E. (1987). Charlie Brown and statistics: An exchange. *Archives of General Psychiatry, 44*, 192–195.

Star, S. (1955). *The dilemmas of mental illness.* Unpublished manuscript.

Stone, A. A. (1990). Law, science, and psychiatric malpractice: A response to Klerman's indictment of psychoanalytic psychiatry. *American Journal of Psychiatry, 147*(4), 419–427.

Strauss, D. H., Spitzer, R. L., & Muskin, P. R. (1990). Maladaptive denial of physical illness: A proposal for DSM-IV. *American Journal of Psychiatry, 147*(9), 1168–1172.

Strauss, J. S. (1982). Comments on Blashfield's article. *Schizophrenia Bulletin, 8*(1), 8–9.

Strauss, J. S. (1986). Psychiatric diagnosis: A reconsideration based on longitudinal processes. In T. Millon & G. L. Klerman (Eds.), *Contemporary directions in psychopathology: Toward the DSM-IV* (pp. 257–264). New York: Guilford Press.

Strober, M., Green, J., & Carlson, G. (1981). Reliability of psychiatric diagnosis in hospitalized adolescents. *Archives of General Psychiatry, 38,* 141–145.

Stuart, R. B. (1970). *Trick or treatment: How and when psychotherapy fails.* Champaign, IL: Research Press.

Szasz, T. S. (1960). The myth of mental illness. *American Psychologist, 15*(February), 113–118.

Szasz, T. S. (1961). *The myth of mental illness.* New York: Hoeber-Harper.

Talbott, J. (1980). An in-depth look at DSM-III: An interview with Robert Spitzer. *Hospital and Community Psychiatry, 31,* 25–32.

Task Force on DSM-IV. (1991). *DSM-IV options book: Work in progress.* Washington, DC: American Psychiatric Association.

Taylor, C. B. (1983). DSM-III and behavioral assessment. *Behavioral Assessment, 5,* 5–14.

Tetlock, P. E. (1981). Pre- to postelection shifts in presidential rhetoric: Impression management or cognitive adjustment? *Journal of Personality and Social Psychology, 41*(2), 207–212.

Thomas, L. (1979). *The medusa and the snail.* New York: Viking.

Thompson, J. D. (1967). *Organizations in action.* New York: McGraw-Hill.

Torrey, E. F. (1974). *The death of psychiatry.* New York: Penguin.

Uebersax, J. S. (1987). Charlie Brown and statistics: An exchange. *Archives of General Psychiatry, 44,* 192–195.

Vaillant, G. (1984). The disadvantages of DSM-III outweigh its advantages. *American Journal of Psychiatry, 141,* 542–545.

Vitiello, B., Malone, R., Buschle, P. R., Delaney, M. A., & Behar, D. (1990). Reliability of DSM-III diagnoses of hospitalized children. *Hospital and Community Psychiatry, 41*(1), 63–67.

Wakefield, J. C. (1992a). Disorder as harmful dysfunction: A conceptual critique of DSM-III-R's definition of mental disorder. *Psychological Review, 99,* 2, 232–247.

Wakefield, J. C. (1992b). The concept of mental disorder: On the boundary between biological facts and social values. *American Psychologist, 47,* 3, 373–388.

Walker, L. (1986). Masochistic personality disorder, take two: A report from the front lines. *Feminist Therapy Institute Interchange*(January), 1–2.

Washington Post (1973). Doctors rule homosexuals not abnormal. December 12, p,. 1.

Watson, J. (1968). *The double helix.* New York: Mentor Books.

Webb, L., Gold, R., Johnstone, E., & Diclemente, C. (1981). Accuracy of DSM-III diagnoses following a training program. *American Journal of Psychiatry, 138,* 376–378.

Weisner, C., & Room, R. (1984). Financing and ideology in alcohol treatment. *Social Problems 32*(2), 167–184.

Werry, J., Methuen, R., Fitzpatrick, J., & Dixon, H. (1983). The interrater reliability of DSM-III in children. *Journal of Abnormal Child Psychiatry, 11,* 341–354.

Widiger, T. A. (1988a). *DSM-IV methods/applications conference synopsis* (November 29, 30, mimeo).

Widiger, T. A. (1988b). *DSM-IV literature reviews: Synopsis of purpose and process* (December 22, mimeo).

Widiger, T. A., Frances, A., Pincus, H., Davis, W., & First, M. (1991). Toward an empirical classification for the DSM-IV. *Journal of Abnormal Psychology, 100*(3), 280–288.

Williams, J. B. W. (1981). DSM-III: A comprehensive approach to diagnosis. *Social Work, 26,* 101–106.

Williams, J. B. W. (1985). The multiaxial system of DSM-III: Where did it come from and where should it go? II. Empirical studies, innovations and recommendations. *Archives of General Psychiatry, 42,* 181–186.

Williams, J. B. W., Gibbon, M., First, M., Spitzer, R. L., Davies, M., Borus, J., Howes, M., Kane, J., Pope, H., Rounsaville, B., & Wittchen, H. (in press). The structured clinical interview for DSM-III-R (SCID) II: Multi-site test-retest reliability. *Archives of General Psychiatry.*

Williams, J. B. W., & Spitzer, R. L. (1982). Focusing on DSM-III's multiaxial system. *Hospital and Community Psychiatry, 33,* 891–892.

Williams, J. B. W., & Spitzer, R. L. (1983). The issue of sex bias in DSM-III: A critique of "A woman's view of DSM-III" by Marcie Kaplan. *American Psychologist, 38,* 793–798.

Williams, J. B. W., & Spitzer, R. L. (1988). DSM-III and DSM-III-R: A response. *Harvard Medical School Mental Health Letter, 5*(4), 3–6.

Wilson, M. (1990). *DSM-III: The transformation of American psychiatry.* Paper presented at the annual meeting of the APA, New York, May.

Wing, J. K., Cooper, J. E., & Sartorius, N. (1974). *The measurement and classification of psychiatric symptoms.* London: Cambridge University Press.

Wing, J., & Nixon, J. (1975). Discriminating symptoms in schizophrenia: A report from the international pilot study of schizophrenia. *Archives of General Psychiatry, 32,* 853–859.

Work Group to Revise DSM-III. (1985). *DSM-III-R in development.* Washington, DC: American Psychiatric Association. (Draft, October 5.)

Work Group to Revise DSM-III. (1986). *DSM-III-R in development.* Washington, DC: American Psychiatric Association. (Second draft, August 1.)

World Health Organization (1977). *Manual of the international classification of disease, injuries and causes of death.* 9th revision. Geneva: Author.

Zigler, E., & Phillips, L. (1961). Psychiatric diagnosis: A critique. *Journal of Abnormal and Social Psychology, 63,* 607–618.

Zilboorg, G. (1941). *A history of medical psychology.* New York: Norton.

Zimmerman, M. (1988). Why are we rushing to publish DSM-IV? *Archives of General Psychiatry, 45,* 1135–1138.

Zimmerman, M. (1990). Is DSM-IV needed at all? *Archives of General Psychiatry.* 47(October), 974–976.

Zimmerman, M., Jampala, V., Sierles, F., & Taylor, M. (1991). DSM-IV: A nosology sold before its time? *American Journal of Psychiatry, 148*(4), 463–467.

Zubin, J. (1978). But is it good for science? *Clinical Psychologist, 31*(2), 1.

INDEX